SURGICAL SECRETS

Charles M. Abernathy, M.D.
Department of Surgery
University of Colorado School of Medicine
Denver, Colorado

Brett B. Abernathy, M.D.
Department of Surgery
University of Texas Health Sciences Center
Parkland Memorial Hospital
Dallas, Texas

**With Members of the Department of Surgery,
University of Colorado School of Medicine**

HANLEY & BELFUS, INC./Philadelphia
THE C.V. MOSBY COMPANY/St. Louis•Toronto•London

Publisher: HANLEY & BELFUS, INC.
                210 S. 13th Street
                Philadelphia, PA 19107

North American and worldwide sales and distribution:

                THE C.V. MOSBY COMPANY
                11830 Westline Industrial Drive
                St. Louis, MO 63146

In Canada: THE C.V. MOSBY COMPANY
                120 Melford Drive
                Scarborough, Canada M1B 2X5

SURGICAL SECRETS   ISBN 0-932883-00-1

Library of Congress catalog card number   85-081928

Last digit is the print number: 9 8 7 6 5

"It doesn't matter that everything has already been said.
No one was listening."

André Gide

CONTRIBUTORS

Brett B. Abernathy, M.D.
Department of Surgery, University of Texas Health Sciences Center; Parkland Memorial Hospital, Dallas, Texas

Charles M. Abernathy, M.D.
Assistant Professor of Surgery, University of Colorado Health Sciences Center, Denver; Montrose Memorial Hospital, Montrose, Colorado

M.A. Ammons, M.D.
Department of Surgery, Veterans Administration Medical Center, Denver

Edward J. Bartle, M.D.
Assistant Professor of Surgery, University of Colorado Health Sciences Center, Denver

Bruce Robert Barton, M.D.
Chief Resident and Instructor, Department of Surgery, University of Colorado Health Sciences Center, Denver

Paul A. Bunn, Jr., M.D.
Professor of Medicine, University of Colorado Health Sciences Center; Head, Division of Medical Oncology, University Hospital, Denver

Athleo Louis Cambre, M.D.
Chief Resident and Instructor in Surgery, University of Colorado Health Sciences Center, Denver

David N. Campbell, M.D.
Assistant Professor of Surgery, Section of Cardiovascular Thoracic Surgery, University of Colorado Health Sciences Center, Denver

Lale Douglas Cowgill, M.D.
Associate Cardiovascular Surgeon, Marshfield Clinic, and St. Joseph's Hospital, Marshfield, Wisconsin

Deborah Davis, M.D.
Resident in Surgery, University of Colorado Health Sciences Center, Denver

Theodore C. Dickinson, M.D.
Assistant Clinical Professor of Surgery, University of Colorado Health Sciences Center, Denver; Montrose Memorial Hospital, Montrose, Colorado

Ben Eiseman, M.D.
Professor of Surgery, University of Colorado Health Sciences Center; Chairman, Department of Surgery, Rose Medical Center, Denver

Richard C. Fisher, M.D.
Assistant Professor, Department of Orthopedics, University of Colorado Health Sciences Center, Denver

Mark Gibson, M.D.
Fellow, Pediatric Anesthesia, The Children's Hospital, Denver

L. Michael Glode, M.D.
Associate Professor of Medicine, University of Colorado Health Sciences Center, Denver

Stephen K. Greenholz, M.D.
Chief Resident in General Surgery, University of Colorado Health Sciences Center, Denver

Joseph Charles Greer, M.D.
Assistant Clinical Instructor, University of Colorado Health Sciences Center, Denver

Cordell E. Gross, M.D.
Associate Professor of Neurosurgery, University of Colorado Health Sciences Center, Denver

Michael Grosso, M.D.
Resident in Surgery, University of Colorado Health Sciences Center, Denver

Roberta J. Hall, M.D.
Resident in General Surgery, University of Colorado Health Sciences Center, Denver

Alden H. Harken, M.D.
Professor and Chairman, Department of Surgery, University of Colorado Health Sciences Center, Denver

Gilbert Hermann, M.D.
Clinical Professor of Surgery, University of Colorado Health Sciences Center; Attending Surgeon, Rose Medical Center, Denver

Alejandro M. Hernandez-Cano, M.D.
Instructor in Surgery, and Pediatric Surgery Research Fellow, University of Colorado Health Sciences Center, Denver

Mark Hilberman, M.D.
Associate Professor of Anesthesia, University of Colorado Health Sciences Center, Denver

Benjamin Honigman, M.D.
Assistant Professor, University of Colorado Health Sciences Center; Director, Emergency Department, University Hospital, Denver

Michael R. Johnston, M.D.
Assistant Professor of Surgery, University of Colorado Health Sciences Center, Denver

Frederick (Fritz) M. Karrer, M.D.
Instructor in Surgery, and Pediatric Surgical Research Fellow, University of Colorado Health Sciences Center, Denver

Glenn L. Kelly, M.D.
Associate Clinical Professor of Surgery, University of Colorado Health Science Center, Denver

R. Dale Liechty, M.D.
Profesor of Surgery and Associate Dean of Graduate Medical Education, University of Colorado Health Sciences Center, Denver

John R. Lilly, M.D.
Professor of Surgery, and Chief of Pediatric Surgery, University of Colorado Health Sciences Center, Denver

Hamilton Lokey, M.D.
Montrose Memorial Hospital, Montrose, Colorado

Joyce A. Majure, M.D.
Assistant Clinical Professor, University of Colorado Health Sciences Center, Denver

Luis Alberto Martinez-Frontanilla, M.D.
Assistant Clinical Professor of Pediatric Surgery, University of Colorado Health Sciences Center, Denver

Michael R. Mill, M.D.
Chief Resident and Instructor in General Surgery, University of Colorado Health Sciences Center, Veterans Administration Hospital, Denver

Mary Bernadette Mockus, Ph.D.
Medical Student, University of Colorado School of Medicine, Denver

Ernest E. Moore, M.D.
Associate Professor of Surgery, University of Colorado Health Sciences Center; Chief, Department of Surgery, Denver General Hospital, Denver,

Frederick A. Moore, M.D.
Assistant Clinical Professor, University of Colorado Health Sciences Center, Denver

George Moore, M.D.
Professor of Surgery, University of Colorado Health Sciences Center; Director and Chief of Surgical Oncology, Denver General Hospital, Denver

James A. Narrod, M.D.
Fellow in Cardiovascular Surgery, New York University Medical Center, New York, New York

G. Richard Neely, M.D.
Assistant Clinical Professor, University of Colorado Health Sciences Center, Denver

William R. Nelson, M.D.
Associate Clinical Professor of Surgery, University of Colorado Health Sciences Center, Denver

Lawrence W. Norton, M.D.
Professor and Vice-Chairman, Department of Surgery, University of Colorado School of Medicine; Chief of Surgery, Denver VA Hospital; Chief of General Surgery, University of Colorado Health Sciences Center, Denver

Robert Papadopoulos, M.D.
Chief Resident, General Surgery, University of Colorado Health Sciences Center, Denver

Richard K. Parker, M.D.
Attending Staff, Presbyterian-St. Luke's Medical Center and Mercy Medical Center, New York, New York

William H. Pearce, M.D.
Assistant Professor of Surgery, University of Colorado Health Sciences Center, Denver

Nathan W. Pearlman, M.D.
Associate Professor of Surgery, University of Colorado Health Sciences Center, Denver

Thomas L. Petty, M.D.
Professor of Medicine, and Director, Webb-Waring Lung Institute, University of Colorado Health Sciences Center, Denver

Robert B. Rutherford, M.D.
Professor of Surgery, and Chief of Vascular Surgery, University of Colorado Health Sciences Center, Denver

Richard J. Sanders, M.D.
Associate Clinical Professor of Surgery, University of Colorado Health Sciences Center; Attending Surgeon, Rose Medical Center, Denver

Robert Sawyer, M.D.
Private Practice, Denver

Scot M. Sedlacek, M.D.
Assistant Professor of Medicine, University of Colorado Health Sciences Center, Denver

Francis L. Shannon, M.D.
Resident in General Surgery, University of Colorado Health Sciences Center, Denver

John Simon, M.D.
Assistant Clinical Professor of Surgery, University of Colorado Health Sciences Center, Denver

Greg Van Stiegmann, M.D.
Assistant Professor of Surgery, University of Colorado Health Sciences Center, Denver

John Hoshyn Sun, M.D.
Research Fellow, University of Colorado Health Sciences Center, Denver

Charles W. Van Way, III, M.D.
Associate Professor of Surgery, University of Colorado Health Sciences Center; Director, Nutritional Support Services, University Hospital, Denver

R.C.A. Weatherley-White, M.D.
Associate Clinical Professor of Surgery (Plastic), University of Colorado Health Sciences Center, Denver

Roger S. Wotkyns, M.S., M.D.
Associate Clinical Professor, University of Colorado Health Sciences Center, Denver

CONTENTS

III: ABDOMINAL SURGERY

IV: ENDOCRINE SURGERY

V: BREAST SURGERY

VI: OTHER CANCER

PREFACE

Surgical Secrets is not intended as a textbook in the traditional sense. It is a pathway of questions from diagnosis to recovery. We first discovered the need for this approach when our students were assigned chapters in a major surgical textbook and then on discussion could not "pull out" the key information. The way we solve this as surgeons is by a series of key questions.

The editors gave the contributing authors wide latitude in style (some are long, some are short) and encouraged them to duplicate the verbal teaching process they use on rounds, in the OR, and on oral exams.

We teach students by asking questions. Knowing "the right question" and its answer is the key to clinical surgery for both a student and the most experienced practitioner. Of the two components of learning surgery, one is experiential and the other didactic, the part that can be written. The only way to learn the experiential component is by long hours of watching, trying and trying again. It takes a *long* time.

But the other part of learning surgery, the "book knowledge," can and should be learned rapidly. A student should learn surgery 101, 202. . .606 all simultaneously, for a patient problem is almost always a complex constellation of decisions, questions, and judgments. To suggest that a student should not learn the ins and outs of aortic grafts, and instead be exposed only to fundamental wound healing concepts, is to belittle the student's ability to handle complicated concepts. Surgery, unlike calculus, is not abstract and can be learned (insofar as the didactic information is concerned) in full breadth at an early stage.

This volume is designed to be carried in a coat pocket. We hope it will also be carried in the coat pockets of many experienced surgeons as they ask the "questions of surgical practice" in their daily work.

Surgical Secrets is *not* intended only to be a guide to help pass an examination. Rather, the questions here teach the knowledge a surgeon must know in order to take care of a patient with a particular problem. The questions by themselves trace the thought process a surgeon uses when thinking about the problem.

Socrates was correct. The best way to teach is to question. We hope we have followed his precepts, perhaps providing even more help in finding answers.

Charles M. Abernathy, M.D.
Brett B. Abernathy, M.D.

1. CARDIOPULMONARY RESUSCITATION AND INITIAL TREATMENT OF HEMORRHAGIC SHOCK

MICHAEL GROSSO, M.D, and ALDEN HARKEN, M.D.

AIRWAY AND BREATHING

1. **The first and foremost priority! Why?**
   Blood oxygen saturation in the unventilated patient falls to approximately 85% with 40 to 90 seconds of apnea and decreases sharply from then on.

2. **Is there an immediate need for an oral, nasopharyngeal, or S tube airway?**

   No. Although they serve a useful function to maintain a patent airway and also serve as bite block to facilitate suctioning, they may induce vomiting or vocal cord spasm in the stuporous or semiconscious patient.

3. **What is the most effective method for removing a foreign body obstructing an airway?** *Controversial*

   Many techniques are cited. For a completely obstructed airway in the unconscious patient, a back blow will deliver 35 mm Hg of airway pressure, and an abdominal thrust will deliver 15 mm Hg of airway pressure. The recommended technique is four successive back blows followed by four successive abdominal thrusts. For a partially obstructed airway (patient is able to phonate), an abdominal thrust will generate 2200 ml of flow/sec as compared with 200 ml/sec for a back blow.

4. **What is the most common cause of airway obstruction in the unconscious patient?**

   The base of the relaxed tongue against the posterior pharyngeal wall (relieved by head tilt, jaw thrust, or chin lift).

5. **How do you establish an airway in the patient with a suspected neck injury?**
   Of the three basic maneuvers, head tilt, chin lift, and jaw thrust, the jaw thrust requires the least amount of cervical hyperextension.

6. **Is endotracheal intubation required in all cases of respiratory arrest?**
   No. With minimal skill and training, mouth-to-mouth resuscitation can deliver 16 to 18% inspired oxygen with adequate tidal volumes. The use of bag and mask along with an oxygen supply can deliver 95 to 100% oxygen. These are relatively safe and effective techniques for ventilatory support. Airway control by endotracheal intubation can be attempted once additional skilled personnel arrive.

7. **What are the disadvantages of ventilatory support without endotracheal intubation?**
   Positive-pressure breathing (mouth-to-mouth or bag and mask) can be associated with significant delivery of air to the stomach. Gastric distention can impair diaphragmatic movement and therefore limit ventilation. Additionally, increased pressure may cause regurgitation and, worse, aspiration. These can be prevented by proper airway positioning and avoiding excessive tidal volume with ventilation.

1

8. **How do you deal with gastric distention?**
    Do not attempt direct abdominal pressure. This can actually promote
    regurgitation and aspiration, and cause gastric rupture. Normal intragastric
    pressure is 7 cm H2O. Regurgitation is likely with pressures greater than 20 cm
    H2O. Gastric distention is quickly alleviated with placement of a nasogastric tube
    and by applying suction.

9. **You decide to intubate the patient. What size tube?**
    For an average-sized adult, an 8.0 or 8.5 mm internal diameter endotracheal tube
    is recommended. A guideline often used: select a tube with an internal diameter
    approximately equal to the width of the patient's thumbnail.

10. **Is the endotracheal tube in proper position?**
    It is imperative that proper tube placement be confirmed. Four quick and relatively
    reliable techniques can confirm proper tracheal position of the tube: (1)
    auscultation of both lung fields should yield equal breath sounds, (2) observation
    of symmetric chest rise with each ventilation, (3) absence of auscultated air
    sounds over the epigastrium during ventilation, and (4) observation of pink rather
    than cyanotic mucous membranes and extremities. Even the presence of all of
    these criteria does not negate the need for confirmation of tube placement by
    chest x-ray as soon as possible.

11. **Oral or nasal intubation?**
    Oral intubation is the preferred method. The tube is directly visualized through
    the vocal cords, ensuring proper placement. Nasal intubation is a "blind
    technique" relatively contraindicated in patients with maxillofacial trauma (risk of
    intracranial placement of the tube through an anterior fossa fracture) and in
    patients with known or suspected coagulopathy (because nasal mucosa is well
    vascularized, intubation can cause major epistaxis). However, in the patient with a
    suspected cervical spine injury, nasal intubation can be accomplished while
    maintaining cervical immobilization and therefore is the preferred method in this
    setting (unless the patient is apneic).

12. **What is the role of esophageal obturator airway (EOA)?** *Controversial*
    The EOA was adopted to eliminate the problem of gastric dilatation as well as to
    provide a reliable technique for regulation of ventilation. The tube can be placed
    quickly and safely; successful attempts range from 96 to 99%. The major
    drawbacks are risk of esophageal perforation (low, 0.2 to 2%) and inadvertent
    tracheal placement preventing ventilation. No data indicate that the device is safe
    in patients with cervical spine injury; therefore, at present, it is not recommended
    in the trauma patient. Also, the technique probably has no role in in-hospital
    resuscitation since other methods of airway control are accessible. At the present
    time, it provides an effective and efficient *temporary* alternative to endotracheal
    intubation in the *field* in non-trauma arrest victims.

CIRCULATION
13. **What is the proper method of external chest compression?**
    The rescuer should be positioned beside the patient's chest. The compression
    point is located by identifying the xiphoid-sternal junction and measuring two
    fingerbreadths toward the head. The heel of one hand is placed here. The heel
    of the second hand is placed over the first. The fingers may be interlocked.
    Keep the arms straight and the shoulders directly over the victim's sternum. The
    compression depth should be 4 to 5 cm. Maintain hand position on the sternum
    at all times. With one rescuer: 15 compressions followed by 2 ventilations, repeat
    cycle. With two rescuers: 5 compressions, 1 ventilation. Compression rates: one

rescuer, 80/minute; two rescuers, 60/minute. Monitor the carotid pulse for effectiveness of CPR and to assess return of spontaneous pulses.

14. What are the essentials of external chest compressions?
The key to effective CPR is to produce blood flow. Typically, one can produce a pulse and a systolic blood pressure with any adequate chest compressions. However, to produce blood flow and, in turn, tissue perfusion, requires prolonging the compression phase. Increasing the compression phase from 30 to 50% more than *doubles* the flow. Compression rate is relatively unimportant. Rates between 40 and 80/minute all produce comparable flows.

15. What are the complications of external chest compressions?
Complications of CPR are multiple and frequent. Rib and sternal fractures range from 40 to 80%. Major cardiac or pericardial injuries are rare but may occur (lacerations). Bone marrow and fat emboli are common, 80% in one series. Additionally, damage to intraabdominal organs has been reported, including lacerations, contusions, and ruptures of liver, spleen, kidneys, colon, stomach, and diaphragm. Strict attention to the details of hand placement and compression depth will minimize complications.

16. Is a "central line" the best access to the venous systemic circulation? *Controversial*
The "central line," i.e., internal jugular or subclavian vein catheter, appears, at first glance, to be part of any successful resuscitation. It is a technique that is mastered relatively early in one's surgical career. Its role in resuscitation, however, is somewhat dubious. Contrary to popular belief, administration of large volumes of fluid to the venous system can be more quickly delivered via large-bore peripheral venous catheters. A 14-gauge, 5-cm catheter (peripheral) can deliver twice the flow of a 16-gauge, 20-cm catheter (central). Additionally, central line placement is associated with significant complications, including pneumothorax, air embolus, and puncture of large arteries. Finally, the placement of a central line may require interruption of CPR. Adequate venous access can therefore be easily achieved by the placement of peripheral catheters via the percutaneous or cutdown approach. However, central venous catheters do offer the ability to obtain a central venous pressure (CVP) once a rhythm is restored and can identify the presence of cardiac tamponade. Additionally, in shock, especially hypovolemia, the peripheral venous system may be collapsed, making cannulation extremely difficult.

17. When should/should not the MAST suit be used? *Controversial*
The military antishock trouser (MAST) suit is an inflatable three-compartment garment that surrounds the abdomen and both lower extremities. When inflated, the suit provides an increase in peripheral resistance. This combination leads to increased blood pressure (increased venous return, increased stroke volume, increased cardiac output; BP = CO x TPR, i.e., both CO and TPR are increased with the MAST suit). Indications for use include trauma arrest, systolic blood pressure less than 80 mm Hg secondary to hypovolemic shock, continued retroperitoneal hemorrhage from pelvic fractures, hemorrhage requiring direct pressure for control, and femoral shaft fractures requiring immobilization. *Contraindications:* pulmonary edema, evisceration of abdominal contents, pregnancy, and decreased pulmonary function, i.e., pneumothorax. The controversy concerns the patient in deep shock after trauma in the field. Application of the MAST suit is theoretically sensible in this setting. However, these patients are often losing blood at very rapid rates and are possibly suffering from tension pneumothorax or pericardial tamponade. The time spent to apply

the suit may be better spent rapidly transporting the patient to an emergency facility where appropriate, definitive, life-saving measures can be applied.

18. **Colloid or crystalloid resuscitation fluid?** *Controversial*
There are data to support both sides. Colloid advocates claim the solutions remain primarily in the intravascular space and thereby are more effective in elevating blood volume. Crystalloid advocates state that capillaries will leak albumin in the shock state. Many studies have shown that resuscitation with crystalloid is safe, especially with respect to pulmonary complications. Given its availability, low cost, and safety, crystalloid solution (lactated Ringer's) is at present the choice for initial fluid resuscitation.

19. **When is blood needed?**
For the patient in hemorrhagic shock, if hypotension remains after infusion of 2 L of crystalloid fluid, a blood transfusion should be started. Type-specific blood is appropriate while waiting for complete cross-match. Whole blood is preferable to packed cells because it provides additional volume. Keep in mind that banked blood is low in factors V and VIII and platelets. Most authors recommend fresh frozen plasma for every 5 to10 units of transfused blood to avoid dilutional coagulopathy. Cold (4°C) bank blood should pass through blood warmers/filters to avoid acidosis and prevent microcirculation clogging secondary to increased viscosity.

20. **Open or closed chest cardiac compression?** *Controversial*
In the nontraumatic cardiac arrest victim, closed-chest cardiac compression can be instituted immediately, is relatively safe, and if performed correctly, can provide adequate tissue perfusion. Open, direct cardiac compression requires training and experience in performing thoracotomy and open massage. With the chest open, respiratory support is mandatory. Complications are many, including laceration of the lung, myocardium, or coronary arteries, phrenic nerve damage, and sepsis. In most instances, open-chest cardiac massage *will not* succeed where closed-chest compression, combined with drug therapy and ventilation, has failed. Indications for thoracotomy will be presented later in the chapter.

21. **What are the common causes of electromechanical dissociation (EMD) and how are they best treated?**
EMD is typified by the presence of an orderly electrical rhythm but with marked absence of detectable blood pressure. In the arrest setting, initial treatment consists of intravenous calcium chloride (see question 23). Keep in mind the potentially correctable situations that commonly cause EMD: (1) pneumothorax tension, alleviated rapidly by placement of a large-bore needle into the pleural space on the side of the collapsed lung (diagnosis: hyperresonant chest, decreased breath sounds, chest x-ray), (2) pericardial tamponade (diagnosis: Beck's triad–distant heart sounds, distended neck veins/elevated CVP, and hypotension) relieved by pericardiocentesis or thoracotomy with pericardiotomy (controversial, see question 25). Also, EMD is associated with hypovolemia (should already have been corrected!), ventricular rupture (traumatic or secondary to myocardial infarction), pulmonary embolism, and pump failure secondary to massive MI.

22. **Can one assist failing circulation mechanically?** *Controversial*
At present, mechanical assistance of circulatory failure consists of the intraaortic balloon counterpulsation pump (IABP) and left ventricular assist devices (LVAD). The latter are currently undergoing clinical trials. The former is a technique to assist circulation in patients with cardiogenic shock not responsive to fluid therapy

or pressors. The device increases coronary perfusion during diastole (with balloon inflated, aortic diastolic pressure increases and coronary perfusion pressure increases) and decreases left ventricular work during systole (with balloon deflated, "afterload" or impedence to left ventricular ejection decreases). The IABP has been widely used following coronary artery or valve surgery. Its role in cardiogenic shock following acute arrest is still being investigated. In this setting its use is considered experimental. Left ventricular assist devices, of which there are many types, provide a means of either partially or totally bypassing the heart on a temporary basis. A tremendous amount of research is currently being conducted on this subject. The role in arrest situations is not yet known.

DRUG THERAPY

23. **What are the common drugs used during resuscitation and the appropriate dosages?**

Oxygen – to reverse hypoxia, 100%; toxicity not a hazard in the initial resuscitation period.

Sodium bicarbonate ($NaHCO_3$) – to reverse acidosis (hypoxia-induced anaerobic metabolism leads to acid accumulation, ventilatory failure leads to carbon dioxide retention–acidosis). Initial dose is 1 mEq/kg. One ampule (50 ml) of a 7.5% solution contains 44.6 mEq of sodium bicarbonate. It should be noted that bicarbonate combines with H^+ (hydrogen ions) to form carbon dioxide and water. Thus, adequate ventilation will be required for bicarbonate therapy to be fully effective. Overzealous use can result in hypokalemia (alkalosis shifts K^+ ions intracellularly) and hypernatremia/hyperosmolality (each HCO_3^- is accompanied by a Na^+ ion).

Epinephrine – alpha, beta agonist. IV dosage (5 to 10 ml of a 1:10,000 solution), short duration, repeat dose after 5 minutes may be necessary. Inactivated by alkali–do no mix with bicarbonate solutions! Although enhancing myocardial performance, epinephrine greatly increases myocardial oxygen demand (ventilate!).

Atropine – parasympatholytic (vagolytic), thereby increasing the discharge rate of the sinus node. Useful in treating sinus bradycardia associated with hemodynamic compromise. Dose of 0.5 mg IV is repeated at 5-minute intervals until a desirable rate is achieved (60 beats/minute). Supplied as a 0.1 mg/ml solution – 5 nl or 0.5 ng/ml solution – 1 ml. Increased heart rate increases myocardial oxygen demand; atropine should be used only if the bradycardia causes hemodynamic compromise, to avoid unnecessary increase in heart rate.

Lidocaine – a local anesthetic, known to suppress ventricular arrhythmias (automatic and re-entrant). One mg/kg IV bolus is followed by infusion at 2 to 4 mg/min IV. An additional IV bolus can be given at 10 minutes after initial dose if arrhythmias persist. Toxicity is limited to the CNS: serious side effects include focal and grand mal seizures (treat with Valium, 5 mg IV).

Bretylium tosylate – a postganglionic adrenergic blocker with positive inotropic and antiarrhythmic effects. Elevates ventricular fibrillation threshold (as does lidocaine). For v-tachycardia, 500 mg over 8 to 10 minutes. Controversy exists surrounding its most effective use (see question 24).

Verapamil –a slow-channel (calcium) blocking agent used to treat paroxysmal supraventricular tachycardia, causing hemodynamic compromise. Dose: 0.075 to 0.15 mg/kg (maximum 10 mg) IV bolus over 10 minutes (2-ml ampule contains 5.0 mg to 2.5 mg/ml). Repeat dose after 30 minutes if not effective. The drug reduces systemic vascular resistance; therefore blood pressure should be closely monitored during its use. A well-known property of the drug is its direct depression of cardiac contractility, yet *cardiac output* usually remains unchanged secondary to reflex sympathetic response.

Calcium chloride – positive inotropic agent. Calcium ions bind to regulatory proteins which inhibit the formation of cross-bridges between muscle contractile filaments (release of this inhibition by calcium binding allows cross-bridge formation, tension generation, and finally fiber shortening). Used when electrical rhythm is present but effective ejection of blood is absent (electromechanical dissociation; question 21). Dose: 2.5-5.0 ml of a 10% solution of calcium chloride (10% solution contains 1.36 mEq/ml). Do not mix with bicarbonate-will precipitate.

24. Lidocaine or bretylium for ventricular arrhythmias? *Controversial*
For treatment of ventricular fibrillation/ventricular tachycardia, lidocaine combined with electroshock therapy has long been the gold standard. Bretylium has a prolonged onset of action in the treatment of ventricular tachycardia, approximately 20 minutes or more. Lidocaine is the initial drug of choice for ventricular tachycardia; for refractory or recurrent ventricular tachycardia, bretylium may then be tried. Data indicate, however, that bretylium is as effective as lidocaine in the treatment of ventricular fibrillation. For ventricular fibrillation, its apparent onset of action is within a few minutes; 5 mg/kg given in IV bolus, followed by electrical defibrillation. More data are presently being compiled.

EMERGENCY SURGICAL PROCEDURES
25. When should emergency thoracotomy be performed?
Emergency thoracotomy is a dramatic, life-saving technique; however, strict guidelines should govern its use. It is indicated in patients with *trauma* who: (1) present in cardiac arrest, (2) remain hypotensive despite adequate fluid therapy, (3) exhibit signs of massive intraabdominal bleeding without response to blood or fluid challenge. It is also indicated for use to perform cardiac massage on patients in whom chest wall deformities preclude external chest compressions. The open chest allows direct cardiac compression, direct defibrillation, control of cardiac or thoracic hemorrhage, repair of exsanguinating hemorrhage sites, direct relief of cardiac tamponade, and aortic cross-clamping to control extrathoracic hemorrhage. Despite anecdotal reports on small series of survivors, judicious use is required in trauma patients arriving at the emergency room in extremis. In a large consecutive series of 400 patients, there were no survivors, despite thoracotomy, in patients with absent vital signs or absent signs of life in the field.

BIBLIOGRAPHY
1.   Gordon, A.S., et al.: Mouth-to-mouth versus manual artificial respiration. J.A.M.A., 167: 320, 1958.
2.   Gordon, A.S., et al.: Emergency management of foreign body obstruction. In Safar, P.: Advances in Cardiopulmonary Resuscitation. New York, Springer Verlag, 1977.
3.   Graber, D., et al.: Catheter flow rates updated. J.A.C.E.P., 6:518, 1977.
4.   Guildner, C.W.: Resuscitation: Opening the airway. J.A.C.E.P., 5:588, 1976.
5.   Haynes, R.E., et al.: Randomized comparison of bretylium and lidocaine in resuscitation of patients from out-of-hospital ventricular fibrillation. Circulation (SupplI):11-177, 1978.
6.   Jackson, C., et al.: Pulmonary and cerebral fat embolism after closed chest cardiac massage. Surg. Gynecol. Obstet., 120:25, 1965.
7.   McIntyre, K.M., and Lewis, F. (eds.): Textbook of Advanced Cardiac Life Support. American Heart Association, 1983.
8.   McIntyre, K.M., et al.: Standards and guidelines for cardiopulmonary resuscitation and cardiac care. J.A.M.A., 244:453, 1980.
9.   McSwain, N.E.: Pneumatic trousers and mangement of shock. J. Trauma, 17:719, 1977.
10.   Moore, E.E., et al.: Rationale for selective application of emergency department thoracotomy in trauma. J. Trauma, 23:453-459, 1983.
11.   Moore, E.E., Eiseman, B., and VanWay, C.W.: Critical Decisions in Trauma. St. Louis, C.V. Mosby, 1984.
12.   Rosen, P., and Baker, F.J. (eds.): Emergency Medicine: Concepts and Clinical Practice. St. Louis, C.V. Mosby, 1983.

13. Spence, A.A., et al.: Observations on intragastric pressure. Anaesthesia, 22:249, 1967.
14. Trunkey, D.T., and Lewis, F.R. (eds.): Current Therapy in Trauma. St. Louis, C.V. Mosby/B.C. Decker, 1984.
15. Weisfeldt, M.L.: Prolonging compression duration resulting in greater forward-flow index at all compression rates studied. N. Engl. J. Med., 296:516, 1977.

2. NUTRITIONAL ASSESSMENT AND ENTERAL NUTRITION
CHARLES W. VAN WAY, M.D.

1. **Who should receive nutritional support?**
   Anyone who is malnourished or who is going to be unable to eat adequately for more than 5 to 7 days. After a large operation or major injury, no one should go without nutritional support for more than 5 days. There is evidence that immediate nutritional support is best.

2. **How do you classify malnutrition?**
   There are two classic categories: marasmus is protein and calorie malnutrition; kwashiorkor is protein malnutrition, which may coexist with obesity. Kwashiorkor-marasmus mix is a combination of the two.

3. **What is nutritional assessment?**
   Nutritional assessment is the measurement of somatic and visceral proteins, cell-mediated immunity, and nitrogen balance.

4. **What are the measurements of somatic protein?**
   Somatic protein is assessed by weight and height, creatinine-height index, arm muscle circumference, triceps skin fold thickness, and the (calculated) mid-arm muscle circumference.
   Creatinine–height index = Actual creatinine/ideal creatinine (from table)
   Mid-arm muscle circumference = Mid-arm circumference (cm) – 0.314 x triceps skin fold thickness (mm)

5. **How is the visceral protein status assessed?**
   Visceral protein status includes serum albumin, serum transferrin, and total lymphocyte count. Serum albumin should be over 3.5 gm/dl. Between 3 and 3.5 is mild malnutrition, 2.5-3 is moderate, and less than 2.5 is severe. Transferrin should be over 200 mg/dl; less than 160 indicates severe malnutrition. Total lymphocyte count should be over 1800/ml; less than 900 is characteristic of severe malnutrition. However, total lymphocyte count may be affected by any condition that increases white blood cell count, including operation, infection, and injury.

6. **How is cell-mediated immunity assessed?**
   A battery of skin tests, usually including *Candida albicans*, mumps, PPD and coccidioidin, is given; these are read in usual fashion. Most patients respond to at least two of the four. Response to one or none is considered anergy.

7. **What is nitrogen balance?**
   Nitrogen balance is the difference between nitrogen input, as calculated from the dietary intake, and nitrogen output, as calculated from total urinary nitrogen. An approximation commonly used is a 24-hour urine urea nitrogen (UUN), which is somewhat less than the total nitrogen output. To approximate the nitrogen output: Total nitrogen output = UUN + 4 or Total nitrogen output = UUN x 1.25

8. **What is the difference between grams of nitrogen and grams of protein?**
Most high quality-protein is about 16% nitrogen, by weight. To obtain grams of protein, multiply grams of nitrogen by 6.25: Gm protein = (gm nitrogen) x   6.25

9. **What is the normal value for nitrogen balance?**
Less than 12 gm/day. If a fasting adult with no protein intake receives 500 calories or less, the negative nitrogen balance (nitrogen loss) will be 6 to 8 gm/day. Following a major operation, this may rise to 12 gm/day. After a major injury, with multiple long bone fractures, nitrogen loss will be 15 to 20 gm/day. After a major burn, nitrogen loss may be as high as 40 gm/day.

10. **Which enteral diet is best?**
Two kinds of diet are generally available. Most common are milk- or egg-based formulas. These contain 0.80 to 0.85 kcal of carbohydrates/ml, 25 to 60 gm of protein/L, plus varying amounts of fat, electrolytes, trace elements, and vitamins. These are available in a variety of flavors, formats, and osmolalities. They are used for nutritional supplement, nasogastric feeding, and feeding through small-diameter nasogastric or nasointestinal tubes. They can be used for gastrostomy feedings. They are not suitable for catheter jejunostomies. If given directly into the small bowel, an isotonic solution should be used rather than the cheaper hypertonic solutions.
Elemental diets are glucose, amino acids, electrolytes, and vitamins. Because of the presence of the amino acids, they taste terrible. While basically undrinkable, they can be given into the stomach or directly into the small bowel through a catheter jejunostomy. Elemental diets are 5 to 10 times as expensive as milk-based diets. Some specialized elemental diets are applicable to a specific disease process, such as diets for renal failure and hepatic failure, and high branched-chain diets for use in injured patients. These diets have amino acid mixtures tailored for particular disease processes. Their efficacy is controversial.

11. **What are normal calorie and protein requirements?**
Recommended minimum daily allowance for an adult human is 50 gm of protein and 1800 kilocalories (25 kcal/kg). However, in critically ill patients, requirements are higher: 25 to 40 kcal/kg/day of nonprotein calories, and 1.2 to 1.8 gm of protein (0.2 to 0.3 gm of nitrogen)/kg/day.

12. **Do children have different requirements?**
These requirements hold for children down to about 20 kg in body weight. Below this, calorie and protein requirements per kilogram increase.

13. **What are the complications of enteral nutrition?**
Mechanical: gastroesophageal reflux, aspiration, tube displacement, tube obstruction, gastrostomy/jejunostomy leaks, and pneumatosis intestinalis from catheter jejunostomy. *Digestive*: diarrhea, bloating, and lactose intolerance. *Metabolic*: hyperglycemia and hyponatremia.

CONTROVERSIES
14. **Should patients receive enteral or parenteral nutrition?**
Enteral nutrition is preferable for three reasons: (1) normal digestion by the GI tract is more physiological, whatever that means; (2) there are fewer metabolic or mechanical complications from enteral nutrition; and (3) the cost of enteral nutrition is one tenth that of parenteral nutrition. If patients can eat, they should eat. If they can be fed by a tube in the GI tract, that should be done.

Parenteral nutrition is faster, surer, more controlled, and must be given if patients cannot eat. Attempted enteral feeding, if unsuccessful, may waste several critical days.

15. What is the best method of GI access?

A nasogastric tube provides easy access to the stomach but may also produce discomfort, sinusitis, gastroesophageal reflux, and aspiration. Small Silastic nasogastric tubes can be used for gastric feeding, and produce very little discomfort and few complications. A nasojejunal tube can be passed through the pylorus into the duodenum. This is useful if stomach empties poorly. Surgical gastrostomy can be done through a relatively small incision under local anesthesia. Percutaneous gastrostomy, using a gastroscope, is promising, although the complication rate is high. Catheter jejunostomy: A 16-gauge catheter is placed in the proximal jejunum, threaded for 20 or 30 cm, and brought out through the abdominal wall, fixing the jejunum at that point to prevent displacement of the catheter. This is best done at laparotomy. Its applicability is greatest following abdominal operations. The small catheter can be pulled out without risking a leak. There is some restriction on what sort of diet may be used, since the fluid must be thin enough to pass through the thin catheter. Elemental diets such as Vivonex or Vivonex HN must be used.

16. Should nutritional support be used perioperatively?

For: In malnourished patients, nutritional support before, during, and after operation is probably beneficial. In injured patients, there is some evidence that nutritional support should be started immediately following injury.

Against: In adequately nourished patients, there is no evidence that nutritional support helps. If the patient can eat within 5 to 7 days, the brief period of inadequate nutrition is not harmful.

BIBLIOGRAPHY

1. Buzby, G.P., Mullen, J.L., and Matthews, D.C.: Prognostic nutritional index in gastro-intestinal surgery. Am. J. Surg., 139:160, 1980.
2. Cerra, F.B.: Pocket Manual of Surgical Nutrition. St. Louis, C.V. Mosby, 1984.
3. Detsky, A.S., and Jeejeebhoy, K.N.: Cost effectiveness of preoperative parenteral nutrition in patients undergoing major gastrointestinal surgery. J.P.E.N., 8:632-637, 1984.
4. Fischer, J.E. (ed.): Surgical Nutrition. Boston, Little, Brown, 1983.
5. Harvey, K.J.B., Ruggiero, J.A., Regan, C.S., et al.: Hospital mortality-morbidity risk factors using nutritional assessment. J. Clin. Nutr., 26:581, 1978.
6. Jeejeebhoy, K.N., et al.: Total Parenteral Nutrition in the Hospital and at Home. Boca Raton, Florida, CRC Press, 1983.
7. Kaminski, M.V., Fitzgerald, M.J., and Murphy, R.J.: Correlation of mortality with serum transferrin and anergy. J.P.E.N., 1:27, 1977.
8. Moore, E.E., Dunn, E.L., and Jones, T.N.: Immediate jejunostomy feeding. Arch. Surg., 116:681-684, 1981.
9. Mullen, J.L., Buzby, G.P., and Matthews, D. C.: Reduction of operative morbidity and mortality by combined preoperative and postoperative nutritional support. Ann. Surg., 192:604, 1980.
10. Page, C.P., Carlton, P.K., Andrassy, R.J., et al.: Safe, cost-effective postoperative nutrition: Defined formula diet via needle-catheter jejunostomy. Am. J. Surg., 138:939-945, 1979.

3. TOTAL PARENTERAL NUTRITION
EDWARD BARTLE, M.D.

1. **What is total parenteral nutrition (TPN)?**
   TPN refers to delivery of all necessary nutrients by central or peripheral vein. The fluid infused is composed of a high dextrose solution mixed with an amino acid solution of varying concentrations of essential and nonessential amino acids. Fats can be infused separately.

2. **What else is included in a TPN solution?**
   Besides amino acids and glucose, electrolytes, calcium, magnesium, and phosphorus as well as acetate as a buffer are included. It is also probably essential to include the trace elements zinc, manganese, copper, chromium, and selenium for long-term TPN. Multivitamins and folate are also routinely added, whereas vitamin K should be given separately.

3. **How is TPN delivered?**
   Usually TPN is delivered via a central vein so that a high glucose solution can be used (25% dextrose in water). TPN is also used peripherally with a solution of 5% dextrose in water and glucose, and should be delivered continuously with fats in order to decrease the incidence of phlebitis.

4. **Which is the best way to deliver TPN?**
   More non-protein calories as glucose can be delivered centrally and usually more than twice the amino acids can be delivered centrally as compared with peripherally. Despite vein sparing by the fat solutions, commonly the peripheral veins do not last long. It is difficult to deliver enough peripherally to do much in excess of protein-sparing alone.

5. **Are fats or glucose better to supply non-protein calories?**
   They are equally good sources of calories; however, prices will vary and it may be less expensive to use glucose. The main advantage of fats is their ability to reduce the respiratory quotient. This is the amount of carbon dioxide produced per substrate (or oxygen) oxidized. A patient on a ventilator or with chronic obstructive pulmonary disease may have lower production of carbon dioxide (decreased minute ventilation) if fats are used as the main non-protein calorie source.

6. **When should TPN be used?**
   Common indications include (1) nothing by mouth for longer than 7 days, (2) enterocutaneous fistulas, including Crohn's, (3) short gut syndrome, (4) neonatal periods, (5) trauma, and (6) burns. Questionable indications are (1) pancreatitis, (2) hepatic failure (branched-chain amino acids) (see Controversies), and (3) cancer cachexia (see Controversies).

7. **What can be done for a patient with uncontrolled hyperglycemia?**
   There are two ways to treat this problem. Insulin can be directly added to the hyperalimentation solution in the pharmacy (up to 100 units per 1000 ml possible). If this does not work, then fats should be used as the main non-protein calorie source. Fats usually are delivered separately, but recently there have been attempts to use fat admixture systems to deliver fats directly. This has not yet gained widespread acceptance.

8. **What are the complications of TPN?**
    The complications can be divided into mechanical (line) and metabolic (solution) problems. *Mechanical:* all the complications associated with insertion of a central line including pneumothorax, carotid stick, line infection, great vein thrombosis, etc. *Metabolic:* Acidosis is common and alkalosis will occasionally be seen. Hyperosmolar nonketotic coma is uncommon (1 to 4%) but associated with a high mortality (30%), and glucose levels must be constantly watched. Levels of electrolytes, calcium, phosphorus, and magnesium must be monitored continuously. Sepsis with associated glucose and insulin intolerance is a constant worry.

9. **What is the cost of TPN?**
    TPN costs approximately $100 per day for solutions and $50 to $100 daily for standard laboratory tests. This compares with $8 to $10 daily to use a nonelemental diet such as Ensure Plus or Sustacal.

10. **What about branched-chain amino acids (BCAA)?**
    BCAA include leucine, isoleucine, and valine. They have the advantage that they can be metabolized peripherally in the muscles as an energy source. They may be beneficial in liver failure, trauma, and sepsis but this is still controversial.

CONTROVERSIES
11. **TPN and cancer.**
    For: (1) Nutritional status is usually poor, and TPN will decrease anergy and perioperative morbidity. (2) Logical, especially when albumin level is 2.5 g/dl.
    Against: (1) Morbidity of TPN. (2) Feed the patient, feed the cancer, especially in patients with metastatic disease. (3) Lack of prospective randomized study to support the use of TPN in patients with cancer.

12. **Use of BCAA.**
    For: (1) Logical, decreases peripheral autocannibalism. (2) Patients with sepsis, trauma, or liver failure have increased needs for amino acids in general.
    Against: (1) Expense: 2 to 4 times as costly as standard solutions. (2) Lack of clinical studies to support their use.

BIBLIOGRAPHY
1.   Bawer, R.H., Kern, K.A., and Fischer, J.E.: Use of branched chain amino acid enriched solutions in patients under metabolic stress. Am. J. Surg., 149:266, 1985.
2.   Bozzetti, E., Migliavacca, S., Scotti, A., et al.: Impact of cancer, type, site, stage and treatment on the nutritional status of patients. Ann. Surg., 196:170, 1982.
3.   Buzby, G.P., Mullen, J.L., Matthews, D.C., et al.: Prognostic nutritional index in gastrointestinal surgery. Am. J. Surg., 139:160, 1980.
4.   Cerra F.B., Siegel, J.H., Cole, B., et al.: Septic autocannibalism: A failure of exogenous nutritional support. Ann. Surg., 192:570, 1980.
5.   Chandra, R.K.: Nutrition, immunity, and infection: Present knowledge and future directions. Lancet, 1983, p. 688.
6.   Christou, N.V., Rode, N., Larsen, D., et al.: The walk in anergic patient: How best to assess the risk of sepsis following elective surgery. Ann. Surg., 199:438, 1984.
7.   Daly, J.M., Massar, F., Giacco, G., et al.: Parenteral nutrition in esophageal cancer patients. Ann. Surg., 196:203, 1982.
8.   Detsky A.S., Mendelson, R.A., Baker, J.P., et al.: The choice to treat all, some or no patients undergoing gastrointestinal surgery with nutritional support: A decision analysis approach. J.P.E.N., 8:245, 1984.
9.   Dudrick, S.S., Wilmore, D.W., Vars, H.M., et al.: Can intravenous feeding as the sole means of nutrition support growth in the child and restore weight loss in an adult? An affirmative answer. Ann. Surg., 169:974, 1969.
10. Harvey, K.B., Moldawer, L.L., Bistrian, B.R., et al.: Biological measures for the formulation of a hospital prognostic index. Am. J. Clin. Nutr., 34:2013, 1981.

11. Koretz, R.L.: Parenteral nutrition: Is it oncologically logical? J. Clin. Oncol., 2:534, 1984.

12. Mullen, J.L., Buzby, G.P., Matthews, D.C., et al.: Reduction of operative morbidity and mortality by combined preoperative and postoperative nutritional support. Ann. Surg., 192:604, 1980.

13. Mullen, J.L., Crosby, L.O., and Rombeau, J.L. (eds.): Symposium on Surgical Nutrition. Surg. Clin. North Am., 61:61-90, 1981.

14. Nehme, A.E.: Nutritional support of the hospitalized patient. The team concept. J.A.M.A., 243:1906, 1980.

15. Padberg, F.T., Ruggiero, J., Blackburn, G.L., et al.: Central venous catheterization for parenteral nutrition. Ann. Surg., 193:264, 1981.

16. Starker, P.M., Lasala, P.A., Askanazi, J., et al.: The response to TPN: A form of nutritional assessment. Ann. Surg., 198:720, 1983.

17. Superina, R., and Meakins, J.L.: Delayed hypersensitivity, anergy, and the surgical patient. J. Surg. Res., 37:151, 1983.

18. Warnold, I., and Lundholm, K.: Clinical significance of preoperative nutritional status in 215 noncancer patients. Ann. Surg., 199:299, 1984.

19. Weinsier, R.L., Jane Bacon, P.H., and Butterworth, C.E.: Central venous alimentation: A prospective study of the frequency of metabolic abnormalities among medical and surgical patients. J.P.E.N., 6:421, 1982.

4. FLUIDS AND ELECTROLYTES
HAMILTON LOKEY, M.D.

1. **How much sodium is in normal saline?**
    154 mEq/L.

2. **What are the daily maintenance intravenous requirements for adults?**
    a. Volume   2500 to 3000 ml
    b. Sodium   80 mEq (~1mEq/kg)
    c. Potassium   40 mEq (~1/2 mEq/kg)

3. **Does the average postoperative patient need**
    a. Potassium chloride added to the intravenous solution?   No
    b. A routine postoperative electrolyte test?   No

4. **Which intravenous solution closely approximates nasogastric tube losses?**
    (D5) 1/2 NS + 20 KCl/liter

5. **What are the components of Ringer's lactate?**
    Na^+, 130 mEq/L; K^+, 4 mEq/L; Ca^{++}, 3 mEq/L; Cl^-, 110 mEq/L; lactate, 28 mEq/L.

6. **Estimate the daily outputs of the stomach, bile, and pancreas.**
    Stomach–2000 ml; bile–up to 1000 ml; pancreas–1500 to 2500 ml.

7. **How do you compute intravenous fluid rates for pediatric patients?**
    0 to 10 kg–100 ml/kg/24hr; plus 10 to 20 kg–75 ml/kg/24 hr; plus 20+ kg–50 ml/kg/24hr

8. **Which electrolyte is most useful in correcting hypokalemic metabolic alkalosis?**
    Chloride.

9. **What are the two most sensitive clinical indicators of a patient's volume status postoperatively?**
Blood pressure and urinary output.

10. **What is the minimum satisfactory adult postoperative urinary output?**
30 ml/hr (~1/2 ml/kg/hr)

11. **How do you manage postoperative patients with low urinary outputs?**
Most patients will need additional volume. Only rarely will a patient be overloaded. Patients with congestive heart failure or those on a regimen of chronic diuretics may occasionally require small doses of furosemide (Lasix).

12. **What does central venous pressure measure?**
Only the filling pressure of the right side of the heart.

13. **What does a Swan-Ganz catheter measure?**
The pulmonary wedge pressure closely parallels left atrial filling pressure and is much more useful than central venous pressure in monitoring volume status. Cardiac output and various other cardiovascular parameters can also be measured.

14. **What is "third spacing"?**
Pathophysiologic processes frequently seen in surgical patients (shock, ischemic injury, trauma, peritonitis, and bowel obstruction) result in rapid accumulations of fluid in tissues and hollow viscus spaces. This fluid is drawn from vascular space, resulting in functional volume depletion requiring additional fluid replacement.

15. **What is the "two-unit transfusion rule"?**
Cardiovascular dynamics *usually* permit blood losses up to 1000 ml (trauma, surgery) with maintenance of vital signs through adequate crystalloid replacement. It has been traditionally considered "inappropriate" to give only a single-unit transfusion. The risks and costs inherent probably exceed the benefits.

16. **How do MAST trousers work?**
Military antishock trousers (MAST) probably do not autotransfuse the patient. Rather, they increase peripheral vascular resistance. This issue is controversial.

17. **What is autotransfusion?**
Special equipment is available to harvest a patient's shed blood during major surgery (especially after trauma), filter it, and transfuse immediately.

18. **What is autologous transfusion?**
Patients undergoing major elective surgery with anticipated transfusion needs may have their own blood drawn preoperatively. This blood is banked and transfused into the patient during surgery, avoiding some complications of homologous blood.

19. **What are the complications of massive blood transfusions?**
Coagulopathies, hypothermia, transfusion reactions, pulmonary insufficiency, hepatitis, electrolyte disturbance (increased K^+, decreased Ca^{++}), and acquired immune deficiency syndrome (AIDS).

CONTROVERSIES
20. **Colloid vs. crystalloid in hemorrhagic shock.**
Colloid *For:* Adequately restores intravascular volume; faster; maintains osmotic pressure. *Against:* Cost.

Crystalloid *For:* Adequately restores intravascular volume; replaces extracellular fluid losses. *Against:* Large volumes and lowered osmotic pressure *may* predispose to acute respiratory distress syndrome.

Current Consensus
Treatment of severe hemorrhage (20 to 25% blood volume): (a) Replace blood cc for cc. (b) Crystalloid, several liters. Acute respiratory distress syndrome related to "sepsis," not to volume or type of fluid. (c) Colloid accomplishes same end, no advantage, increased cost.

21. **Should packed cells be used instead of whole blood?**
    For: More efficient use of blood components. Clinically, there is no evidence of increased coagulopathy or pulmonary dysfunction.
    Against: Larger volumes of crystalloid are required to maintain wedge pressure. Osmotic presure is decreased.

BIBLIOGRAPHY

1. Kaback, K. R., et al.: MAST suit update. J.A.M.A., 252:2598, 1984.
2. Mengoli, L.: Excerpts from the history of postoperative fluid therapy. Am. J. Surg., 111:311, 1971.
3. Poole, G.V., et al.: Comparison of colloids and crystalloids in resuscitation from hemorrhagic shock: Collective review. Surg. Gynecol. Obstet., 154:577, 1982.
4. Shackford, S.R., et al.: Whole blood vs. packed-cell transfusions. Ann. Surg., 193:337, 1981.
5. Shires, T., et al.: Acute changes in extracellular fluids associated with major surgical procedures. Ann. Surg., 154:803, 196l.
6. Shires, T., et al.: Fluid resuscitation in the severely injured. Surg. Clin. North Am., 53:1341, 1973.
7. Shoemaker, W. C., et al.: Comparison of the relative effectiveness of colloids and crystalloids in emergency resuscitation. Am. J. Surg., 142:73, 1981.
8. Thurer, R., et al.: Autotransfusion and blood conservation. Curr. Probl. Surg., 19 (3), 1982.
9. Virgilio, R.W., et al.: Crystalloid vs colloid resuscitation: Is one better? Surgery, 85:129, 1979.

---

5. PROPHYLACTIC ANTIBIOTICS
CHARLES ABERNATHY, M.D.

---

1. **What is the infection rate in intraabdominal surgery without use of prophylactic antibiotics? With prophylactic antibiotics?**

	Without	With
Gastroduodenal surgery	22–63%	0–5%
Hepatobiliary surgery	1.4–17%	0–3%

2. **What factors make a patient "high-risk" for operations on the biliary tract?**
   Age over 70 years; jaundice at operation; stress within one week of operation; emergency operation; operation within 4 weeks before emergency admission; previous biliary operation; stones in bile duct; bile duct obstruction.

3. **When should prophylactic antibiotics be given?**
   Most recent studies have found that the antibiotic should be given just prior to surgery for maximum benefit.

4. **How long should prophylactic antibiotics be continued?**
    No benefit appears to accrue if antibiotics are continued beyond 24-36 hours. For grossly contaminated or dirty cases, antibiotics are continued longer; however, in these cases antibiotics are considered to be early therapy rather than prophylaxis.

5. **What type of antibiotics should be used for prophylaxis in intraabdominal surgery?**
    For elective intraabdominal (includes gastroduodenal, hepatobiliary):
    Piperacillin–2 gm prior to surgery; then 2 gm q 6 hr for no more than 24 hr
    (use cefoxitin or another cephalosporin for penicillin-allergic patients).

6. **Should prophylactic antibiotics be used in appendicitis?**
    Yes. A wide variety of preoperative antibiotics have been used in both perforated and nonperforated appendicitis, including ampicillin, metronidazole, and cephalosporins. Virtually all studies have shown significant reduction in the infection rates with antibiotic prophylaxis.

7. **Are antibiotics given for a ruptured appendix really "prophylactic"?**
    The semantics are difficult, but in grossly contaminated settings, the terms "preventive" or "early therapy" are more appropriate than "prophylactic."

8. **In penetrating intraabdominal trauma, which factors appear to affect the infection rate most?**
    Distal ileal or colon injuries consistently correlate with high infection rates. Other factors such as shock, degree of contamination, and increased age are important but difficult to correlate directly with infection rates.

9. **In elective vascular surgery, should prophylactic antibiotics be used?**
    Two well-controlled studies have shown antibiotic prophylaxis to be of benefit in vascular surgery. Certainly, where prosthetic grafts are to be used, antibiotic prophylaxis is mandatory.

BIBLIOGRAPHY
1. Baker, R.J., et al.: A prospective double-blind comparison of piperacillin, cephalothin, and cefoxitin in the prevention of postoperative infections in patients undergoing intra-abdominal operations. Surg. Gynecol. Obstet., 161:409-415, 1985.
2. Conte, J.E., Jacob, L.S., and Polk, H.C.: Antibiotic Prophylaxis in Surgery: A Comprehensive Review. Philadelphia, J. B. Lippincott, 1984.

---

6. PULMONARY INSUFFICIENCY, RESPIRATORY FAILURE, AND PULMONARY EMBOLUS
THOMAS L. PETTY, M.D.

PART I: Pulmonary Insufficiency and Respiratory Failure

1. **What is meant by pulmonary insufficiency and respiratory failure?**
    Pulmonary insufficiency can occur in a wide variety of insults to airways, alveoli, and the respiratory pump, meaning the diaphragm and chest wall. Pulmonary insufficiency covers a broad spectrum of severity ranging from increased effort of breathing to overt acute respiratory failure defined by blood gas abnormalities. We define respiratory failure as inadequate arterial oxygenation, inadequate carbon dioxide elimination, or both.

2. **When are pulmonary insufficiency and respiratory failure present?**
Pulmonary insufficiency is present when tachypnea and labored breathing begin. Respiratory failure is present when the arterial PO_2 while breathing air is less than 60 mm Hg and/or the PCO_2 is more than 50 mm Hg. It is even easier to remember the 50-50 rule, i.e., PO_2 less than 50 (an oxygen saturation of about 80%) and PCO_2 of more than 50.

3. **How is an exact diagnosis made? The word EXACT is the tipoff.**
E = Examine the patient. Count the respiratory rate. Tachypnea, i.e., a respiratory rate more than 20, is the first sign of pulmonary insufficiency. Notice the patient's appearance. Does he/she look distressed, appear anxious, and have diaphoresis? Is he/she using the accessory muscles of respiration? Is cyanois present (generally an unreliable sign)?
X = X-ray of the chest. Here use your A & P check list. A = aspiration, A = atelectasis, P = pneumonia, P = pleural effusion, P = pneumothorax, P = pulmonary embolus (although x-ray signs of pulmonary embolization are not reliable). See Part II of this chapter on Pulmonary Embolus.
A = Arterial blood gases (ABGs). Remember that blood gases are only a "snapshot" of what is going on. ABGs should be interpreted in light of the clinical state. They tell you what the patient is doing but not how hard he/she is working to accomplish oxygen transfer and carbon dioxide elimination. Interpret blood gases in the light of the inspired oxygen, i.e., room air, oxygen by nasal cannula, oxygen by mask, or oxygen delivered by mechanical ventilation. What is the inspired oxygen fraction in relation to the arterial oxygen tension (a crude estimate of oxygen transfer across the lung)? Is PEEP being used to augment oxygen transfer? What is the pH? Are we dealing with acidemia, i.e., pH less than 7.35, or alkalemia, i.e., pH more than 7.45? Compensated states are called "acidosis" and "alkalosis," respectively, with a pH within the range of 7.35 to 7.45.
C = Capacity. Here we mean *vital capacity,* which is the capacity to live and survive in the postoperative period. Forced vital capacity (FVC) is the volume of air exhaled from fully inflated lungs. It is the best predictor of outcome in surgical states. Learn to measure FVC at the bedside with a disposable spirometer. Also, time expiration. If expiratory airflow requires more than 6 seconds as you listen over the trachea, airflow obstruction or limitation is present. Think only in terms of volume and flow in capacity tests of lung function. The FVC is the volume test, and the forced expiratory volume in the first second (FEV1) and peak flow are tests of expiratory airflow. Peak flow is also a simple bedside airflow test. It roughly parallels the FEV1. You can also estimate flow by timing it. Bedside spirometry should also be available in your hospital. Learn to use a spirometer and to interpret the results of FVC and FEV1 in your surgical patients.
T = Think. Think and correlate what the clinical signs, underlying disease state, chest x-ray, vital capacity, FEV1 or peak flow, and arterial blood gases tell you. They will help you decide whether the problem is in the airways, the parenchyma, the respiratory pump, or combinations of these.

4. **What conditions require PEEP?**
PEEP is often helpful in increasing arterial oxygenation in ARDS. PEEP should be used at 5 to 15 cm if the FIO_2 requirements are > 0.6.

5. **What are the criteria for endotracheal intubation/mechanical ventilation?**
Inability to spontaneously maintain blood gases with PO_2 > 50 and PCO_2 < 50 with pH of 7.35 while breathing supplemental oxygen; progressive respiratory muscle fatigue; apneic states.

6.   **When can the patient be taken off mechanical ventilation?**
     When the patient can comfortably do what the ventilator has been doing.
     Checklist: rate ≤ 20; FIO2 ≤ 0.4 or off PEEP; minute ventilation < 10 L/min.; vital
     capacity 1000 cc; awake and alert; wants off ventilator.

7.   **Should all patients with FVC and/or FEV1 abnormalities receive bronchodilators?**
     The answer to this question as to most other questions of surgical judgment is, "It
     all depends." Certainly a trial course of an inhaled beta agonist, such as albuterol
     (Proventil or Ventolin) or bitolterol (Tornalate) is wise. It will help determine
     whether improvements in airflow occur as judged by FEV1. Two puffs inhaled
     slowly from a metered dose inhaler are all that is needed. Repeat both the FVC
     and FEV1 and look for improvement; 15% above baseline is considered signifi-
     cant. Cardiac arrhythmias are rarely stimulated by inhaled beta agonists. The use
     of systemic bronchodilators becomes another consideration. Theophylline is a
     potent long-acting oral bronchodilator. It also strengthens respiratory muscles
     and helps prevent respiratory muscle fatigue. It may have a small but beneficial
     effect on cardiac output and is a modest respiratory stimulant. Since it is a cardiac
     stimulant, theophylline should not be administered to patients suffering serious
     arrhythmias. Theophyllines also stimulate gastric secretions and relax the
     gastroesophageal physiological sphincter, and thus should not be used in
     patients suffering gastroesophageal reflux or in those with peptic ulcer disease.

8.   **What about corticosteroids?**
     They are not bronchodilators. They do augment the effect of inhaled beta
     agonists by restoring beta receptor activity but may interfere with wound healing if
     used in large doses.

9.   **Are there guidelines for determining the potential for thoracic surgery that are useful in clinical practice?**
     Guidelines are only crude estimates and must be applied to the individual patient,
     considering each patient in total. However, Table 1 provides crude criteria for
     determining the potential for common thoracic surgical procedures for a
     60-year-old man.

Table 1
Determining Potential for Thoracic Surgery for a 60-Year-Old Man

	Approximate % of Predicted *FEV_1	Approximate *FEV_1 (L/sec)
Candidate for pneumonectomy	45	1.6
Candidate for lobectomy	35	1.2
Candidate for thoracotomy for wedge biopsy only	25 to 35	0.9
No thoracic surgery possible	20	0.7

*For a 6-foot man, aged 60, predicted FEV1 is 3.6 L/sec. Exceptions to these
rough guidelines must be individualized.

10. **Which criteria determine normal ventilatory function (FVC and FEV1)?**
     As first defined by a surgeon, John Hutchinson, who introduced the spirometer
     into clinical medicine in 1846, normal values are based on age, sex, and height.

These have been refined over the past 140 years, and nomograms are widely published.

CONTROVERSIES

11. Many sophisticated physiologists have introduced flow–volume loops and practically more numbers derived therefrom than one can count. Forget them. They tell nothing more than the FVC and FEV1. Other tests, such as measurements of lung compartments and diffusion, do not call for clinical decision making in surgical patients. Only spirometric tests, i.e., FVC and FEV1, and arterial blood gases require decision making.

Remember that the chest x-ray is not a pulmonary function test!

BIBLIOGRAPHY

1. Anders, A.J., Baidwan, B., and Petty, T.L.: An evaluation of the vitometer, a simple method for measuring vital capacity. Respir. Care, 84:1144-1146, 1984.
2. Bagg, L.R., Evans, S.J.W., Empey, D.W., et al.: Analysis of simple pulmonary function screening tests in preoperative assessment before lung resection for bronchiogenic carcinoma. Respiration, 42:1-7, 1981.
3. Boysen, P.G., Block, A.J., and Moulder, P.V.: Relationship between preoperative pulmonary function tests and complications after thoracotomy. Surg. Gynecol. Obstet., 157:813-815, 1981.
4. Gelb, A.F., William, A.J., and Zamel, N.: Spirometry (FEV_1 vs $FEF_{25-75\%}$). Chest, 84:473-474, 1983.
5. Hudson, L.D., Petty, T.L., Baidwan, B., et al.: Clinical evaluation of a new office spirometer. J.A.M.A., 240:2754-2755, 1978.
6. Hutchinson, J.: On the capacity of the lungs and on the respiratory functions with a view of establishing a precise and easy method of detecting disease by the spirometer. Med. Clin. Trans. (London), 29:147, 1846.
7. Kannel, W.B.: The value of measuring vital capacity for prognostic purposes. Trans. Assoc. Life Inst. Med. Dir. Amer., 64:66-81, 1980.
8. Light, R.W., Conrad, S.A., and George, R.B.: The one best test for evaluating the effects of bronchodilator therapy. Chest, 72:512-516, 1977.
9. Morris, J.F.: Spirometry in the evaluation of pulmonary function. West. J. Med., 125:110-118, 1976.
10. Peto, R., Speizer, F.E., Cochrane, A.L., et al: The relevance in adults of airflow obstruction, but not of mucus hypersecretion, to morbidity from chronic lung disease. Am. Rev. Respir. Dis., 128:491-500, 1983.

PART II: Pulmonary Embolus

1. **How important is the diagnosis of a pulmonary embolus?**

    It is extremely important. It is estimated that 200,000 deaths occur annually from major pulmonary emboli. Since this frequent complication in surgical patients can be both prevented and effectively treated, an accurate diagnosis is essential.

2. **In what setting does pulmonary embolism usually occur in surgical patients?**

    Since dehydration resulting in blood "sludging" can occur faster in venous thrombosis, which is the major risk factor for pulmonary embolus, and because the reverse is rehydration of the patient, it seems reasonable to use the mnemonic MOIST.

    M = Malignancy. Pulmonary embolism is known to occur in patients with all forms of malignant disease, particularly intraabdominal cancer. It also occurs in occult malignancies and may be the presenting sign.

O = Orthopedics. Patients who are immobilized for orthopedic injuries, with or without surgery, are at high risk for development of pulmonary embolism.

I = Immobility from any cause. Be concerned about your obese patient lying in bed with venostasis.

S = Surgery, either elective or emergent. Any patient in the postoperative period is at risk for pulmonary embolism.

T = Trauma. Certainly the traumatized patient is at risk for pulmonary embolism as well for a specialized form of embolism, fat embolism, which often follows major fractures of the long bones and pelves.

3.   How is the diagnosis made?   Think *SCAN*.

S = Suspicion. Consider pulmonary embolus in any patient who is suddenly short of breath. Shortness of breath is the most common symptom in pulmonary embolism. The second commonest is chest pain, which often varies with respiration (pleuritic chest pain). Patients with pulmonary embolism, however, may be asymptomatic. Listen to the patient's chest. If you hear a pleural friction rub, consider that it may be associated with a pulmonary embolism.

C = Chest x-ray. A chest x-ray, of course, is not diagnostic of pulmonary embolism, but related findings may be suggestive. A large infiltrate with or without effusion that is not accompanied by chills, fever, or leukocytosis strongly suggests pulmonary embolism. Patients with pulmonary embolism may be febrile, however, and also may have leukocytosis. They rarely have chills unless infectious complications are present.

There may be decreased lung markings from major pulmonary emboli owing to decreased perfusion of localized regions of the lung. You will need the chest x-ray to help interpret radionuclide studies, which are helpful in diagnosing pulmonary embolism (see below).

A = Arterial blood gases. It has been taught that normal arterial blood gases can rule out pulmonary embolism. They can not. Some subtleties, however, may be present. The patient may be hyperventilating with a low PCO_2, i.e., less than 40, but may have a normal PO_2, suggesting ventilation–perfusion abnormalities. This should raise your level of suspicion. Arterial blood gases must be assessed to determine whether oxygen therapy or even mechanical ventilation is required in the face of a major pulmonary embolus.

N = Nuclear medicine. Perfusion and ventilation scans will be very helpful. The following are true: (a) A normal perfusion scan with a normal chest x-ray effectively excludes pulmonary embolus. (b) Mismatched scans, i.e., a perfusion defect where there is normal ventilation, effectively confirm a diagnosis of pulmonary embolism in the proper setting.

Matching of a large ventilation and perfusion defect is not diagnostic of pulmonary embolism but is strongly suggestive if pneumonia can be reasonably excluded. If the patient has not had chills, fever, or leukocytosis but has a matched defect, pulmonary embolism is likely. In time, ventilation–perfusion adjustments occur in pneumonia and in pulmonary embolus, so a matched ventilation–perfusion defect can occur in both.

4.   What is the gold standard for diagnosis?

Today it is the pulmonary angiogram. An angiogram will effectively confirm or exclude pulmonary embolism. It becomes less effective in states of delay. If several days have gone by since pulmonary embolism has occurred, a clot may have been broken up and thus not been detected. Rarely a scan is normal but an angiogram can show a large saddle embolism. Here you need your greatest index of suspicion.

5. **What are the electrocardiographic patterns suggestive of pulmonary embolus?**
    S_I, Q_{III}, T_{III}.

6. **Can a Swan-Ganz catheter help in diagnosing a pulmonary embolus?**
    A limited angiogram "shot" through a Swan-Ganz catheter can reveal a pulmonary embolus. This may be successful at the bedside.

7. **Is the triad of increased LDH, increased bilirubin, and normal SGOT helpful in diagnosing pulmonary embolism?**
    No.

8. **What are Hampton's hump and Westermark's sign?**
    Hampton's hump is an infiltrate with the curvature or hump pointed toward the hilus. It represents central clearing with a vascular distribution.
    Westermark's sign is a localized region of comparable reduced vascularity. This is not a reliable sign on a standard chest x-ray.

9. **Is prophylactic therapy effective?**
    Yes, if properly applied. The early use of low-dose heparin, 5000 units twice daily, can reduce postoperative complications. Coumadin is also useful in prophylaxis but is rarely used for this purpose in surgical patients. Neither low-dose heparin nor coumadin is effective in states of active venous thrombosis resulting in pulmonary embolism. The bottom-line therapy for established pulmonary embolism is intravenous heparinization using a continuous drip. Be guided only by partial thromboplastin times or conventional clotting times.

CONTROVERSIES

10. **Can a diagnosis of pulmonary embolism be made without an angiogram?**
    Yes, in the proper setting. A surgical patient with sudden dyspnea, hypoxemia, and a perfusion scan defect, particularly if the defect is not matched with an equivalent ventilation scan abnormality, *has a pulmonary embolus*. There is no sense procrastinating when you have these types of data. If still in doubt, do the angiogram. Do not hesitate to institute heparin therapy on the basis of a high index of suspicion, especially when the above confirmatory evidence is present.

11. **Name some clinical syndromes that can be marked by acute pulmonary embolus?**
    Fever of unknown etiology, asthma, acute abdomen, and subtle mental aberrations are occasionally mimicked by pulmonary embolism. Of course pneumonia and pulmonary embolism are most frequently confused.

12. **What about streptokinase?**
    It is probably better than heparin in massive pulmonary emboli. It protects the lung and lyses clots faster than heparin. It causes no more bleeding complications than heparin. It should not be used if there is head trauma or recent intracranial surgery, and it is nobody's first choice in the immediate postoperative period.

BIBLIOGRAPHY

1. Alpert, J., Smith, R., Carlson, J., et al.: Mortality in patients treated for pulmonary embolism. J.A.M.A., 236:1477-1480, 1976.
2. Bettman, M.A., and Saltzman, E.W.: Current concepts in the diagnosis of pulmonary embolism. Mod. Conc. Cardiovasc. Dis., 53:1-5, 1984.
3. Halkin, H., Goldberg, J., Modan, M., et al.: Reduction of mortality in general medical in-patients by low dose heparin. Ann. Intern. Med., 96:561-561, 1982.
4. Humphries, J.V., Bell, W.R., and While, R.I.: Criteria for the recognition of pulmonary emboli. J.A.M.A., 235:2011-2012, 1976.
5. Moser, K.M.: Diagnosis and management of pulmonary embolism. Hosp. Pract., 15:57-68, 1980.
6. Moser, K.M., Lemoine, J.R., Nachtwey, F.J., et al.: Deep venous thrombosis and pulmonary embolism (frequency in respiratory intensive care unit). J.A.M.A., 246:1422-1424, 1981.
7. Murray, H.W., Ellis, G.C., Blumenthal, P.S., et al.: Fever and pulmonary thromboembolism. Am. J. Med., 67:232-235, 1979.
8. Nelson, P.H., Moser, K.M., Stoner, K.M., et al.: Risk of complications during intravenous heparin therapy. West. J. Med., 136:189-197, 1982.
9. Potts, P.E., and Sahn, S.A.: Abdominal manifestations of pulmonary embolism. J.A.M.A., 235:2835-2837, 1976.
10. Rossman, I.: True incidence of pulmonary embolization and vital statistics. J.A.M.A., 230:1677-1679, 1974.
11. Sasahara, A.A., Sharma, G.V.R.K., Tow, D.E., et al.: Clinical use of thrombolytic agents in venous thromboembolism. Arch. Intern. Med., 142:684-688, 1982.
12. Wilson, S.E., III, Pierce, A.K., Johnson, R.L., Jr., et al.: Hypoxemia in pulmonary embolism, a clinical study. J. Clin. Invest., 50:481-491, 1971.
13. Windebank, W.J., Boyd, G., and Moran, F.: Pulmonary thromboembolism presenting as asthma. Br. Med. J., 1:90-94, 1973.

---

7. POSTOPERATIVE FEVER
Theodore C. Dickinson, M.D.

---

1. **What temperature is considered a fever?**
    Generally a small elevation about 37ºC is not considered significant, but an elevation greater than 37.5ºC is cause for concern.
    Comment: A temporary elevation is of less concern than a prolonged elevation. Postoperative fevers are categorized into different time frames. Although there is considerable overlap, these time frames aid in the diagnosis of the underlying cause of the fever.

2. **Fever in the immediate postoperative period (within 6 hours) is usually secondary to what?**
    Fever in this setting is usually produced by metabolic abnormalities such as thyroid crisis, adrenocortical insufficiency, or transfusion reaction. An early streptococcal infection should be looked for.

3. **What is the most likely cause of fever during the first three days after surgery?**
    Atelectasis or other pulmonary abnormality is overwhelmingly the most likely cause. It is thought that these changes occur because of inadequate pulmonary expansion during the operation or because of poor pulmonary hygiene (coughing) postoperatively.

4. **Is the fever associated with atelectasis caused by bacteria?**
    Usually not initially. Secondary bacterial infection may arise secondary to the atelectasis.

5. **Which patients are most likely to get postoperative atelectasis?**
    Smokers. Debilitated patients and obese patients are also prone to this complication as are those patients with chronic pulmonary disease.

6. **Which incisions are most likely to be associated with atelectasis?**
    Upper abdominal and chest incisions. There is evidence that transverse abdominal incisions help to protect against this complication.

7. **How do you identify postoperative atelectasis?**
    It is usually associated with tachypnea and tachycardia. Chest findings may include dullness, decreased breath sounds, rales, and rhonchi. A chest x-ray may be useful in following the process but the diagnosis can usually be made without it.

8. **What can be done to prevent postoperative atelectasis?**
    Preoperative pulmonary instruction in combination with postoperative therapy can be of great help. If the patient will stop smoking in anticipation of the operation there will be fewer pulmonary problems.

9. **How do you treat atelectasis?**
    Coughing, deep breathing, postural drainage, incentive spirometry, blow bottles, mist mask, endotracheal suctioning, and, rarely, bronchoscopy can be helpful.

10. **How do you differentiate atelectasis from pneumonia?**
    Chest x-ray is very useful. Sputum Gram stain and culture may be positive for pneumonia. Fever and chest findings that persist for longer than 2 or 3 days usually signal bacterial pneumonia.

11. **What is the most common nonpulmonary cause for positive chest findings associated with fever?**
    Inflammatory process below the diaphragm.
    Comment: A unilateral pleural effusion associated with fever is commonly seen with inflammatory processes below the diaphragm.

12. **What is the most common cause of fever that begins 5 to 7 days after surgery?**
    Wound infection.

13. **What type of cases most commonly develop wound infections?**
    Bowel cases, both infected and clean. Immunosuppressed patients are also prone to wound infections.

14. **If prophylactic antibiotics are used to prevent wound infections, when are they begun and for how long are they used?**
    They must be begun preoperatively and continued for no longer than 72 hours postoperatively.

15. **In what time frame do postoperative urinary tract infections occur?**
    Any time.

16. **What factors predispose to urinary tract infections?**
Urethral catheters, urinary tract instrumentation, and urinary stasis.

17. **What are the most useful tests for the diagnosis of a urinary tract infection?**
Urinalysis and culture.

18. **Are urinalysis and culture more accurate in males or females?**
Males. *Comment:* A clean catch urine in the male is much easier to obtain. Cultures showing greater than 100,000 organisms per ml have a very high probability that a urinary tract infection is present. Cultures showing less than 10,000 organisms/ml have a low probability. The in-between group has a low probability for females and an intermediate probability for males. The presence of many organisms in the culture also lowers the probability. Pyuria and bacteriuria likewise are more significant in males.

19. **Are any x-ray procedures helpful in the diagnosis of urinary tract infection?**
Yes. *Comment:* An intravenous pyelogram (IVP) may be needed. However, the overwhelming majority of cases can be handled without this study. It is usually reserved for recurring infections.

20. **Fever and tachycardia beginning more than 2 weeks after surgery are likely to be secondary to what condition?**
Thrombophlebitis with or without associated pulmonary embolism.

21. **What is the most common physical finding with thrombophlebitis?**
Tenderness along the involved vein.
Comment: The tenderness will be along the course of the saphenous vein if the process is superficial. The tenderness is likely to be along the course of the deep veins (calf, popliteal space, adductor canal, inguinal canal) if the process involves the deep venous system. The physical examination can be very misleading.

22. **What is the most accurate test in diagnosing thrombophlebitis?**
Venography. *Comment:* Noninvasive (Doppler) studies are very helpful if they fit in with the clinical picture. The "gold standard" remains the venogram, however.

23. **Does upper extremity thrombophlebitis lead to pulmonary emboli?**
Very rarely.

24. **What are the most effective means of preventing thrombophlebitis?**
Early ambulation, well-fitting elastic stockings, and prophylactic heparin therapy.

25. **If you have ruled out as the cause of the fever wound infection, urinary infection, thrombophlebitis, and chest causes, what should you next suspect as the cause of the fever?**
Abscess. *Comment:* Abscesses can be extremely difficult to diagnose. Multiple laboratory and x-ray (sonograms, CT scans, and gallium scans) studies may be required to locate the abscess, but abscesses must be suspected with prolonged fevers. Contaminated indwelling venous catheters are another common cause of fever. Blood cultures are frequently useful in the diagnosis of prolonged fever.

8. SHOCK

ROGER S. WOTKYNS, M.D.

1. **What is shock?**
   Shock is an acute, generalized, inadequate perfusion of critical organs which, if unchecked, will produce serious pathophysiologic consequences.

2. **What volume of blood loss is necessary to produce shock?**
   Twenty percent of blood volume is lost in mild shock, 20 to 40% in moderate shock, and 40% or more in severe shock. The blood volume of a man weighing 70 kg is 5000 ml.

3. **How is shock classified?**
   There are four major categories: oligemic (hypovolemic), cardiogenic, obstructive, and distributive.

4. **What is the clinical picture of shock?**
   In *mild shock* there is often normal blood pressure, increased heart rate, postural hypotension, cool clammy skin, flat neck veins, and a clear mental status. *Moderate shock* results in a lowered blood pressure. The patient is pale, cold, thirsty, anxious, apathetic or sleepy, but easily aroused. Urine output is reduced. In *severe shock,* blood pressure is barely perceptible, the pulse is thready, respirations are rapid, the skin is mottled, and the patient is apathetic or comatose.

5. **Summarize the causes and treatment of shock.**

	Causes	*Treatment*
Oligemic (hypo-volemic)	Hemorrhage	Blood
	Intravascular depletion. (vomiting, diarrhea, diabetes, peritonitis, burns, pancreatitis, adrenocortical insufficiency)	Rehydration, electrolyte replacement, medication
Cardiogenic	Arrhythmias	Medication, pacemaker
	Regurgitant lesions (mitral, aortic, septal defect, ventricular aneurysm)	Medication, repair
	Obstruction (mitral/aortic), lesion	Medication, repair
	Cardiomyopathies. Acute MI, CHF	Medication, revascularization, counterpulsation
Obstructive	Cardiac tamponade, constrictive pericarditis, aortic coarctation, pulmonary embolus or hypertension	Repair, medication, anticoagulation

	Causes	Treatment
Distributive	Sepsis, respiratory failure, renal failure, acid/base problems. Endocrine disorders. Microcirculatory problems (polycythemia, sickle cell, fat emboli). Neurologic problems, anaphylaxis	Medication, ventilation, dialysis

CONTROVERSIES

There is certainly no controversy about oxygen administration, adequate venous access, and emergency measures to stabilize life-threatening problems. Common to all types of shock is inadequate blood flow. Controversies arise as to the most efficacious and efficient ways of monitoring and treating the problems.

Monitoring. Systemic arterial monitoring of right-sided and left-sided heart pressures guides the rational plan. In patients with normal hearts, cuffs and CVP lines may be safe. If response to treatment is not dramatic, consider direct arterial monitoring and a left ventricular filling pressure monitor (Swan-Ganz catheter).

Volume Replacement. Volume-expanding fluids should be given to raise the CVP to 12 to 16 cm of water or pulmonary wedge pressure (PWP) of 18 to 20 mm Hg. If rapid infusion results in a rise of 3 to 4 mm Hg (PWP) and stays such without clinical improvement, persistence is not likely to be helpful. The type of fluid replacement depends on the situation: blood or packed cells for hemorrhage, crystalloids for GI losses, and colloid for plasma losses. Packed cells should probably be used in replacement of blood losses of less than 4 units and when the loss has not been rapid. Crystalloid solutions should be designed to replace fluid and electrolyte losses. Colloid losses are replaced by albumin or plasma. Artificial plasma expanders such as Hespan can be used and are cost-effective.

Correction of Acidosis and Hypoxia. The administration of intravenous sodium bicarbonate to raise the arterial pH to 7.3 or higher. Oxygen administration or ventilation may be necessary to correct arterial PO_2.

Medication. Catecholamines, vasodilators, antibiotics, diuretics, digitalis, and corticosteroids are some of the medications used in the situations listed above. Choosing a specific drug in a particular setting is often controversial and a matter of fine judgment. To underscore the controversy, a list of choices follows:

Catecholamines	Dopamine. A vasoconstrictor that increases renal blood flow.
Vasodilator	Inprecisely defined. In septic or hemorrhagic shock that progresses despite adequate volume replacement, there may be improvement in cardiac output by reducing left ventricular end-diastolic pressure. A very short-acting drug such as nitroprusside is the drug of choice.
Antibiotic	If the sensitivity of the organism is known, a specific antibiotic. If the organism is unknown, gram-positive and gram-negative organism coverage should initially be instituted (example: gentamicin, Cleocin).

Diuretic	If oliguria persists after volume restoration, furosemide (Lasix) may be useful in initiating high urine flow. Correct electrolyte and acid-base problems. It may be necessary to accept intrinsic renal insufficiency, not produce fluid overload, and to consider dialysis.
Digitalis	Ordinarily, digitalis is not of value in treatment of shock.
Corticoids	Their role is not clearly defined (question vasodilation or inhibition of prostaglandin synthesis).

BIBLIOGRAPHY

1. Shires, G.T., Carrico, C.J., and Cannizaro, P.C.: Shock. Philadelphia, W. B. Saunders Co., 1973.
2. Sobel, B.E.: Cardiac and noncardiac forms of an acute circulatory collapse (shock). In Braunwald, E. (ed.): Heart Disease: A Textbook of Cardiovascular Medicine. Philadelphia, W. B. Saunders Co., 1980.
3. Walt, A.J., and Wilson, R.F.: The treatment of shock. Adv. Surg., 9:1, 1975.
4. Zweifach, B.W., and Fronek, A.: The interplay of central and peripheral factors in irreversible hemorrhagic shock. Prog. Cardiovasc. Dis., 18:147, 1975.

9. PERIOPERATIVE MYOCARDIAL INFARCTION
MARK HILBERMAN, M.D.

1. **Why be concerned about perioperative myocardial infarction?**
    Perioperative myocardial infarction (MI), though infrequent, substantially increases the incidence of death following operation. The risk of MI is quite high (up to 40%) in patients with a recent MI and is also increased in those with coronary artery disease. Furthermore, the risk has remained unchanged except when intensive perioperative hemodynamic management regimens are employed or preoperative coronary revascularization is performed.

2. **What is the magnitude of the problem in individuals who have previously had an MI?**
    For patients undergoing noncardiac operations, the risk of reinfarction is 25 to 40% in the first 3 months after infarction and has been associated with a mortality rate of 50 to 100%. From 4 to 6 months, the risk of reinfarction is around 15%, and thereafter plateaus at 6 to 7% with a mortality rate of 30 to 50%.

3. **What is the nature of the problem in people who have previously had an MI?**
    Major vascular, intrathoracic, and intraabdominal procedures are associated with a higher incidence of reinfarction than "other" operations. While the incidence of reinfarction is lower following minor surgery, minor operations are performed more frequently and thus are a significant part of the overall problem. The incidence of operative therapy appears to be approximately the same in those with prior MI as in the general population.

4. **Can this gloomy outlook be altered?**
   Yes. (See below.)

5. **What factors, besides prior MI, identify the patient at risk?**
   (1) Symptoms or signs of congestive heart failure, (2) diffuse arteriosclerotic cardiovascular disease (scheduled for vascular operation), (3) use of anti-anginal medications (nitroglycerin, beta-blockers, calcium antagonists), (4) age (over 60), (5) evidence of coronary artery disease (CAD), (6) hypertension, and (7) the combination of CAD and hypertension.

6. **Is type of operation more important than the underlying cardiac disease?**
   The available data suggest that both the magnitude of the surgical stress and the risk factors identified above are critical determinants of outcome. Thus, while approximately half of patients who sustain their first MI are not clinically identifiable, the same does not appear to be true of patients who sustain a perioperative MI. Exercise stress testing and dipyridamole (Persantine)-thallium imaging of the heart can be used to identify the subset of individuals whose risk for MI exceeds 40%. Thus while patients undergoing high-risk procedures should receive more detailed evaluation, it does seem warranted to focus on identification of the individual patient and heart at risk.

7. **What are the risks associated with different operative procedures in patients whose cardiac disease is not rigorously identified or treated?**
   The risk of MI following aortic aneurysm operations appears to be 3 to 5% compared with 0.2% in patients undergoing biliary tract procedures. The mortality from MI following ophthalmologic surgery approximates 0.02%. Data on reinfarction suggest the risk to ophthalmic surgical patients approaches 0, compared with an overall risk of 6%. However, reinfarctions have been reported, and it is wise to consider patients individually.

8. **What is the incidence of significant CAD in patients presenting for aortic and peripheral vascular operations?**
   Investigators at The Cleveland Clinic, alarmed by the impact of perioperative MI on overall mortality, have taken a very aggressive approach to this problem, performing routine preoperative angiography in all patients presenting for vascular operations. Their data are invaluable to all of us, though few centers are likely to adopt this approach to preoperative evaluation. Approximately 90% of vascular surgical patients have CAD, and in 25% of these patients it is of sufficient severity and correctability to warrant cardiac revascularization prior to peripheral vascular repair. When patients with no evidence of CAD were compared with those with suspected CAD, the former had 14% normal coronary arteries compared with 4% in the latter; the incidence of "operable" CAD was 14% compared with 34%. Thus a significant subset of this population appears to have a potential for unanticipated perioperative MI.

9. **Since surgical stress appears to be the most common precipitating factor for perioperative MI, can exercise stress testing identify patients at risk?**
   An excellent study by Cutler and colleagues provides two important pieces of information. First, 20% of patients with peripheral vascular disease and normal electrocardiograms had borderline or definite ischemia on exercise electrocardiograms, and an additional 10% had premature ventricular contractions (PVCs). Of the 100 patients studied, 48 came to operation, and all of the periop-

erative infarctions occurred in the 16 patients (34%) with ischemic changes. The incidence of MI was 25% in those with borderline ischemia (8), and no deaths occurred. In the eight patients with definite ischemia, there were four MIs and two of these patients died.

10. **That's very good. Are any better noninvasive tests available?**
Yes. Though data are still preliminary, "redistribution" on dipyridamole-thallium (D-T) imaging is nearly twice as specific as exercise electrocardiographic testing in predicting future ischemic events. Furthermore, though more than twice as expensive, the test does not require the ability to exercise, and thus can be used in high-risk patients not candidates for exercise testing. (Still experimental as of late spring 1985.)

11. **How does D-T imaging work (roughly) and what is this redistribution bit?**
Thallium is a radioactive marker taken up by normal myocardium, which may be turned into a picture by gated nuclear medicine scans of many cardiac cycles. Dipyridamole is a potent vasodilator capable of creating a "steal" whereby normal vessels dilate and fixed stenotic vessels receive a marked reduction in blood flow. Thus when thallium is administered a few minutes after dipyridamole, it will go mostly to myocardium supplied by normal vessels. A "hole" is seen in the early image where dead or poorly perfused myocardium exists. A few hours later repeat scan differentiates these two possibilities. Scar is still represented by a hole; however, poorly perfused myocardium has since had thallium enter and the hole is filled. Thus there is a redistribution of thallium into an area of poorly perfused but viable myocardium--quite a dramatic event to see from outside the body!

12. **How do I apply all this information to the care of my next patient?**
     1.   The risk factors mentioned above should allow identification of the overwhelming number of patients at risk during standard preoperative work-up. If indicated on the basis of clinical severity of the disease, more precise information can be obtained by stress testing or D-T imaging.
     2.   For patients undergoing peripheral vascular surgery, the risk of perioperative MI is sufficient to warrant exercise stress testing or D-T imaging (preferred, if available) in all patients coming to surgery.
     3.   For all patients with significant clinical or test-demonstrated CAD, the risk of dying from a perioperative MI is usually greater than the risk of dying from the primary disease or related operative intervention. This relative risk must always be assessed, and frequently will require discussion with patient and family. In all such patients, but in particular those with impaired left ventricular function or three vessel disease, "prophylactic" coronary revascularization merits consideration.

13. **Can intraoperative anesthetic management alter outcome when, as is most common, the primary operation is performed and coronary surgery not recommended or refused?**
     Probably, though the data are sparse. Several separate aspects of the answer to this question require identification.

     1.   Seventy percent of reinfarctions occur on postoperative days 1 through 5. Alertness during operation alone is insufficient; the period of attentive management must include most of the first postoperative week (true in Tarhan's retrospective review as well as Rao and El-Etr's therapeutic intervention study).

2. Pre-bypass ischemia was the best single predictor of postoperative MI in patients undergoing coronary revascularization (Slogoff and Keats). Tachycardia was the most important hemodynamic abnormality leading to ischemia in this study, although both hypertension and hypotension have been previously identified as hemodynamic states leading to ischemia. Importantly, substantial differences in the incidence of ischemia existed according to anesthesiologists (18 to 45%), and was significantly higher in 2 of the 9 involved. This is the first clear demonstration of a link between individual skill in intraoperative anesthetic management and postoperative MI.

3. Pulmonary artery catheterization is indicated in patients with significant differences in ventricular function, in those with variant angina, and in those in whom substantial blood loss or fluid shifts are anticipated. Avoidance or rapid treatment of tachycardia, hypotension, or hypertension is possible without this monitor, and is probably more important than the monitor per se in the majority of operations performed. Intravenous nitroglycerin, beta-blocking agents, calcium antagonists, antihypertensive agents, and vasodilators are all important in managing these patients, and frequently justify placement of at least a central venous catheter for pressure monitoring and to serve as a dedicated administration line for potent vasoactive drugs.

4. ECG monitoring in these patients should include standard limb leads and a V4 or V5 lead. Preferably two or more leads should be displayed simultaneously; if that is not possible the V lead should be displayed continuously and the limb leads examined at intervals. Paper recording of starting lead configuration should be routine in patients at risk. Monitors that do not possess these capabilities should be replaced as funds permit. A modified V lead may be created by placing the left arm lead over the apex of the heart and recording lead I (R–L arm).

14. Can intensive perioperative management really change outcome?

Yes. Rao et al. reported that "preoperative optimization of the patient's status, aggressive invasive monitoring of the hemodynamic status, and prompt treatment of any hemodynamic aberration. . .decreased perioperative morbidity and mortality in patients with previous myocardial infarction." Although their data combine retrospective analysis with prospective treatment, their results are remarkable: a decrease in perioperative infarctions in patients operated upon 0 to 3 and 4 to 6 months after MI from 36% to 5.7% and 26% to 2.3%, respectively. Though no one is quite sure how they did it, the results seem real, and they have recently reported similar striking success when their treatment groups were quantified by the Goldman-Caldera criteria, rather than by time from the occurrence of MI.

There now exists a richness of both data and techniques which, carefully applied, offer the ability to identify individual hearts and patients at particular risk for perioperative MI. Furthermore, preoperative, intraoperative, and postoperative prophylactic and therapeutic techniques exist which can substantially alter the incidence of reinfarction and risk of operation in patients with CAD. It is clear that the excellent results achieved by some are not simply due to performing operations "today" with "modern techniques of anesthesia and surgery" but require a specific, carefully planned, coordinated, and very active intervention-oriented therapeutic strategy.

BIBLIOGRAPHY

1.   Bonow, R.O., Kent, K.M., Rosing, D.R., et al.: Exercise-induced ischemia in mildly symptomatic patients with coronary-artery disease and preserved left ventricular function–identification of subgroups at risk of death during medical therapy. N. Engl. J. Med., 311:1339-1345, 1984.

2.   Boucher, C.A., Brewster, D.C., Darling, R.C., et al.: Determination of cardiac risk by dipyridamole-thallium imaging before peripheral vascular surgery. N. Engl. J. Med., 312:389-394, 1985.

3.   Brown, O.W., Hollier, L.H., Pairolero, P.C., et al.: Abdominal aortic aneurysm and coronary artery disease. Arch. Surg., 116:1484-1488, 1981.

4.   Cutler, B.S., Wheeler, H.B., Paraskos, J.A., et al.: Assessment of operative risk with electrocardiographic exercise in patients with peripheral vascular disease. Am. J. Surg., 137:484-489, 1979.

5.   Eerola, M., Eerola, R., Kaukinen, S., et al.: Risk factors in surgical patients with verified preoperative myocardial infarction. Acta Anaesthesiol. Scand., 24:219-223, 1980.

6.   Goldman, L., Caldera, D.L., Nussbaum, S.R., et al.: Multifactorial index of cardiac risk in noncardiac surgical procedures. N. Engl. J. Med., 297:845-850, 1977.

7.   Hertzer, N.R., Beven, E.G., Young, J.R., et al.: Coronary artery disease in peripheral vascular patients: A classification of 1000 coronary angiograms and results of surgical management. Ann. Surg., 199:223-233, 1984.

8.   Leppo, J.A., O'Brien, J., Rothendler, J.A., et al.: Dipyridamole-thallium-20I scintigraphy in the prediction of future cardiac events after acute myocardial infarction. N. Engl. J. Med., 310:1014-1018, 1984.

9.   Maher, L. J., Steen, P.A., and Tinker, J.H.: Perioperative myocardial infarction in patients with coronary artery disease with and without aorta-coronary artery bypass grafts. J. Thorac. Cardiovasc. Surg., 76:533-537, 1978.

10. Rao, T.L.K., Jacobs, K.H., and El-Etr, A.A.: Reinfarction following anesthesia in patients with myocardial infarction. Anesthesiology, 59:499-505, 1983.

11. Slogoff, S., and Keats, A.S.: Does perioperative myocardial ischemia lead to postoperative myocardial infarction? Anesthesiology, 62:107-114, 1985.

12. Steen, P.A., Tinker, J.H., and Tarhan, S.: Myocardial reinfarction after anesthesia and surgery. J.A.M.A., 239:2566-2570, 1978.

13. Tarhan, S., Moffitt, E.A., Taylor, W.F., et al.: Myocardial infarction after general anesthesia. J.A.M.A., 220:1451-1454, 1972.

---

10. PERIOPERATIVE HYPOXIA

MARK GIBSON, M.D., and MARK HILBERMAN, M.D.

---

1. Who is at risk for perioperative hypoxia?

Perioperative hypoxia occurs in 5 to 10% of patients undergoing operation and anesthesia, and may develop in patients undergoing even minor procedures.

2. How is hypoxia diagnosed?

Cyanosis on physical examination (lips, nail beds, conjunctiva), confirmed by measurement of arterial PO_2 or hemoglobin saturation. Cyanosis may be difficult to detect in the anemic patient, the elderly, the young, or those with darkly pigmented skin. Bradycardia or hypotension (unexplained by blood loss) must trigger a rapid and thorough search for the etiology of the hypoxia. The signs of hypoxia are variable and include restlessness, tachypnea, dyspnea, cardiac arrhythmias, tachycardia, and hypertension.

3. What identifies the patient at high risk for hypoxia?

(1) Operation proposed, (2) obesity, (3) cigarette abuse, (4) pre-existing lung disease, (5) pre-existing heart or kidney disease, (6) pulmonary function assessment, (7) emergency operation, and (8) race.

4.   **Why do each of these factors increase risk?**
       1.   Operation proposed: (a) Upper abdominal, lateral thoracotomy, midline abdominal, and median sternotomy incisions are associated with splinting to minimize postoperative pain. Tidal volume may fall below functional residual capacity, and coughing is suppressed, which contributes to subsequent atelectasis and/or pneumonia. (b) The patient's position on the operating table may interfere with ventilation or access to the airway. (c) One-lung anesthesia for thoracic operations is frequently indicated but always creates the risk of hypoxia.
       2.   Obesity: The impairment of ventilation caused by obesity is similar to that of incisional pain. When upper abdominal or thoracic operations are performed in the obese patient, postoperative respiratory difficulties are routine.
       3.   Cigarette abuse: (a) Chronic cigarette use impairs pulmonary function. (b) Recent cigarette use impairs ciliary motion, and increased carboxyhemoglobin levels decrease oxygen transport.
       4.   Pre-existing lung disease: (a) The superimposition of postoperative respiratory impairment upon chronic pulmonary disease may be life-threatening, depending upon the severity of each. (b) Impaired gas exchange preoperatively is present only in patients with severe pulmonary disease. Gas exchange postoperatively is generally similar to that observed preoperatively, if the patient is "kept dry" and the operation and incision site do not severely impair ventilation. (c) Chronic airway infection is not infrequent in this population. Interference with ventilation and coughing may result in severe pulmonary infections.
       5.   Pre-existing heart or kidney disease: In both cases the ability to compensate for fluid overload (or underload) may be severely limited and monitoring of central venous or pulmonary artery pressures should be considered.
       6.   Pulmonary function assessment: (a) If no significant abnormalities are detected by careful history and physical examination, further testing is generally not indicated. Auscultation of the chest should be performed carefully; the detection of diminished breath sounds is among the most sensitive indicators of decreased airflow. (b) The forced vital capacity, peak expiratory flow, and maximum breathing capacity are the most sensitive quantitative predictors of postoperative pulmonary dysfunction. A 70-kg adult with a vital capacity of 1 L (15 ml/kg) will experience little change in lung function following bunionectomy or inguinal herniorrhaphy. However, following cholecystectomy vital capacity would be expected to decrease by 30 to 50%. In the latter circumstance, prolonged ventilatory support might be used to avoid postoperative hypoxia, and special techniques in management of postoperative pain may be useful such as thoracic epidural analgesia. (c) Preoperative arterial blood gases are of little predictive value and are measured too frequently.
       7.   Emergency operation: (a) Preoperative evaluation of lung function is usually incomplete. (b) Esophageal intubation and other major anesthetic misadventures are overwhelmingly associated with emergency procedures. (Mental red flag.)
       8.   Race. Dark skin color makes visual colorimetric detection of hypoxia more difficult. Review of medical malpractice claims suggests that blacks have a threefold higher risk of serious hypoxic injury during anesthesia than do whites. (Another mental red flag.) Awareness, careful individual assessment of normal skin hue, and routine pulse oximetry are indicated.

5.   **What are the most important causes of perioperative hypoxia?**
       1.   Hypoventilation due to: (a) Upper airway obstruction. In any obtunded patient the tongue may fall backward, obstructing the airway. (b) Persistent effects of drugs used during anesthesia. (c) Postoperative pain and consequent splinting. Hypoxia and pulmonary complications are usually avoided by appro-

priate pain management, early ambulation, and routine prophylactic pulmonary care. (d) Pneumothorax may occur spontaneously or as a complication of positive pressure ventilation, central line placement, or certain operative procedures. (e) Misplaced endotracheal tubes. A high index of suspicion must be maintained at all times, particularly during and immediately after intubation.

2. Ventilation/perfusion inequalities. An imbalance between ventilation and perfusion to individual alveoli may result in hypoxia. There are data indicating that impaired gas diffusion may also contribute. (a) Atelectasis. Alveolar collapse is common during anesthesia or prolonged mechanical ventilation. In most patients this does not lead to clinical hypoxia. (b) Pulmonary edema. May develop as a result of cardiac or renal insufficiency, or following resuscitation and/or operations in which crystalloid loading is employed to minimize the incidence of hypovolemia or renal failure. (c) Pulmonary embolism. Particularly at risk are patients at bed rest for prolonged periods. (d) Fat embolism. Most frequently associated with major long bone fractures.

3. Hypoxia secondary to inadequate oxygen in the inspired gas. (a) Air may not provide sufficient oxygen in the presence of the conditions discussed above. (b) Oxygen may not be delivered through oxygen supply circuits because of misconnections in anesthesia machines or newly installed oxygen systems. (c) Nitrous oxide is still a standard component of many inhalation anesthetics, and may cause alveolar hypoxia during emergence.

4. Hypoxia secondary to inadequate tissue oxygen delivery. (a) Acute anemia without cardiac compensation will result in systemic hypoxia. Experiments in healthy primates indicate that the limit for cardiac compensation is reached with precipitous hemodynamic deterioration at a hemoglobin of approximately 3.5 gm/100 ml, and the same appears to be true in humans. (b) Hypoxia secondary to inadequate blood flow (shock). These important conditions must be mentioned, but their effects on peripheral oxygen delivery are too complex to discuss here.

6. **How is upper airway obstruction diagnosed and treated?**
Nasal flaring, suprasternal or intercostal retractions, a rocking thoracoabdominal motion (abdomen moving forward and chest backward) with attempted inspiration, a silent airway or respiratory stridor, and the response to therapeutic maneuvers are all important in the diagnosis. The most effective single maneuver is forward thrust of the mandible. Neck extension and lifting the jaw are also useful. A nasal airway may be used to maintain airway patency and is usually better tolerated than an oral airway. Turning the patient to the lateral position allows the tongue to fall forward and usually alleviates such obstruction.

7. **How are the common residual effects of anesthetic drugs assessed and treated?**
Anesthetic drug "overdosage" is usually diagnosed situationally and is best treated by airway support and the passage of time. This is particularly true for the polypharmaceutical anesthetic marvels for which specific reversal agents are not available.

Severe narcotic-induced respiratory slowing (less than 8 breaths per minute) may warrant reversal by naloxone or other narcotic antagonists (or agonist/antagonists). Naloxone should be administered slowly intravenously in 1 to 2 μg/kg increments.

Sensory confusion caused by benzodiazepine or scopolamine may respond to physostigmine.

Residual muscle paralysis has two clinically distinct features: discoordinate motion, particularly of the arms and hands, and the patient's complaint of an inability to breathe (persons who are oversedated or narcotized do not mind their impaired state). The patient's ability to squeeze your hand or to protrude the tongue provides quick, pain-free verification of the diagnosis. The most rapid and effective reversal agent is edrophonium (0.75 to 1.0 mg/kg) mixed with glycopyrrolate (0.01 mg/kg) or atropine (0.02 mg/kg); additional atropine may be warranted if bradycardia develops following administration of this mixture.

8. **What are the diagnostic and treatment steps when a pneumothorax is suspected?**
Auscultation for bilateral breath sounds is the first step. A shift in the point of cardiac impulse should be sought. If the patient is unstable, insertion of a No. 14 IV catheter or chest tube is indicated if physical findings confirm the clinical suspicion of pneumothorax. If the patient is stable, a chest x-ray film provides the definitive diagnosis. Thereafter, a chest tube should be inserted if the pneumothorax is large, the patient is hypoxic, or a continued air leak is anticipated.

9. **How is correct endotracheal tube placement assured?**
(a) Direct visual verification that the endotracheal tube passes between the vocal cords and in front of the arytenoid cartilages is the best single test. (b) Careful observation of normal and symmetrical upper chest motion synchronous with manual, mechanical, or spontaneous ventilation. (c) Auscultation of absolutely normal and symmetrical breath sounds (a and b exclude intubation of a mainstem bronchus). (d) Monitoring carbon dioxide in the airway provides absolute verification of tracheal intubation on the first breath. (e) Monitoring hemoglobin saturation will detect hypoxia due to tube misplacement well before brain or cardiac injury is sustained. (f) Phonation following intubation implies an esophageal intubation!

10. **How are atelectasis, pulmonary edema, and other ventilation/perfusion (V/Q) abnormalities diagnosed and treated?**
Hypoxia in the face of adequate inspired oxygen tension implies a V/Q mismatch, as does any increase in the alveolar-arterial blood oxygen gradient (normally 30 to 50 mm Hg). Atelectasis should be suspected following any anesthetic or thoracic or abdominal operation. Diagnosis is by chest x-ray.

Pulmonary edema is most commonly seen in association with cardiac failure, fluid overload, or renal failure. Diagnosis is by physical examination, chest x-ray, or visualization of frothy secretions in an endotracheal tube.

The mainstays of therapy are increased inspired oxygen tensions, diuresis, and alveolar expansion. In the intubated patient the latter may usually be achieved by sustained mechanical hyperinflation or positive end-expiratory pressure (PEEP). In some patients inspissated material must be removed from the distal bronchi; saline lavage and suction are usually sufficient, although bronchoscopy may be needed. In the spontaneously breathing patient, ambulation, coughing, incentive spirometry, and chest physiotherapy are all useful. Positive end-expiratory pressure may be achieved by application of a tight-fitting face mask.

11. **How is pulmonary embolus diagnosed and treated?**
At particular risk are patients at bed rest for long periods. Symptoms include sudden severe chest pain, pleuritic chest pain, shortness of breath, and tachypnea. If the pulmonary embolus is massive, hypotension accompanied by high central venous and pulmonary artery pressures may be seen. The diagnosis may be confirmed by identification of deep vein thrombosis, by lung scan, by venous angiography, and occasionally by pulmonary arteriography.

Treatment is usually supportive. Anticoagulation is routine. Partial plication of the inferior vena cava or insertion of an "umbrella" is routine if the emboli are recurrent or life-threatening. Surgical removal of pulmonary artery clot and thrombolytic therapy are used infrequently and only in the most severely compromised patients who do not respond to simpler methods.

12.   How is fat embolism usually diagnosed and treated?
The diagnosis is usually situational: a patient develops respiratory distress, without evidence of fluid overload, in the first day or two following major long bone fracture. Treatment is usually supportive and successful.

13.   In which patients is the risk of hypoxia such that postoperative intubation and mechanical ventilation should be anticipated?
The decision not to extubate postoperatively may be made in (a) patients with poor pulmonary function preoperatively in whom the operation is anticipated to have a substantial negative impact on the preoperative pulmonary state; (b) patients undergoing prolonged surgical procedures who are hypothermic; (c) patients with circulatory instability; (d) patients who undergo cardiopulmonary bypass. Fluid shifts are frequent and substantial. An elective period of several hours of postoperative ventilation is a sound routine. (e) patients who have incompletely reversed muscle relaxants, excessive narcotic effects, poor respiratory effort, or low tidal volumes at the end of the procedure; and (f) patients who receive massive transfusions, exhibit cyanosis or hypoxia, or require inspired oxygen tensions in excess of 50% to maintain adequate oxygenation.

14.   How is oxygen best delivered to the patient?
The simplest solution (though frequently not the best) is to keep the trachea intubated. Oxygen, positive pressure, endotracheal toilet, and mechanical ventilation may all be delivered. This is the safest technique for patients who require inspired oxygen tensions over 50% or are otherwise compromised.

15.   What are the options for delivery of oxygen in the extubated patient?
(a) Nasal prongs. Simple but poorly controlled levels of oxygen are achieved due to variable mixing with inspired air. (b) A simple face mask can deliver 40 to 60% oxygen. (c) A partial non-rebreathing mask can achieve 60 to 80% oxygen if flows are high enough to prevent reservoir collapse or entrainment of air on inspiration. (d) Non-rebreathing masks with one-way valves and vents can permit 95% oxygen to be delivered. With the use of straps and a proper expiratory circuit, such masks can also be used to deliver positive end-expiratory pressure or continuous positive airway pressure. (e) Venturi masks are especially useful in patients with chronic pulmonary insufficiency. Accurate inspired oxygen concentrations between 21 and 50% may be delivered at flows of 4-8 L/min.

BIBLIOGRAPHY

1.   Bowe, E.A., and Klein, E.F., Jr.: Postoperative respiratory care. Int. Anesthesiol. Clin., 21:77, 1983. Good list of complications. Short discussion of V/Q mismatch. Treatment is strong suit. Good discussion of ventilators.
2.   Catley, D.M.: Postoperative analgesia and respiratory control. Int. Anesthesiol. Clin., 22:95-110, 1984. Nice review of pulmonary function and analgesic effects on respiration.
3.   Cullen, D.J., and Cullen, B.L.: Postanesthetic complications. Surg. Clin. North Am., 55:987, 1975. Quick overview of respiratory, cardiovascular and metabolic complications.

4. Gibson, R.L., et al.: Actual tracheal oxygen concentration with commonly used oxygen equipment. Anesthesiology, 44:71-73, 1976. Intratracheal catheters placed in only two volunteers, but interesting study and results.

5. Latimer, R.G., et al.: Ventilatory patterns and pulmonary complications after upper abdominal surgery determined by preoperative and postoperative computerized spirometry and blood gas analysis. Am. J. Surg., 122:622, 1971. Impressive findings of increased FVC and FEV1.

6. Leigh, J.M.: Oxygen therapy: Physiological principles, monitoring and administration technique. Crit. Care Int., 3:4-7, 1984. Quick overview and basic introduction.

7. Marshall, B.E., and Wycke, M.Q., Jr.: Hypoxemia during and after anesthesia. Anesthesiology, 37:178-209, 1972. Very complete and a classic reference.

8. Muskin, W.W., et al.: Automatic Ventilation of the Lungs, 2nd ed. Philadelphia, F.A. Davis, 1969.

9. Nunn, J.F., and Payne, J.P.: Hypoxaemia after general anaesthesia. Lancet, 2:631, 1962. The original paper to study the problem. A classic and still timely.

10. Otto, W.: Respiratory morbidity and mortality. Int. Anesthesiol. Clin., 18:85,1980. One of the better recent overviews of respiratory complications.Pathophysiology explained simply.

11. Parfey, P.S., et al.: Pulmonary function in the early postoperative period. Br. J. Surg., 64:384-389, 1977.

12. Spence, A.A.: Postoperative pulmonary complications. In Gray, T.C., et al. General Anesthesia, 4th ed., 1980, pp. 591-608. Good review of topic with emphasis on short gastric aspiration and pulmonary embolism.

13. Tisi, G.M.: Preoperative evaluation of pulmonary function. Am. Rev. Respir. Dis., 119: 293, 1979.

14. Tordo, T.A.: Oxygen delivery services. Crit. Care Int., 3:7-10, 1984. Another simple discussion of the topic.

15. West, J.B.: Ventilation-Blood Flow and Gas Exchange, 3rd ed. Philadelphia, F.A. Davis, 1969.

---

11. CENTRAL VENOUS PRESSURE
ALDEN HARKEN, M.D.

---

1. What is central venous pressure?

Central venous pressure is synonymous with right atrial pressure or right ventricular filling pressure.

2. What does central venous pressure mean?

The heart can increase its cardiac output in two ways: by increasing heart rate and by increasing stroke volume. Central venous or right atrial pressure is the pressure that pushes blood into the right ventricle during diastole. The higher the central venous pressure, the more the blood will flow into the right ventricle during each diastolic filling period. Starling's law indicates that with increasing end-diastolic volume (to a point), more blood will be ejected during systole, thus resulting in an increased stroke volume.

3. What is a normal central venous pressure?

Normally the right ventricle can fill adequately with an astonishingly low central venous pressure, perhaps 3 to 5 mm Hg. A central venous pressure of 3 in a young healthy person with a normal cardiac output is perfectly normal. Conversely, a central venous pressure of 3 in a 55-year-old, cigar-chomping executive with a low cardiac output suggests hypovolemia.

4. Physiologically, how does a failing heart compensate for a decreasing cardiac output?

With a decreasing cardiac output, both the baroreceptors and the juxtaglomerular apparatus promote aldosterone release and a resultant increase in extracellular sodium and water. With this increase in intravascular volume both central venous and left-sided filling pressures increase. Ventricular failure is usually accompanied by a stiffening or loss of compliance of that ventricle. Thus increasing filling pressures are required in order to maintain end-diastolic volume. High central venous pressure characteristically indicates a failing heart.

5. **What causes an elevated central venous pressure?**
    The most common cause of right ventricular failure is left ventricular failure. Florid pulmonary edema may occur in patients with a normal central venous pressure. Most of our patients are limited by their left ventricle, not by their right. In slowly evolving situations the central venous pressure is an adequate reflection of left-sided filling pressure. However, in acute volume changes or with acute myocardial infarction, hemodynamic changes may happen so quickly that the left heart fails, causing pulmonary edema prior to an elevation in central venous pressure.

6. **How do you measure central venous pressure?**
    A tube must be placed in the superior vena cava or right atrium. Because there is a negligible pressure drop between the superior vena cava and the right atrium, either one of these locations is acceptable. Indeed, all intrathoracic veins have essentially the same pressure. The monitoring tube may be threaded in from an antecubital vein cutdown. It is usually easier, however, to access the central venous compartment by percutaneous subclavian vein puncture.

7. **What are the contraindications to percutaneous subclavian vein puncture?**
    The risk of bleeding during subclavian access in a patient with a profound coagulopathy is low but not zero. In a patient whose anticoagulation status is over the therapeutic range or in a patient who is profoundly thrombocytopenic, it may be safer to access the central venous compartment by peripheral cutdown. Similarly a patient with hyperinflated lungs from chronic obstructive pulmonary disease and some respiratory distress might tolerate a pneumothorax very poorly. The incidence of pneumothorax associated with percutaneous subclavian vein puncture is also low but not zero. Inadvertent arterial puncture is generally not a problem unless the patient has coagulopathy.

8. **How do you place a central venous line by direct subclavian vein puncture?**
    With the patient in a mild head-down (Trendelenburg) position, the subclavicular area is prepared with antiseptic solution. Full aseptic precautions must be taken in that placement of a central venous line is a first-class way to make a patient septic if you are sloppy. A skin wheal is made at the mid-point of the undersurface of the clavicle. A No. 21 needle and a 10-ml syringe of 1% lidocaine is then inserted at this wheal half-way down on the clavicle, hugging the undersurface of the clavicle and directed toward the sternal notch. Usually you have to insert the needle right up to the hub before you hit the subclavian vein. As you insert this small needle you may inject small amounts of local anesthestic ahead of you; accomplished in this fashion, this should not be a particularly uncomfortable procedure for the patient. When you hit the subclavian vein with the No. 21 needle, dark blood is easily withdrawn. The small needle is then removed and a No. 16 or 18 needle, again on a 10-ml syringe, is inserted along the same track. Presumably if you found the subclavian vein with a small needle, you should be able to find the subclavian vein with the larger No. 16 needle. When you hit the

vein, dark blood should again be easily withdrawn. The 10-ml syringe is then detached. In a patient with a high central venous pressure (20 to 25 mm Hg), blood may shoot out of this needle and you may think "Oh my gosh, I've hit the artery." This is not a problem. However, in a hypovolemic patient who has a gasping respiration, the central venous pressure may actually become negative during inhalation. It is possible in these circumstances for a substantial amount of air to be sucked into the intravascular venous compartment. This is bad! Be prepared to place a gloved finger over the end of the inserting needle to prevent a large right-sided air embolus. The plastic catheter is easily passed down the access needle.

9. **What is the Seldinger technique?**
An easier and safer method of maintaining intravascular access after you have found the subclavian vein with a small No. 21 needle is to slide a flexible metal stilette down the No. 21 needle after central venous access has been established. The No. 21 needle is then slid back out over the flexible stilette and the No. 16 or 18 catheter then easily slides down over the stilette.

10. **How do you confirm the position of the central venous catheter?**
After placement of the central venous catheter it is mandatory to obtain a chest x-ray film in order to confirm its central location. This can usually be assured by free return of blood from the catheter through a syringe. Once or twice a year on most busy services, however, this catheter is inserted into the intrapleural space, with subsequent infusion of fluids producing a pleural infusion. A confirmatory chest x-ray is invaluable.

11. **How do you place an internal jugular catheter for central venous pressure measurement?**
The patient is placed in a head-down position. The patient's head is turned away from the side that is to be catheterized. Sterile procedures are used. The two heads of the sternocleidomastoid muscle are identified. These two heads attach to the manubrium and the clavicle and then rise to join into one mass of muscle about 2 cm about the clavicle. This forms a triangle. Along the lateral aspect of the triangle (the medial aspect of the clavicular attachment of the sternocleidomastoid muscle), a needle is inserted and directed toward the ipsilateral hip. Interestingly, when placed in this fashion, this probably constitutes a "supraclavicular subclavian vein puncture" rather than an internal jugular catheterization.

12. **How is a central venous pressure line secured?**
When placing any catheter or any tube in any orifice, if you want it to stay there it is imperative to suture it to the skin directly. When a valuable line is placed, it is always nice to know that you can pick the patient up by his catheter.

13. **Are there any advantages of an internal jugular catheter over a subclavian catheter?**
The incidence of pneumothorax is probably slightly higher with subclavian vein puncture, while the incidence of inadvertent carotid artery puncture is slightly higher with internal jugular vein catheterization.

14. **If a patient already has a chest tube in place, on which side do you place a subclavian central venous line?**
Always place the subclavian catheter on the same side as the chest tube, so that if a pneumothorax occurs, you have already treated it.

12. WOUND INFECTION AND WOUND DEHISCENCE
BEN EISEMAN, M.D.

1. **Isn't wound infection a thing of the past in this era of antibiotics and asepsis? Aren't you being old fashioned?**
   No, indeed not. About 7% of all wounds on a surgical service are in some way infected. Over one million operative wounds become infected in the U.S. each year. A wound infection will almost double the length of hospital stay and increase the cost of care. Overall a wound infection will add about 5 extra days of hospitalization and $18,000 in cost. Infection also prolongs the time before a working person can return to the job. Wound infection costs the U.S. about $1.5 billion annually.

2. **How can one predict the probability of wound infection?**
   This is best done by classifying wounds as to the likelihood of infection. This is as follows: total, 7%; clean, 5%; clean-contaminated, 10%; contaminated, 15%; and dirty, 30%. The probability of a hernia wound becoming infected is 1.9%, cholecystectomy 7.0%, appendectomy 11% (see Chapter 47, Appendicitis).

3. **What factors affect the probability of wound infection?**
   Presence of dead tissue, dirt, or foreign body in the wound; contamination of the wound; patient's age; immune defenses of the patient; sterility of the skin prior to incision; sterile technique during the operation; gentleness of the surgeon and surgical team in handling tissue; avoidance of contaminating the field by cutting across a contaminated structure such as the intestinal tract, bile duct, vagina, etc.; and prior administration of antibiotic.

4. **Of these, which is the most and which the least important?**
   Most: Condition of the wound. Is it clean and well vascularized, is it free from blood clots, and when closed are there empty spaces where blood or plasma may collect? *Least:* Antibiotics, age, and general nutrition of the patient.

5. **If a patient has a dirty (contaminated) wound, how can a surgeon minimize the chances of its becoming infected?**
   If seen early enough (within 8 to 18 hours), the wound may be debrided. This involves excising all of the dead tissue back to good healthy tissue which has a good blood supply. All foreign bodies (dirt, gravel, etc.) are removed, and the wound is washed with large amounts of saline.

6. **Why not add some sort of antibacterial substance to this fluid to kill the organisms?**
   Although Galen would not have used the term "organisms" because bacteria had not yet been discovered, he suggested the same thing. It was wrong then and it still is! The antibacterials not only kill bacteria but also depress cell function and resistance. It is far better to clean the wound mechanically, including debridement (which means *excision*), than to try to clean it chemically.

7. **After cleaning the wound, should you close the muscles, fascia, and skin over the wound?**
   This depends on the condition of the wound. If it is well vascularized and very clean, it is best to close the wound. This minimizes disability and scar. However, if the wound is still contaminated, it is safer to leave the skin edges open so that there is no chance for pockets of blood or pus to form and produce a florid infection.

8. **Do you then let the wound heal over?**
   Sometimes, if the wound is very dirty. If, however, on the third to fifth day the wound looks clean, the skin can be brought together and the wound closed. This is called delayed closure.

9. **What are the common organisms that cause wound infection?**
   The most common organism on the skin is staphylococcus. The organism grown from an infected wound depends on the site of the wound and the procedure performed. If the gut was cut, the organisms in the infected wound are probably *E. coli* and Bacteroides. Each area of the body, such as the vagina, urinary tract, etc., has specific organisms that are likely to infect the wound.

10. **What is the role of antibiotics in decreasing wound infection?**
    If given prior to operation or injury they minimize the probability of infection, but if started after the operation they have little value.

11. **How long should antibiotics be administered after operation?**
    If there is no other indication for maintaining antibiotics they can be discontinued within 1 to 2 days.

12. **What is the clinical appearance of an infected wound?**
    Calor (heat or temperature), rubor (red), dolor (painful), and tumor (swollen).

13. **What organism is likely to be present if a wound develops a fruity-odored exudate?**
    Pseudomonas.

14. **What organism is likely to be present if a wound develops a red-brownish exudate in the early postoperative period?**
    Clostridium.

15. **What organism is likely to be present if a wound develops erythema and tenderness of the wound edges in the early postoperative period?**
    Streptococcus.

16. **What should be done when a wound becomes infected?**
    Open it and let out the pus *(ubi pus ibi evacua)* .

17. **What happens if an infected wound is not opened?**
    The patient soon shows systemic signs of infection which may result in generalized bacteremia, multiple abscesses, and multiple organ failure.

18. **Will infection alter the strength of a wound?**
    Yes. This is the usual reason that an abdominal wound breaks down.

19. **What happens when a laparotomy wound breaks down?**
    The first evidence is merely localized tenderness. If the infection is deeper and untreated, it may so weaken the underlying layers that the fascia will not hold the wound together. If the skin holds together and the patient gets over the infection, postoperative incisional hernia may occur. However, if the infection spreads down through all layers, the entire wound may break down and the intestine break through to or even through the skin. This is a wound dehiscence.

20. **What are the clinical signs and symptoms of a wound dehiscence?**
Between the third and seventh day after operation the patient may feel the wound give way. Alternatively there may at first be nothing to signal this catastrophe except a thin serous discharge from the wound. The patient usually soon becomes toxic and shows signs of peritonitis.

21. **What should the surgeon do then?**
The wound should be inspected carefully and palpated with a sterile glove. If there is any suspicion of dehiscence the patient should be taken to the operating room before removing one or two stitches and palpating the wound with a sterile glove. If there is indeed a dehiscence, the patient should be given general anesthesia, and wound area sterilely prepared, and the wound entirely reopened and closed with retention sutures.

22. **Can a wound dehiscence be treated conservatively (i.e., not re-closed in the operating room?**
The safest method is to take the patient to the operating room as soon as possible, open the entire incision from top to bottom, and re-close with retention sutures leaving the skin partially unclosed. Some surgeons actually pack a highly infected wound open, which, in essence, is a controlled "dehiscence." This however implies that the gut will remain confined. The simple answer to the question is "no"—don't rely on nonoperative means; re-close the abdominal wall.

23. **Should retention sutures be used in re-closure?**
Figure-of-8 interrupted sutures enclosing all layers of fascia and muscle (excluding the peritoneum if you wish) can be used leaving the skin open for delayed closure. An alternative is interrupted heavy retention sutures that also include the skin. These are left in 3 weeks.

24. **What are the choices of suture material in an abdominal closure?**
Choices, of course, are almost infinite including absorbable versus nonabsorbable material, different caliber and different material. There is even wide variation in choice for closing a clean elective laparotomy.

25. **Should the peritoneum be closed separately?**
Although many surgeons close the peritoneum separately with a light absorbable suture, there are neither experimental nor clinical data to prove its need. Closing the fascia and muscle and perhaps skin over the incision apposes the peritoneum which quickly is sealed. Omitting separate closure of the peritoneum does not increase the probability of infection.

26. **Are vertical incisions stronger than tranverse, and/or less prone to infection?　To dehiscence?**
There is no good answer to this question. There are as many articles and clinical advocates for vertical as for horizontal incisions. Most senior surgeons have strong feelings about which one they use but there is no overall proof that a horizontal incision is less likely to disrupt or to become infected than a vertical incision.

BIBLIOGRAPHY

1.　Altemeier, W.A.: Manual on Control of Infection in Surgical Patients, 2nd ed. American College of Surgeons, Philadelphia, J.B. Lippincott Co., 1984.

13. ESOPHAGEAL FOREIGN BODY
BENJAMIN HONIGMAN, M.D.

1. **What is the immediate concern or threat to life in a patient with an esophageal foreign body?**
(1) To ensure that the airway is clear and that the foreign body is not in the upper airway or trachea. (2) To rule out esophageal perforation, which is evidenced by presence of fever, subcutaneous air, severe chest pain on physical examination, pneumomediastinum on chest x-ray, or soft tissue air on neck films.

2. **Where do esophageal foreign bodies usually lodge?**
Over 90% lodge below the level of the cricopharyngeal muscle. The four most common areas are : (1) at the level of the cricopharyngeal muscle; (2) at the level of the aortic arch and left mainstem bronchus; (3) at the esophageal gastric junction; and (4) at pathologic sites of narrowing such as Zenker's diverticulum and esophageal strictures.

3. **What are the foreign bodies that are usually found?**
Adults: Bones comprise 60 to 70%; other objects include meat bolus, fruit pits, and aluminum can tops. *Children:* Coins, buttons, toys, and mercury disc batteries.

4. **Are some foreign bodies more dangerous than others?**
Yes. Sharp objects such as fish bones cause esophageal perforation. Dentures are difficult to remove and iatrogenic perforation occurs frequently. Mercury disc batteries have corrosive capabilities after a 4 to 6 hour period in the esophagus; immediate removal is necessary if lodged in the esophagus.

5. **What are the predisposing factors?**
Patient type: children (the highest incidence occurs in the first decade of life), the mentally handicapped, and denture wearers in adults. *Pathology:* The possibility of underlying pathology such as rings, strictures, and carcinoma should be considered in every case in an adult.

6. **What is the clinical presentation?**
Chest or throat pain is the most common. Dysphagia and odynophagia are also common. Drooling and profuse salivation increase the likelihood of finding a complete obstruction. Patients with long-term unrecognized foreign bodies may present with respiratory symptoms or with signs of esophageal perforation.

7. **Is a patient's localization of pain accurate in assessing exact location of foreign body?**
No, since sensory innervation of the esophagus is not specific for location; pain from the lower esophagus may be referred to the upper chest, although the reverse does not usually happen. Sensation of a foreign body in the pharynx or larynx is, however, more specific.

8. **Is clinical presentation similar in children?**
Children also report pain or discomfort and may have drooling. The very young, however, may manifest an esophageal foreign body only by refusing to take feedings. Some young children may present with recurrent respiratory symptoms secondary to an unrecognized esophageal foreign body that has been lodged for weeks to months.

9. **What are the complications of foreign bodies?**
   (1) Esophageal perforation or abscess formation occurs in 0.6 to 1%, and is generally caused by sharp objects or prolonged impaction, or is iatrogenically produced secondary to removal. Minor complications such as esophageal abrasions and lacerations occur in 1%. (2) Airway obstruction usually occurs in children only when a large bolus is impacted, causing compression of the posterior portion of the trachea, which is softer and more compressible in children. (3) Aspiration pneumonia usually occurs in children or mentally handicapped with unrecognized long-standing impaction that produces aspiration and subsequent respiratory symptoms.

10. **How is the diagnosis made?**
    In most instances, by history. The patient reports something being "stuck"; physical examination reveals drooling or inability to swallow in complete obstruction.

11. **How is the diagnosis confirmed?**
    X-ray films (chest, neck) may reveal a radiopaque substance; a xeroradiogram is preferable when the foreign body is lodged in the hypopharynx or upper esophagus. X-rays should be obtained if a patient has the sensation of a foreign body. Coins appear in the coronal plane if they are in the esophagus, and in the sagittal plane if they are in the trachea. Barium swallow examination confirms the diagnosis in most instances of significant foreign bodies. Swallowing cotton pledgets with the barium sometimes is helpful since cotton will get "hung up" at the site of obstruction.

12. **What are the indications for a barium study?**
    Symptomatic patients with obvious clinical history (drooling, inability to swallow); symptomatic patients with questionable history (i.e., chest pain and symptoms indicating potential for obstruction); and patients who have ingested dangerous foreign bodies such as chicken bones or sharp objects that do not appear on plain films (see Controversies).

13. **When should barium not be used?**
    When perforation is suspected, Gastrografin is advised. Barium allows better visualization of the foreign body but, unlike Gastrografin, may be toxic to the mediastinal structures.

14. **Are there any noninvasive means of removal?**
    Yes. Glucagon provided intravenously may be effective in meat impactions of the lower esophagus. Glucagon acts by relaxing the lower esophageal sphincter. It does not appear to be effective in upper or mid-esophageal foreign bodies. It also does not affect peristalsis once the sphincter is relaxed. The weight of the object itself or the barium (if a barium study is done) along with normal peristalsis pushes the foreign body through the esophageal sphincter. Papain and other "digestive agents," on the other hand, should not be used.

15. **What are the indications for endoscopy?**
    Immediate endoscopy is indicated in any patient with a confirmed foreign body in the esophagus. Immediate removal of sharp or pointed objects and mercury disc batteries is essential. Endoscopy is also indicated in patients with symptoms that continue for 12 to 24 hours when the results of x-rays and barium studies are negative.

CONTROVERSIES

16. **Is endoscopy preferred over barium swallow?** (For patients who have obvious history and clear physical findings, some would go directly to endoscopy.)
For: Endoscopy facilitates removal without exposure to x-ray.
Against: Endoscopy may subject the patient to an invasive procedure unnecessarily if there is no foreign body; also exposes the patient to anesthesia.

17. **Should a barium swallow study be done immediately in mildly symptomatic patients?**
For: Will detect almost all foreign bodies lodged in the esophagus.
Against: Many patients have the sensation of a foreign body without a foreign body being present. In mildly symptomatic patients, observation for 12 to 24 hours to see if symptoms improve is advocated by some.

18. **Is glucagon a safe and effective means of removal?**
For: Glucagon is relatively harmless and free of complications; other invasive maneuvers can be performed if glucagon is ineffective.
Against: There are no controlled studies indicating effectiveness of glucagon, only anecdotal ones.

19. **What about papain?**
For: Papain enzymatically reduces the size of the foreign body, thereby facilitating ingestion, which precludes maneuvers for invasive removal.
Against: Papain has produced esophageal perforation in 2% of patients, thus increasing morbidity and mortality.

20. **What are the best methods of removal?**
Hypopharynx: Laryngoscope with pediatric Magill forceps. Esophagus: endoscopy with rigid scope for some items (larger meat bolus, large coins, sharp objects, unusual shapes). Alternative methods of removal: flexible endoscopy and Foley catheter.

21. **What are the pros and cons of using a rigid scope?**
For: You can remove almost any foreign body.
Against: There is an increased risk of perforation due to traction on the presenting part of the foreign body.

22. **Is flexible endoscopy effective?**
For: Decreased chance of perforation (1.3 in 1000 cases) includes all complications for all procedures; also more applicable in patients with severe cervical arthritis in whom a rigid scope cannot be used.
Against: A flexible scope is unable to remove all types of objects owing to varied sizes and unusual shapes.

23. **Should a Foley catheter be used?**
For: A Foley catheter is good for removing coins or other small smooth objects, is noninvasive, does not require general anesthesia, and works well in children.
Against: Is useful only for foreign bodies lodged in the cervical esophagus, and then is appropriate only for coins and buttons; there is no direct visualization, therefore no direct control.

24. **Are there any changes in the management of children who swallow a foreign body?**

Since the majority of foreign bodies are swallowed by children in the first decade of life, the following guidelines for management are recommended: (1) X-rays are required for all asymptomatic children over age 2 who swallow an object larger than a penny. (2) In any child under age 2 who swallows any foreign body, an x-ray is required for localization of the object.

For: Most children swallow radiopaque objects; therefore it is possible to determine whether the object has passed the gastroesophageal junction. Once in the stomach, most of these objects will pass uneventfully. Unrecognized buttons or coins can lodge in the esophagus and go on to perforate or produce chronic respiratory symptoms secondary to aspiration in small children.

Against: X-rays are unnecessary since most children who swallow objects will pass them uneventfully.

BIBLIOGRAPHY

1. Campbell, J.B., Quattromani, F.L., and Foley, L.C.: Foley catheter removal of blunt esophageal foreign bodies: Experience with 100 consecutive children. Pediatr. Radiol., 13:116-118, 1983. Successful in 98%. Advocates use in children who swallow round foreign bodies and who arrive between 24 and 48 hours of ingestion.

2. Cavo, J.W., Koops, H.J., and Gryboski, R.A.: Use of enzymes for meat impactions in the esophagus. Laryngoscope, 87:630-634, 1977. Case report using papain.

3. Friedland, G.W.: The treatment of acute esophageal food impaction. Radiology, 149:601-602, 1983. Anecdotal use of tartaric acid and sodium bicarbonate for digestion of foreign body.

4. Glauser, J., Lilja, G.P., Greenfeld, B., et al.: Intravenous glucagon in the management of esophageal food obstruction. J.Am.Coll.Emerg.Phys., 8:228-231, 1979. Review of successful glucagon use in meat impactions.

5. Handal, K.A., Riordan, W., and Siese, J.: The lower esophagus and glucagon. Ann. Emerg. Med., 9:577-579, 1980. Case report of successful use of glucagon.

6. Hernanz-Schulman, M., and Naimark, A.: Avoiding disaster with esophageal foreign bodies. Emerg. Med. Rep., 133-140, 1984. American Medical Reports, San Francisco, CA. Review of topic; advocates early endoscopy after barium swallow; Foley catheter for round objects.

7. Litovitz, T.L.: Button battery ingestions: A review of 56 cases. J.A.M.A., 249:2495-2500, 1983. Review of large number of cases; advocates immediate removal if lodged in esophagus; can let them pass spontaneously if beyond the gastroesophageal junction with very close observation.

8. Nahman, B.J.: Asymptomatic esophageal perforation by a coin in a child. Ann. Emerg. Med., 13:672-629, 1984. Long term complications of unrecognized esophageal foreign body lodged for six months.

9. Nandi, P., and Ong, G.B.: Foreign body in the esophagus: Review of 2394 cases. Br. J. Surg., 65:5-9, 1978. Excellent review of diagnosis and management of large numbers of cases.

10. Temple, D.M., and McNeese, M.C.: Hazards of battery ingestion. Pediatrics, 71:100-103, 1983. Strongly advocates immediate removal via endoscopy or surgery since there is high danger of corrosive necrosis or systemic mercury toxicity.

---

14. TRACHEAL FOREIGN BODY
BENJAMIN HONIGMAN, M.D.

---

1. **What is the major life threat?**
   Complete airway obstruction with respiratory arrest.

2. **Is there a role for a surgical airway?**

Only if obstruction is proximal to the proposed surgical incision, i.e., cricothyroid-otomy or tracheostomy. Neither procedure will be effective if a foreign body is in the trachea since the air will still not bypass the object to get to the lungs.

3. **Are there immediate maneuvers that can be performed if a foreign body in the trachea is producing complete obstruction, and bronchoscopy is either not available or would take too long?**
Attempt to push the foreign body distally into one of the mainstem bronchi with an endotracheal tube; then intubate the opposite lung with an endotracheal tube, thus aerating at least one lung.

4. **How can you differentiate between complete and incomplete airway obstruction?**
Complete: Patient becomes acutely dyspneic, unable to talk, cough, or breathe, and becomes rapidly cyanotic. *Incomplete:* Patient becomes acutely dyspneic and has coughing paroxysms, but can usually talk and breathe, although with difficulty.

5. **How can you differentiate clinically between upper and lower airway obstruction?**
Upper: Usually acute in onset with rapid development of labored respirations and respiratory failure; stridor is present. *Lower:* Bronchial foreign bodies present with more subacute and insidious course. Initial coughing spell and dyspnea may occur. Wheezing may develop with asymmetric breath sounds, i.e., unilateral decreased breath sounds; history of aspiration is usually present (85%); if the foreign body has been present for a period of time, signs and symptoms of pneumonia will develop.

6. **What age groups are commonly affected by upper and lower airway obstruction?**
Children: Ages 1 to 3. *Adults:* Cafe coronary usually occurs in adults older than 45 years of age with a history of eating associated with alcohol ingestion and sudden aspiration of food bolus.

7. **How is the diagnosis of lower respiratory tract obstruction by a foreign body confirmed?**
If the foreign body is radiopaque, a chest film will confirm the diagnosis. If the foreign body is not radiopaque, inspiratory and expiratory films may show indirect evidence of foreign body: (a) mediastinal or tracheal shift away from the side of obstruction on forced expiration; (b) unilateral high-riding diaphragm; and (c) presence of atelectasis. Fluoroscopy is a better technique in children because they cannot usually cooperate sufficiently to obtain a good expiratory film. Diagnosis can be confirmed in over 70% of bronchial foreign bodies by looking for paroxysmal mediastinal shifts on fluoroscopy.

8. **How do you manage the airway of an adult with complete airway obstruction?**
Laryngoscopy and bronchoscopy are definitive methods with manual removal. If instruments are not immediately available, then use an abdominal thrust, followed by back blows if the manual thrusts are not successful. An alternative method is to use back blows prior to manual thrusts, as recommended by the American Heart Association and the American Academy of Pediatrics.

9. **How do you manage the airway of a pediatric patient with complete airway obstruction?**

Laryngoscopy and bronchoscopy are the definitive methods with manual removal; however, if instruments are not immediately available, back blows followed by chest thrusts may dislodge the foreign body. One can then remove the object with the fingers. Never do a blind finger sweep in children. Chest thrusts are preferred over abdominal thrusts in children.

10. **How is a tracheal foreign body removed?**
Bronchoscopy with the fiberoptic scope is the procedure of choice once the patient is hospitalized and the foreign body is too distal for removal by a laryngoscope.

11. **What are the complications of bronchoscopy?**
Death secondary to cardiac arrest is the most serious complication. In experienced hands the incidence of death is less than 1%. Bradycardia is common. Hypoxia may occur if the patient is not ventilated adequately during the procedure or if a foreign body becomes lodged in the upper airway upon removal. With repeated bronchoscopic attempts or prolonged bronchoscopy, laryngeal edema can occur.

12. **When should bronchial foreign bodies be removed?**
In cases of vegetable matter (such as a peanut) or if there is moderate to severe respiratory distress, remove immediately. In mild distress and nonvegetable matter (such as hard candy, button, etc.), 12 to 24 hours of vigorous respiratory therapy and postural drainage can be attempted to remove the object.

CONTROVERSIES

13. **Are manual thrusts effective for complete airway obstruction in adults?**
For: Manual thrusts produce a more sustained increase in pressure and airflow; anecdotal evidence supports this method.
Against: Manual thrusts may produce complete airway obstruction if only partial obstruction is present; solid visceral organ damage may result from thrusts that are too vigorous.

14. **Should back blows be used in complete airway obstruction in adults?**
For: Back blows produce a more instantaneous rise in pressure, which will expel the foreign body.
Against: Anecdotal evidence finds this method unsuccessful in most cases.

15. **Are chest thrusts preferred over abdominal thrusts in children with complete airway obstruction?**
For: Similar effects are obtained regarding sustained pressure from both maneuvers and there is a lower incidence of visceral organ damage with a chest thrust.
Against: Anecdotal evidence is accumulating that abdominal thrusts may be just as safe in children as in adults and that the incidence of organ damage is not increased.

16. **Are fiberoptic scopes preferred over rigid scopes?**
For: Fiberoptic scopes give flexibility and maneuverability, allowing the operator to get into narrow airways; the fiberoptic scope can be used through an endotracheal tube, thus reducing the incidence of aspiration.
Against: Rigid scopes make it easier to remove larger objects.

17. Is it acceptable to defer removal of bronchial foreign bodies?
For: Waiting 12 to 24 hours in stable patients or in patients who have not aspirated a vegetable material may obviate the need for an invasive procedure under general anesthesia with its associated morbidity; postural drainage is successful in 50 to 60% of cases.

Against: Once the diagnosis is confirmed, the object should be removed immediately to prevent potential complications such as break-up of the object and pneumonia. The incidence of pneumonia is 20% when the object is left in place for 24 hours compared with less than 8% if it is removed immediately.

BIBLIOGRAPHY

1.   Abman, S.H., Fan, L.L., and Cotton, E.K.: Emergency treatment of foreign body obstruction of the upper airway in children. J. Emerg. Med., 2:7-12, 1984. Review of controversy; recommends guidelines of AHA: back blows followed by chest thrusts in children.

2.   American Heart Association: Standards and guidelines for cardiopulmonary resuscitation (CPR) and emergency cardiac care (ECC). J.A.M.A., 244:453-509,1980. American Heart Association's recommendations include combination of back blows and thrusts.

3.   Aytac, A., Yurdakul, Y., Ikizler C., et al.: Inhalation of foreign bodies in children: Report of 500 cases. J. Thorac. Cardiovasc. Surg., 74:145-151,1977. Early bronchoscopy favored; postural drainage felt to be dangerous; vegetable matter fragments, if left in place for a short time, increase difficulty of removal and increase incidence of pneumonia.

4.   Blazer, S., Naveh, Y., and Friedman, A.: Foreign body in the airway: A review of 200 cases. Am. J. Dis. Child., 134:68-71,1980. Pediatric patients; favors early bronchoscopy; repeat bronchoscopy if symptoms do not clear since other "missed" foreign bodies may be present.

5.   Brady, P.G., and Johnson, W.F.: Removal of foreign bodies: The flexible fiberoptic endoscope. South Med. J., 70:702-704,1977. Arguments for fiberoptic endoscopy for removal of foreign bodies.

6.   Brown,T.C.K.: Bronchoscopy for removal of foreign bodies in children. Anaesth. Intens. Care., 1:521-523,1973. Anesthetic procedures described for bronchoscopy.

7.   Burrington, J.D., and Cotton, E.K.: Removal of foreign bodies from the tracheobronchial tree. J. Pediatr. Surg., 7:119-122,1972. Postural drainage compares favorably with bronchoscopy.

8.   Chatterji, S., and Chatterji,P.: The management of foreign bodies in air passages. Anesthesia, 27:390,1972. Classic article describing pathophysiologic changes associated with foreign bodies. Anesthetic techniques are also described; general anesthesia with bronchoscopy favored.

9.   Cohen, S.R., Herbert, W.I., Lewis, G.B., Jr., et al.: Foreign bodies in the airway: Five-year retrospective study with special reference to management. Ann. Otol., 89:437-442,1980. Bronchoscopy and anesthesia methods for small airway foreign bodies.

10. Day, R.L., Crelin, E.S., and DuBois, A.B.: Choking: The Heimlich abdominal thrust vs. back blows: An approach to measurement of inertial and aerodynamic forces. Pediatrics, 70:113-119,1982. Attempted to analyze air pressures generated in airways by back blows and thrusts with various mechanical measurements; found thrusts to produce higher pressures.

11. Greensher, J., and Mofenson,H.C.: Emergency treatment of the choking child. Pediatrics, 70:110-112,1982. Review of recommendations of American Academy of Pediatrics. Advocates chest thrusts and back blows for pediatric patients.

12. Harris, C.S., Baker, S.P., Smith, G.A., et al.: Childhood asphyxiation by food: A national analysis and overview. J.A.M.A., 251:2231-2235,1984. Epidemiologic data; occurs in kids under the age of 5; objects found were hot dogs, round candy, grapes. Hot dogs were associated with highest mortality.

13.   Heimlich, H.: A life-saving maneuver to prevent food choking. J.A.M.A., 234:398-401, 1975. One of the first articles describing the thrust maneuvers by Heimlich.

14.   Heimlich, H.J.: First aid for choking children: Back blows and chest thrusts cause complications and death. Pediatrics, 70:120-125,1982. Heimlich's defense of his maneuver; excellent bibliography.

15.   Kim, I.G., Brummitt, W.M., Humphry, A., et al.: Foreign body in the airway: A review of 202 cases. Laryngoscope, 83:347-354,1973. Description of clinical findings in children associated with bronchial foreign body, i.e., cough, wheezing, decreased unilateral air entry is common triad; management with bronchoscopy.

16.   Law, D., and Kosloske, A.M.: Management of tracheobronchial foreign bodies in children: A reevaluation of postural drainage and bronchoscopy. Pediatrics, 58:362-367,1976. Postural drainage in intensive care unit advocated for 24 hours when (1) patient has recently aspirated foreign body, i.e., less than 24 hours prior to therapy; (2) there is only mild to moderate respiratory distress. Bronchoscopy advocated for severe distress if postural drainage unsuccessful.

17.   Mittleman, R.E., and Werti,C.V.: The fatal cafe coronary. J.A.M.A., 247:1285-1288,1982. Demographic data; most occur secondary to meat ingestion in elderly adults associated with alcohol use; institutional aspiration secondary to soft foodstuffs. Witnesses present in 85% of cases; strong advocate of education to recognize cafe coronary.

18.   Redding, J.S.: The choking controversy: Critique of evidence on the Heimlich maneuver. Crit. Care Med., 7:475-479,1979. Historical perspective of controversy up to 1976; recommends both back blows and thrusts in combination.

19.   Torrey, S.B.: The choking child: A life-threatening emergency. Clin. Pediatr., 22:751-754, 1983. Review of the controversy. Stresses need for further studies. With present data recommends combination of maneuvers.

20.   Vauthy, P.A., and Reddy, R.: Acute upper airway obstruction in infants and children: Evaluation by the fiberoptic bronchoscope. Ann. Otol., 89:417-418,1980. Diagnostic, but not therapeutic, use of fiberoptic bronchoscope.

21.   Visintine, R., and Baick, C.: Ruptured stomach after Heimlich maneuver. J.A.M.A., 234:415,1975. First reported complication of Heimlich maneuver; patient had esophageal obstruction and airway obstruction.

22.   Votteler, T.P., Nash, J.C., and Rutledge, J.C.: The hazards of ingested alkaline disk batteries in children. J.A.M.A., 249:2504-2506,1983. Advocates of early endoscopic or surgical removal no matter where in the GI tract.

---

15. ACUTE ABDOMEN
JAMES NARROD, M.D.

---

1.   **What is the critical question a surgeon must answer in evaluating a patient with an acute abdomen?**
     The responsibility of the surgeon seeing a patient with an acute abdomen is to decide if the patient has a "nonsurgical" abdomen (e.g., ureteral calculi, pyelonephritis, pancreatitis, hepatitis, myocardial infarction, porphyria, mesenteric adenitis, Crohn's disease, lead poisoning, ketoacidosis, etc.) or a "surgical" abdomen (see schematic diagram on opposite page).

2.   **What questions in the history are critical?**
     1. Age? Certain diseases are more common in different age goups. Infants and children: intussusception, Meckel's diverticulitis, mesenteric adenitis, appendicitis. Adults: cholecystitis, gynecologic disorders, perforated ulcers. Elderly: diverticulitis, colon cancer, ruptured aneurysm.

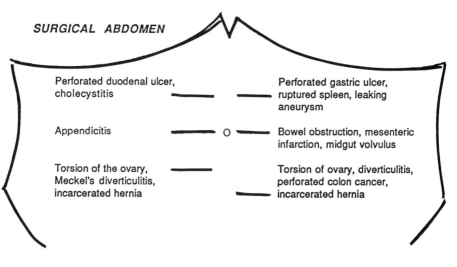

SURGICAL ABDOMEN

Perforated duodenal ulcer, cholecystitis

Perforated gastric ulcer, ruptured spleen, leaking aneurysm

Appendicitis

Bowel obstruction, mesenteric infarction, midgut volvulus

Torsion of the ovary, Meckel's diverticulitis, incarcerated hernia

Torsion of ovary, diverticulitis, perforated colon cancer, incarcerated hernia

2. What are the time and mode of onset? Perforated ulcer: sudden severe onset after waking the patient. Bowel obstruction: intermittent crampy pain. Appendicitis: gradual onset.

3. Quality of pain? Burning, eroding ulcer; sharp and constricting, cholecystitis; crampy, intestinal obstructions or related calculi; tearing, dissecting aneurysm; dull and constant, pyelonephritis; agony, pancreatitis.

4. Gynecologic history? Pelvic inflammatory disease, or common around the time of menstrual period. A missed menstrual period suggests possibility of an ectopic pregnancy.

3. What is Mittelschmerz?
This is intramenstrual pain often associated with ovulation.

4. What is Kehr's sign?
Intense pain, beginning in the left upper quadrant and radiating to the top of the left shoulder, caused by diaphragm irritation. This may be present with a ruptured spleen.

EXAMINATION

5. What are "peritoneal signs"?
When inflammation extends to the parietal peritoneum, the patient will manifest peritoneal signs that include localized tenderness, involuntary guarding, rebound tenderness, and returned pain.

6. What is Rovsing's sign?
Palpation of the left lower quadrant causes pain in the right lower quadrant in patients with appendicitis.

7. Does afebrile status exclude a surgical abdomen?
No. Fever is often a late occurrence. Elderly and immunocompromised patients often are afebrile despite frank peritonitis.

8. What is the significance of bowel sounds?
High-pitched rushes, bowel obstruction; decreased bowel sounds, peritonitis. This is an unreliable sign.

9.   What is the significance of palpation of the abdomen?
This is the most important portion of the abdominal examination because it allows detection of localized tenderness, guarding, referred pain, as well as diffuse peritonitis. Remember, in a patient with localized right lower quadrant pain, appendicitis may be present despite a normal leukocyte count and normal body temperature temperature.

10.   What is a psoas sign?
Inflammation around the psoas muscle will cause pain on extension of the thigh.

11.   What is the obturator sign?
Inflammation around the obturator internus muscle will cause pain upon rotation of the flexed thigh (especially internal rotation).

DIAGNOSTIC TESTS

12.   Should urinalysis be done?
Yes. Glucose and ketones may be detected, suggesting diabetic ketoacidosis. White cells may be seen in pyelonephritis. Hematuria may suggest ureteral calculi. Unfortunately, appendicitis may cause both red and white blood cells in the urine.

13.   What is the value of a complete blood count?
An elevated and shifted differential leukocyte count is unreliable. Commonly, the elderly do not have leukocytosis. In appendicitis, the leukocyte count is a late change. Leukocyte counts greater than 20,000 are unusual in appendicitis and cholecystitis.

14.   Should an abdominal three-way x-ray be done?
While only 10% of gallstones are radiopaque, 90% of urinary calculi can be visualized. Free air may be seen under the diaphragm in a chest x-ray film (upright view) or over the liver in a left lateral decubitus view. Air-fluid level may suggest a bowel obstruction, whereas an absent psoas shadow suggests retroperitoneal irritation.

15.   What is a sentinel loop?
In localized inflammatory conditions, a loop of bowel adjacent to the lesion may become distended with gas. This is commonly seen in pancreatitis.

SURGERY

16.   Is a negative laparotomy ever justified?
Yes. An exact diagnosis cannot always be made and it is better to have a negative laparotomy than to miss appendicitis or an infarcted piece of bowel.

17.   What incision should be used?
If the diagnosis is in doubt, a midline incision allows access to the entire peritoneal cavity.

BIBLIOGRAPHY

1.   Schwartz, S.I., and Storer, E.H.: Manifestations of gastrointestinal disease. In Schwartz, S.I., Shires, T.G., et al. (eds.): Principles of Surgery. New York, McGraw-Hill Book Company, 1984.
2.   Silen,W.: Cope's Early Diagnosis of the Acute Abdomen. New York, Oxford University Press, 1979.

16. MULTIPLE TRAUMA

DEBORAH DAVIS, M.D., and ERNEST E. MOORE, M.D.

Initial evaluation and treatment of the multiply injured patient require simultaneous physical examination, resuscitation, and diagnostic testing. The priority of procedures depends on the nature and severity of injuries.

1. **What is the "golden hour"?**
The "golden hour" is the 60 minutes from the time of injury in which rapid triage, transport, and treatment can effectively change the patient's outcome.

2. **What information from the scene is important?**
Blunt trauma: (1) mechanism of injury: speed of vehicles, damage to car; (2) vital signs at the scene: hypotension at the scene is important despite stable vital signs in the emergency room; (3) witnessed loss of consciousness; (4) use or non-use of seat belts; (5) integrity of windshield and steering wheel: if damaged, suspect head and chest injury. *Penetrating trauma:* (1) nature of weapon: length of knife and depth of penetration; (2) velocity of missile: high- or low-caliber bullet.

3. **Which lines and catheters are required for resuscitation?**
Peripheral Intravenous. Large-bore, 14-gauge, at least two. Avoid injured extremities; use saphenous vein cutdown if no other lines are available or if massive fluid resuscitation is required. *Central Line.* If blood pressure does not respond to vital fluid resuscitation or if tamponade is suspected. *Nasogastric Tube.* Bleeding via nasogastric line suggests injury to stomach or duodenum: decompresses stomach to prevent aspiration in comatose patient; used prior to peritoneal lavage. *Foley Catheter.* Check prostate and urethral meatus for blood prior to placement; used to follow urine output in treatment of shock.

4. **What are the methods used to stabilize the cervical spine?**
Position sandbags beside the head and tape forehead to the stretcher. Place a Philadelphia or four-poster collar if injury is suspected or if the patient is to be moved prior to clearing.

5. **What are the initial priorities, the ABC's of resuscitation?**
Airway, Breathing, Circulation (treatment of shock).

6. **What features of the physical examination are important?**
Vital signs: including temperature. *Head:* presence of fractures, lacerations, hemotympanum, facial injuries. *Neck:* neck veins, tenderness of cervical spine. *Chest:* breath sounds, crepitus or palpable rib fractures, sucking chest wounds. *Cardiac:* presence of pulses, sternal tenderness, evidence of tamponade. *Abdomen:* tenderness, heme-positive stools. *Pelvis:* stability. *Genitourinary:* position of prostate, blood at urethral meatus. *Extremities:* fractures and soft tissue injury, pallor of nail beds. *Neurologic:* mental status, presence of ethyl alcohol, localizing signs, rectal tone.

7. **What initial diagnostic tests are required?**
Cervical spine: cross-table lateral film identifies 98% of injuries. *Chest x-ray:* best screen for hemo-pneumothorax, aortic injury. *Pelvic x-ray:* if suspected injury or unexplained blood loss. *Electrocardiogram:* identifies arrhythmias, ST changes associated with myocardial contusion.

8. **What initial laboratory tests are required?**
    Hematocrit; crossmatch; arterial blood gases to monitor hypoxemia in pulmonary contusion and hyperventilation in patients with head injuries, and to monitor acidosis in shock; urinalysis: if dipstick is heme-positive a specimen is spun for red blood cell count (hematuria suggests renal/bladder injury).

9. **What are the methods of establishing an airway?**
    Passive management: jaw thrust and oral airway. *Active management:* nasotracheal intubation, contraindicated in maxillofacial trauma; orotracheal intubation, contraindicated if the status of the cervical spine is unknown or injury is present; cricothyroidotomy, if nasotracheal or orotracheal intubation is not possible; tracheostomy, only in tracheolaryngeal injury.

10. **How does one optimize ventilation?**
    Supplemental FiO_2 for hypoxemia; assisted ventilation for hypercapnia; chest tube for hemo-pneumothorax; cover sucking chest wounds.

11. **How is external hemorrhage best treated?**
    External compression is best. Tourniquet or blind clamping of vessels in a wound is rarely necessary. Hemorrhage from head wounds is treated by injection of lidocaine with epinephrine, and suturing.

12. **What are the two factors involved in shock?**
    Hypovolemia and pump failure.

13. **What are causes of pump failure in trauma?**
    Tension pneumothorax, treat with chest tube. Pericardial tamponade, treat with pericardiocentesis or thoracotomy. Myocardial contusion. Myocardial infarction. Coronary air embolization (rare) occurs with pulmonary injury. Air embolized into the pulmonary veins and into the coronary arteries (treated with thoracotomy and by cross-clamping the pulmonary hilum).

14. **What are MAST pants, their use and contraindications?**
    Military anti-shock trousers (MAST) are pneumatic compression pants; they may provide autotransfusion of blood from the lower extremities and abdomen to increase venous return (controversial) and increase peripheral resistance. They are contraindicated in pulmonary edema, pregnancy, and abdominal evisceration.

15. **Which fluids should be used in volume resuscitation?**
    Crystalloid (lactated Ringer's) is used initially, 1000 to 2000 ml. Blood is used to maintain hematocrit > 30%: (1) crossmatched: ideal in stable patient; requires 15 to 20 minutes from blood bank; (2) type-specific: non-crossmatched; risk of transfusion reaction < 1% in men, < 2% in parous women; available in 5 minutes; and (3) O-negative: for use in major hemorrhage requiring immediate resuscitation; risk of transfusion reaction is low but may make later crossmatch more difficult.

16. **What are the second priorities in evaluation of the multiply injured patient?**
    Neurologic examination. Orthopedic examination: splint fractures, document neurovascular injury. Identify occult hemorrhage. Definitive diagnostic x-ray if patient is stable (CT scan, IVP, angiography, other x-rays as indicated).

17. **Which diagnostic tests or procedures are used to identify occult hemorrhage?**

Chest x-rays, peritoneal lavage, and pelvic x-ray.

18. Does ethyl alcohol intoxication change the overall outcome of a patient with multiple trauma?
No.

19. What are the contraindications to doing a rectal examination on the traumatized patient?
If the patient has no anus.

CONTROVERSIES

20. What is the meaning of "scoop and run"?
Some trauma specialists now recommend rapid transport to a designated trauma center rather than placing intravenous lines, etc., in the field.

21. Crystalloid versus colloid for fluid resuscitation?
Crystalloid: inexpensive and readily available. Colloid: thought to be more physiologic to increase oncotic pressure, prevents pulmonary edema; has not been shown to be more effective than crystalloid and is expensive. (See chapter 1 for further discussion.)

BIBLIOGRAPHY

1. American College of Surgeons Committee on Trauma: Treatment protocol for prehospital management of the trauma patient. Bulletin of the American College of Surgeons, February 1980, pp. 23-27. An outline of management procedures in the field.
2. Chan, R.M.W.: Diagnostic failures in the multiply injured. J. Trauma, 20:684-687,1980.
3. Light, T.R.: Diagnosis and management of fractures in the multiply injured patient. Surg. Clin. North Am., 60:1121-1131, 1980. Describes the commonly associated orthopedic injuries and other system injury as a result of specific mechanisms of injury.
4. Lindsey, D.: Teaching the initial management of major multiple system trauma. J.Trauma, 20:160-162, 1980. A simple summary of the stepwise physical examination and thought processes involved in evaluating the multiply injured patient.
5. Moore, E. E.: Resuscitation and evaluation of the injured patient. In Zuidema, G., Ballinger, W., and Rutherford, R. (eds.): Management of Trauma. Philadelphia, W.B. Saunders Co., 1985. An overview of the initial management of the critically injured patient.
6. Shafton, G.W.: The initial evaluation of the multiple trauma patient. World J. Surg., 7:19-25,1983. A succinct summary of the priorities in resuscitation and physical examination of multiply injured patients.
7. Shaw, R.K.: Modifications in the treatment of the multiple injured patient. J. Trauma, 17:30-33, 1977. Describes changes in management when multiple injuries include thermal injury.
8. Trunkey, D.: Symposium on Trauma. Surg. Clin. North. Am., 62:February 1982. An entire edition dealing with the specifics of trauma medicine including basic physiology.

17. BLUNT ABDOMINAL TRAUMA
JAMES NARROD, M.D.

1. What is the central problem in blunt abdominal injury?
Diagnosis: ascertaining if the patient is injured intraabdominally and, if so, how severely.

2. **What are common injuries associated with blunt abdominal trauma?**
    Head trauma, chest trauma, and fractures.

3. **What organs are most commonly injured in blunt abdominal trauma?**
    The spleen, followed by the liver.

HISTORY AND PHYSICAL EXAMINATION

4. **What are the key questions in the history?**
    Mechanism of injury (often alerts one to potential seriousness, e.g., high-speed, rollover motor vehicle accident). A memory aid for asking the right history questions is AMPLE, i.e., an ample history. *A* = Allergies, *M* = Medications, *P* = Past medical history, *L* = Last meal, and *E* = Events leading up to the accident.

5. **Is the physical examination reliable?**
    No. The physical examination has false-negative and false-positive rates of 10 to 20% each.

6. **What is Kehr's sign?**
    The patient with a ruptured spleen has left shoulder pain from blood irritating the diaphragm.

7. **What else should be examined besides the abdomen?**
    Associated injuries are common. The first priority is the respiratory system. The patient must be able to protect his own airway or it must be protected for him. Pneumothorax may be caused by fractured ribs.

8. **What do distended neck veins suggest?**
    Cardiac tamponade is manifested by distended neck veins, tachycardia, distant heart sounds, and eventually decreased blood pressure. An elevated central venous pressure confirms the diagnosis and pericardiocentesis should be performed.

9. **If the patient is initially lucid and then has a progressive loss of consciousness, what needs to be ruled out?**
    In epidural hematoma, the patient has an initial lucid interval for a few minutes to hours followed by progressive loss of consciousness. A skull fracture over the middle meningeal artery is a common finding. A CT scan of the head will confirm the diagnosis. Don't forget to look at the back! A patient often arrives at the emergency room strapped on a board and no one examines the back. Serious injuries may be missed.

10. **Is the abdominal examination reliable in a comatose or intoxicated patient?**
    No.

11. **Why perform a rectal examination?**
    Blood in the rectum suggests a colorectal injury. A high-riding prostate suggests a urethral tear. Absent rectal tone suggests a spinal cord injury.

DIAGNOSTIC TESTS

12. **If the hematocrit is normal, can the patient have significant blood loss?**

It takes 6 hours for the hematocrit to equilibrate after blood loss; therefore, hematocrit may be normal on arrival at the emergency room despite loss of several units of blood. However, a hematocrit should be done initially (it may already be low) and repeated often (1 to 2 hours) if indicated.

13. What x-rays should be obtained in those involved in high-speed automobile accidents?
A lateral film of the cervical spine to rule out a cervical fracture; chest x-ray to look for a wide mediastinum, pneumothorax, and rib fracture; and a pelvic film to look for a pelvic fracture. Additional x-rays are suggested by the physical examination.

14. What is the role of peritoneal lavage?
Because the physical examination is unreliable, irrigating the peritoneal cavity with 10 to 15 ml/kg of Ringer's lactate solution and looking at the cell count have been found to detect abdominal injuries. The sensitivity and specificity are over 95%.

15. What are the criteria for a positive peritoneal lavage?
RBC > $100,000/mm^3$, WBC > $500/mm^3$, the fluid coming out of a chest tube or Foley catheter, and bile or bacteria on the Gram stain. An easy bedside rule is that if you can read newsprint through the tubing with the pink/red lavage in it, it is probably negative.

16. Can the lavage be normal in the presence of a significant injury?
Yes. The peritoneal lavage is not 100% sensitive; therefore patients should be observed for 24 hours, and serial examinations performed after peritoneal lavage is done.

17. If a patient is in hemorrhagic shock from obvious intraabdominal bleeding, should peritoneal lavage be performed?
No. A patient with an obvious abdominal injury should be taken to the operating room.

18. If a pelvic fracture is present, should peritoneal lavage be done?
Yes. There is a 15% incidence of associated intraabdominal injury. The lavage should be done above the umbilicus in order to avoid the pelvic hematoma. Normally the lavage is done just inferior to the umbilicus.

19. What are the relative contraindications to peritoneal lavage?
Previous abdominal surgery, an unemptied urinary bladder, and pregnancy.

20. What is the role of a Gastrografin study?
If a duodenal injury is suspected, a Gastrografin study should be done. Because the duodenum is retroperitoneal, the injury is difficult to detect by peritoneal lavage and physical examination. The mortality rate associated with a perforated duodenum is over 50% if it is overlooked for 24 hours.

21. What are the roles of a CT scan, liver-spleen scans, and angiograms for abdominal injuries?
The CT scan is neither as sensitive nor as specific as peritoneal lavage. In a stable patient a few hours after injury, these tests may occasionally prove helpful. An angiogram is useful in detecting a suspected renal artery injury.

SURGERY

22. Is a negative laparotomy dangerous?

The risks from a negative laparotomy are few. There is a low incidence of bowel obstruction secondary to adhesion as well as complications from a general anesthetic.

23. **What is the "seat belt syndrome"?**
While seat belts have dramatically reduced serious injuries, the bowel is occasionally crushed between the seat belt and the vertebral column when sudden deceleration occurs.

BIBLIOGRAPHY

1.   Blaisdell, W.F., and Trunkey, D.D.: Trauma Management. Vol. 1: Abdominal Trauma. New York, Thieme-Stratton, Inc., 1982.
2.   Zuidema, G.D., Rutherford, R.B., and Ballinger, W.F. (eds.): The Management of Trauma. Philadelphia, W.B. Saunders Co., 1985.

---

18. PENETRATING ABDOMINAL TRAUMA
ROBERT PAPADOPOULOS, M.D.

INITIAL RESUSCITATION

1. **What are the major priorities in resuscitation of the trauma patient with penetrating abdominal wounds?**
Resuscitation of these patients should be based on physiologic principles with the goal being to maximize oxygen supply to the tissues. Priorities are based on a physiologic ABC schedule. (1) *A* for maintaining an effective airway, (2) *B* for breathing, and (3) *C* for circulation, representing control of hemorrhage and restoration of an adequate intravascular volume. Resuscitation of the patient must proceed simultaneously with the initial evaluation. Important history that should be obtained from paramedics or family include the type of weapon used, blood loss at the scene, and time interval since injury. A rapid but thorough physical examination is performed with particular emphasis on areas often neglected such as inspection of the flanks, back, perineum, and axilla, rectal examination, neurologic assessment, and evaluation of peripheral pulses. A nasogastric tube should be inserted to decompress the stomach and to look for occult blood. A Foley catheter should be inserted to empty the bladder and check for hematuria. A nasogastric tube and Foley catheter are always inserted prior to peritoneal lavage to prevent iatrogenic injury.

2. **What preoperative studies should be done?**
A chest x-ray is mandatory to rule out intrathoracic bleeding and to check the position of central lines and endotracheal, nasogastric, and chest tubes. Other studies that should be considered in the stable patient are biplanar abdominal films, which are useful in visualizing bullet fragments and foreign bodies but are generally not useful in stab wounds. Sigmoidoscopy should be performed for injuries with proximity to the rectum. Intravenous pyelography should be performed in patients with hematuria. Initial laboratory tests should include a baseline hematocrit, white blood cell count, blood sample for type and crossmatching, and a urinalysis as a bare minimum.

3. **When should thoracotomy in the emergency department be utilized in the resuscitation of patients with penetrating abdominal trauma?**

Thoracotomy should be utilized in patients presenting with cardiac arrest or hypotension (systolic blood pressure < 60 mm Hg) refractory to initial resuscitative measures. The physiologic rationale in severely hypotensive patients is that resuscitative thoracotomy allows proximal vascular control via the descending aorta prior to release of the abdominal wall's tamponade effect during definitive laparotomy. In patients who present in cardiac arrest, thoracotomy allows access to the heart for internal cardiac massage. For the patient in extremis with a penetrating wound in proximity to the heart, thoracotomy allows release of a pericardial tamponade and access to cardiac hemorrhage.

STAB WOUNDS

4. **What has been the traditional approach to stab wounds to the abdomen?**

Following military experience, exploratory laparotomy was considered mandatory for all patients with abdominal stab wounds. This approach led to a negative celiotomy rate of 30 to 60% in civilian practice with substantial morbidity and cost. A selective approach to managing these injuries has subsequently evolved.

5. **What are the indications for immediate exploratory laparotomy?**

Patients with signs of hemorrhagic shock, peritonitis, or significant evisceration should undergo rapid resuscitation followed by immediate celiotomy. All other patients should be selectively managed.

6. **How accurate is physical examination in ascertaining intraperitoneal injury?**

Bull and Matheson have noted false-positive results in 18% of patients and false-negative results in 23%.

7. **What adjunctive methods are available to ascertain penetration of the peritoneum?**

The procedure of choice is exploration of the wound under local anesthesia in the emergency room. Twenty to thirty percent of these patients will have unequivocally negative wound explorations and can be discharged from the emergency room with local wound care. Sinography, the injection of radiopaque contrast material, was used in the past with a high incidence of both false-positive and false-negative results and is no longer recommended.

8. **What are the management options for patients with proven or suspected peritoneal penetration?**

Exploratory laparotomy and diagnostic peritoneal lavage (DPL). Most authorities recommend DPL, although this is controversial. While two thirds of the stab wounds penetrate the peritoneum, only one half of those will inflict significant visceral injury.

9. **What constitutes a positive DPL?**

Initial aspiration of more than 10 ml of gross blood or fluid containing bile, feces, or particulate matter constitutes a positive lavage necessitating immediate exploration. A negative aspirate is followed by infusion of 1000 ml of normal saline (15 ml/kg in children), which is drained by gravity and then analyzed. The most useful test for predicting visceral injury is the red blood cell count (RBC), although the minimum level for mandatory celiotomy is controversial. Recent experience confirms that > 100,000 RBC/mm^3 is the most accurate predictor of intraabdominal injury. Interpretations of white blood bell count (WBC) and enzymes are also controversial, with the current recommendations being that isolated WBC elevations > 500/mm^3 or elevations of enzymes such as amylase or alkaline phosphatase should mandate exploration.

10. **How should patients with a negative DPL be managed?**
These patients should be admitted to the hospital and followed clinically for 24 hours. Approximately 5% of patients with RBC levels < 100,000 will require laparotomy. Most of these patients will have hollow viscus perforation of the small bowel, stomach, or colon.

GUNSHOT WOUNDS TO THE ABDOMEN

11. **Should patients with civilian gunshot wounds undergo selective management?**
No. Current data document peritoneal penetration in > 80% of patients with gunshot wounds to the abdomen, and > 95% of these will have significant visceral injury. Therefore, all patients with intraperitoneal penetration should undergo exploratory laparotomy.

12. **What other studies are indicated?**
Biplanar roentgenograms, coupled with physical examination, are useful in estimating missile trajectory and predicting intraperitoneal penetration. Wound exploration is technically impractical and never indicated. Physical examination alone is unreliable in determining visceral injury, with a false-negative rate of up to 20%.

13. **How should asymptomatic patients with tangential missile tracts or equivocal missile penetration be managed?**
Many authorities would continue to recommend exploratory laparotomy, although another option is diagnostic peritoneal lavage. The RBC criteria for exploration in this setting is reduced to > 5000 RBC/mm^3, with the rationale that this quantity of intraperitoneal blood cannot be due to the lavage procedure and must represent missile penetration of the peritoneum. Since > 95% of gunshot wounds that violate the peritoneum cause significant visceral injury, this is an absolute indication for exploratory laparotomy. Patients with a negative DPL are admitted to the hospital and followed clinically for 24 hours to rule out a hollow viscus injury or delayed injury secondary to extraperitoneal blast effect.

PENETRATING WOUNDS TO THE LOWER CHEST

14. **What is the incidence of significant intraabdominal injury with penetrating wounds to the lower chest?**
The lower chest is defined as the area between the fourth intercostal space (ICS) anteriorly, the seventh ICS posteriorly, and the costal margins. Diaphragmatic excursion during full expiration may reach the fourth ICS, placing upper abdominal organs at risk. The experience at Denver General Hospital documents a 15% incidence of significant intraabdominal injury with stab wounds and a 46% incidence with gunshot wounds.

PENETRATING WOUNDS TO THE BACK OR FLANK

15. **Why do penetrating wounds of the back or flank present diagnostic problems?**

These patients may develop injuries that may become tamponaded or contained anatomically in the retroperitoneum and present with minimal physical findings. Physical examination alone is inaccurate in 10 to 20% of these patients.

16. What is the incidence of significant visceral injury with stab wounds to the back or flank?
The risk for stab wounds to the back is 10%, whereas for stab wounds to the flank it is approximately 25%. This relatively low risk of injury justifies a selective approach to exploratory laparotomy in such wounds. Such an approach can reduce the negative laparotomy rate to approximately 10%.

17. What other adjunctive studies are useful in assessing these injuries?
In patients without absolute indications for laparotomy, diagnostic peritoneal lavage is useful in predicting intraabdominal injury, although this modality may miss significant retroperitoneal injuries. Intravenous pyelography should be performed in patients with hematuria or with wounds in proximity to the kidney. CT scan is currently the diagnostic modality of choice for evaluation of the retroperitoneum.

18. Should gunshot wounds to this region be selectively managed?
Data are sparse for isolated flank or back wounds, although the high incidence of significant visceral injuries mandates laparotomy for all gunshot wounds with fascial penetration.

INITIAL OPERATIVE MANAGEMENT

19. What type of incision is preferred for abdominal exploration?
A long, midline incision is generally used. This provides rapid entry and wide access. It can also be extended into a median sternotomy or into either side of the chest if necessary.

20. What is the initial operative approach to intraabdominal injury?
Evisceration is quickly performed and intraperitoneal blood rapidly evacuated. Laparotomy packs are used temporarily to control any bleeding that is present. The abdomen is quickly examined, with the major source of hemorrhage identified and controlled first. Next, gross contamination from hollow viscus injury is identified and temporarily controlled with Babcock or Allis clamps. Once the major abdominal injuries have been controlled, the entire abdominal cavity is systematically explored.

BIBLIOGRAPHY

1. Bill, J.C., and Matheson, C.: Exploratory laparotomy in patients with penetrating wounds of the abdomen. Am. J. Surg., 116:223-228, 1968.
2. Feliciano, D.V., Bitondo, C.G., Steed, G., et al.: Five hundred open taps or lavages in patients with abdominal stab wounds. Am. J. Surg., 148:772-777, 1984.
3. Moore, E.E., and Marx, J.A.: Penetrating abdominal wounds: Rationale for exploratory laparotomy. J.A.M.A., 253:2705-2708, 1985.
4. Peck, J.J., and Berne, T.V.: Posterior abdominal stab wounds. J. Trauma, 21:298-306, 1981.
5. Shaftan, G.W.: Indications for operation in abdominal trauma. Am. J. Surg., 99:657-664, 1960.
6. Thal, E.R.: Evaluation of peritoneal lavage and local exploration in lower chest and abdominal stab wounds. J. Trauma, 17:642-648, 1977.
7. Thompson, J.S., Moore, E.E., Moore-Van Duzer, S., et al.: The evolution of abdominal stab wound management. J. Trauma, 20:478-484, 1980.

19. SPLENIC TRAUMA
FREDERICK A. MOORE, M.D.

1. What is a typical history for splenic trauma?
Because the spleen is the second most commonly injured intraabdominal organ, any history is consistent. Localized trauma to the left upper quadrant or lower left chest with associated fractures of the eleventh or twelfth ribs or hematuria should arouse suspicion. Delayed hypotension following blunt trauma occasionally occurs when a perisplenic hematoma ruptures.

2. How is splenic trauma diagnosed?
Peritoneal lavage, though not organ-specific, determines significant hemoperitoneum and leads to laparotomy in the vast majority of cases of splenic trauma. Overall accuracy is roughly 98%. Alternatives that are organ-specific include technetium scanning, selective arteriography, ultrasound, and CT scanning. Accuracy falls in the range of 90 to 95%. The limitations of these methods are time, expense, and failure to rule out hollow visceral injuries, thus restricting their use to those patients with localized trauma or delayed presentation.

3. What is overwhelming post-splenectomy sepsis (OPSS)?
A typical scenario is abrupt onset of fever, chills, nausea, and vomiting following a mild upper respiratory tract infection. This progresses over 12 to 24 hours to fulminant sepsis associated with shock, disseminated intravascular coagulation, and adrenal insufficiency. Mortality rates vary from 40 to 70%, and although the mortality rate is 50% within one year, the syndrome has been reported to occur as long as 37 years after splenectomy. In 70% of patients with OPSS, the responsible organism is an encapsulated bacterium such as pneumococcus, *H. influenzae*, or meningococcus. In the remaining cases of OPSS, nonencapsulated bacteria, viruses, and protozoa have been incriminated.

4. In whom does OPSS develop?
In 1952 King and Shumacker made a startling observation. Five children who underwent splenectomy within the first six months of life all developed severe sepsis, and two·died. This stimulated a healthy debate over the spleen's role in infection. Some believed that the increased risk of sepsis was caused by the underlying disease. It was not until 1973, when Singer analyzed a series of 24 asplenic patients, that the clear risk of OPSS became apparent. The incidence of severe sepsis was related to the indication for splenectomy. In healthy individuals, and in those with trauma or incidental splenectomy, the risks were 1.5% and 2.1%, respectively. In those with hematologic disorders, the incidence varied from 2.0 to 7.5%. The incidence is also greater in children under 4 years of age by a factor of 2.5. Everyone agrees that children are at increased risk, but a debate continues about adult trauma. Recent reviews confirm this risk to be in the range of 1 to 2%.

5. What is the immunologic role of the spleen?
The spleen represents 25% of the reticuloendothelial system, being perfused with 200 ml of blood per minute. Ninety percent of this is forced through the cords of Billroth, where fixed macrophages phagocytize particulate matter. As such it represents a major immunologic filter. Its second role is that of an immunologic factory, i.e., the site of IgM, tuftsin, and properdin production. These are

critical in opsonization, and thus play a major role in phagocytosis of intravascular antigens. Finally, there is some evidence that the spleen may modulate the ratio of helper T cells to suppressor T cells.

6. **Can splenic trauma be managed nonoperatively?**
Transfusions and supportive care have been effectively utilized in selected cases of pediatric trauma. In children the spleen is less protected and therefore vulnerable to minor blunt injuries in which associated injuries to intraabdominal organ are infrequent. The pediatric spleen has a thicker capsule which contracts to promote hemostasis. Nonoperative management of adult splenic trauma has been proposed, but most feel that the risk of associated injuries is too high. It is therefore limited to those adults presenting in a delayed fashion who are hemodynamically stable and in whom associated injuries seem unlikely.

7. **When should the spleen be salvaged?**
In many cases, the spleen can be saved with simple, temporary packing or topical hemostatic agents. If additional techniques are required, it is wise to proceed with splenectomy in the unstable patient with multiple associated abdominal injuries and in patients with extraabdominal trauma such as closed head injuries or a widened mediastinum in whom treatment is uncertain. Obviously some injuries are quite extensive and repair would be unsafe. It must be kept in mind that the risk of repair should not exceed the risk of the asplenic state.

8. **How often can the spleen be salvaged and at what risk?**
Using the above guidelines, splenic salvage is possible in roughly one half of acute injuries. The only morbidity appears to be postoperative bleeding, which occurs in less than 3%. This tends to happen in the early postoperative period, when the patient is under close supervision. It is easily detected and therefore easily managed without significant risk of hemorrhagic mortality.

9. **What are splenic implants?**
They involve autotransplantation of splenic tissue into an omental pouch, which offers a rich blood supply. In both animals and humans these implants survive and are found to increase in size with time.

10. **Do splenic implants work?**
Numerous animal studies have confirmed the immunologic benefits of splenic implantation; however, the extent is variable. Data from studies in humans are limited. Follow-up studies show that IgM, platelet counts, and complement levels normalize. Uniform implant viability is demonstrated by technetium scanning. Target cells and Howell-Jolly bodies disappear. However, more sophisticated studies are needed to confirm whether these implants protect against OPSS.

11. **What advice should be given to asplenic patients?**
They should be warned of the lifelong risk of OPSS. They should seek medical attention for any lingering infections; early aggressive therapy markedly decreases mortality. Pneumococcal vaccination is recommended, but does not give full protection against OPSS. Pneumococcus is the responsible organism in only one half of the cases and the vaccine does not cover all serotypes. Penicillin prophylaxis may be of benefit in the immunocompromised host.

BIBLIOGRAPHY

1.   Dickerman, J.D.: Traumatic asplenia in adults: A defined hazard. J. Trauma, 116:361, 1981. A review of the cases of OPSS in the trauma literature; 50% occurred in adults, 70% of these died. This confirms the occurrence of OPSS in adult trauma.

2.   King, H., and Shumacker, H.B.: Splenic studies. Ann. Surg., 136:239, 1952.
3.   Moore, F.A., et al.: Risk of splenic salvage after trauma. Am. J. Surg., 148:800, 1984.
4.   Sherman, R.: Perspectives in management of trauma to the spleen. J. Trauma, 20:1,
     1980. Excellent review of the history and rationale of the present approach to the
     traumatized spleen.
5.   Singer, D.B.: Postsplenectomy sepsis. Perspect. Pediatr. Pathol., 1:285, 1973. A
     review of 24 series of splenic patients; quantitates the risk of sepsis according to
     age and indication for splenectomy and confirms the risk of OPSS in healthy adults.
6.   Wara, D.W.: Host defense against *Streptococcus pneumoniae*: The role of the spleen.
     Rev. Infect. Dis., 3:299, 1981. Outlines the present knowledge concerning the
     spleen's role in preventing overwhelming pneumococcal sepsis.
7.   Wessen, D.E., et al.: Ruptured spleen: When to operate? J. Pediatr. Surg., 16:324,
     1981. Nonoperative treatment of splenic injuries in children can, in selected cases
     and under ideal circumstances, reduce the need for operation, thus avoiding splen-
     ectomy with little risk to the patient.

20. LIVER TRAUMA

FRANCIS L. SHANNON, M.D., and ERNEST E. MOORE, M.D.

1. **Why is the liver the second most frequently injured abdominal organ?**
   Despite its protection by the lower rib cage, the liver is frequently lacerated by both blunt and penetrating mechanisms because of its large size and relative inelasticity.

2. **What is the major difference between splenic and hepatic injuries in terms of their relative need for surgical repair?**
   The liver has a unique ability to establish spontaneous hemostasis after superficial laceration. At laparotomy, therefore, approximately 50% of liver injuries have stopped bleeding and require no further treatment. In contrast, splenic fractures continue to hemorrhage and require operative repair or splenectomy.

3. **What are the major determinants of mortality following acute liver injury?**
   Mechanism of injury and number of associated abdominal organ injuries are the major determinants of mortality. Liver stab wounds have a 1 to 2% mortality, gunshot wounds a 15% mortality, and blunt injuries have an average 25% mortality. Isolated hepatic injuries incur a 5% mortality; the mortality with each additional organ injury doubles such that four associated injuries result in a 50% mortality.

DIAGNOSIS

4. **What historical facts and physical signs suggest acute liver injury?**
   Any patient sustaining blunt abdominal trauma with hypotension must be assumed to have a liver injury until proved otherwise. Specific signs that increase the likelihood of a hepatic injury are right lower rib fractures (especially posterior fractures of ribs 9 to 12) and penetrating injuries to the right lower chest (below the fourth intercostal space), flank, and upper abdomen.

5. **What diagnostic tests are helpful in confirming acute liver injury?**

Physical signs of hemoperitoneum are absent in one third of patients. Diagnostic peritoneal lavage is the most sensitive test for hemoperitoneum resulting from liver laceration (98% sensitivity). Abdominal CT scan is also useful in identifying and characterizimg hepatic parenchymal lacerations in the stable patient with blunt abdominal trauma.

6. **What is the role of hepatic angiography and radionucleotide biliary excretion scans in the diagnosis of liver injury?**
    The primary purpose of these procedures is to identify delayed complications of liver injuries (i.e., arteriovenous fistulas, hepatic artery pseudoaneurysms, hemobilia).

SURGICAL ANATOMY OF THE LIVER

7. **How many anatomic lobes are present in the liver and what is their topographic boundary?**
    The liver is divided into two anatomic lobes, the right and left. Their boundary lies in an oblique plane extending from the gallbladder fossa anteriorly to the inferior vena cava posteriorly.

8. **What is the blood supply to the liver and relative contribution of each structure to hepatic oxygenation?**
    The hepatic artery supplies approximately 30% of the blood flow to the liver and 50% of its oxygen supply. The portal vein provides 70% of its blood flow and 50% of its oxygen.

9. **What are the most common variations in hepatic arterial supply to the right and left lobes of the liver?**
    In most people, the common hepatic artery originates from the celiac axis and divides into right and left hepatic arterial branches within the porta hepatis. In 10% of patients, however, the right hepatic artery originates from the superior mesenteric artery and is the sole arterial supply to the right lobe. In a similar number of patients, the left hepatic artery originates from the left gastric artery and is the sole arterial supply to the left liver lobe.

10. **What is the venous drainage of the liver?**
    The right, middle, and left hepatic veins are the major venous tributaries, leaving the liver to enter the inferior vena cava below the right hemidiaphragm.

OPERATIVE MANAGEMENT OF LIVER INJURY

11. **How are acute liver injuries classified?**
    Liver wounds are generally graded on a scale of I to V according to the depth of parenchymal laceration and involvement of the hepatic veins or retrohepatic portion of the inferior vena cava. Optimal methods of obtaining hemostasis vary with the graded severity of the liver injury.

12. **What is the Pringle maneuver?**
    The Pringle maneuver is an initial means of controlling major liver bleeding by digital or vascular clamp compression of the hepatic artery and portal vein within the hepatoduodenal ligament. Failure of the Pringle maneuver to control liver hemorrhage suggests that a retrohepatic inferior vena cava or hepatic vein injury is present or that the liver receives arterial supply from an aberrant right or left hepatic artery.

13.   What is the role of selective hepatic artery ligation in securing hemostasis in a major liver injury?
Deep lacerations of the right or left hepatic lobes may result in bleeding that cannot be completely controlled by suture ligation of specific bleeding points within the liver parenchyma. In this situation, either the right or the left hepatic artery can be ligated with control of the bleeding and little risk of ischemic necrosis. Selective hepatic arterial ligation fails in about one third of patients.

14.   How frequently is hepatic lobectomy required for acute liver injury?
Only 1 to 2% of major liver injuries require formal hepatic lobectomy. The mortality for this procedure in trauma is 50%.

15.   Why is retrohepatic vena caval laceration lethal?
The retrohepatic portion of the inferior vena cava is difficult to expose because it is enveloped by the liver and therefore requires right hepatic lobectomy for successful repair. The large caliber of this vessel and high blood flows result in prohibitive hemorrhage while surgical exposure is being obtained.

16.   What is the physiologic rationale for use of an atriocaval shunt in attempted repair of retrohepatic vena caval injuries?
Hemorrhage control requires maintaining venous return to the heart from the lower body while both antegrade and retrograde bleeding through the laceration is stopped. These requirements are met by shunting blood through a tube spanning the laceration between the right atrium and lower inferior vena cava.

17.   What are the indications for packing the perihepatic area and closing the abdominal incision in a patient with major liver trauma?
Liver packing with planned reoperation for definitive hemorrhage control and liver debridement is necessary for patients with a refractory coagulopathy from massive blood loss, extensive bilobar liver injuries, and massive lobar injury requiring hepatic lobectomy.

POSTOPERATIVE COMPLICATIONS AFTER LIVER TRAUMA

18.   What are the most common complications following major liver injury that are life-threatening?
Postoperative hemorrhage due to refractory coagulopathy occurs in 5 to 10% of patients in the early postinjury period. The usual causes of this coagulopathy are massive blood transfusion, hypothermia, and acidosis. Sepsis due to an intraabdominal abscess occurs in 5% of patients following liver trauma. Associated hollow viscus injuries and major liver injury contribute to an increased incidence of abscess by providing a bacterial inoculation of residual blood and bile collections around the injured liver.

19.   What are the metabolic complications of hepatic resection for trauma?
Hypoglycemia, hypoalbuminemia, and hyperbilirubinemia are the most common consequences of major hepatic resection. Treatment of hypoglycemia with a 10% dextrose infusion is usually sufficient. Hypoalbuminemia usually appears by the second postoperative day and rarely requires replacement if early positive nitrogen balance can be achieved. Hyperbilirubinemia is usually mild (total bilirubin less than 10 mg/dl), appears on the third postoperative day, and peaks within one week of injury in uncomplicated cases.

20.   What is the utility of T-tube drainage of the common bile duct following liver injuries without extrahepatic bile duct involvement?
Routine T-tube drainage was originally advocated to prevent bile leaks following major liver injury. A controlled, prospective study of Lucas et al., however, showed that the incidence of complications is greater with T-tube drainage while the incidence of biliary fistulas is low (1%).

21.   What is the role of routine external drainage of superficial liver injuries?
Retrospective studies have shown that the incidence of perihepatic abscess and bile peritonitis is no different between patients with superficial liver injuries that are drained and those whose injuries are not drained. Furthermore, the high incidence of abdominal sepsis (25%) following major hepatic fractures was not reduced by the placement of perihepatic external drains.

BIBLIOGRAPHY

1.   Carmona, R.H., Lim, R.C., and Clark, G.C.: Morbidity and mortality in hepatic trauma: A 5 year study. Am. J. Surg., 144:88-94, 1982. Review of the results of conservative management of 443 liver injuries with emphasis on treatment and injury factors associated with increased morbidity.

2.   Defore, W.W., Mattox, K.L., et al.: Management of 1590 consecutive cases of liver trauma. Arch. Surg., 111:493-497, 1976. Historical perspective of the changing patterns of liver injury, overall morbidity of liver trauma and the impact of associated abdominal organ injuries on survival.

3.   Feliciano, D.V., Mattox, K.L., and Jordan, G.L.: Intra-abdominal packing for control of hepatic hemorrhage: A reappraisal. J. Trauma, 21:285-289, 1981. Description of the maneuvers used to control life-threatening hemorrhage from major liver injuries and merits of temporary packing in salvaging these otherwise moribund patients.

4.   Fischer, R.P., O'Farrell, K.A., and Perry, J.F.: The value of peritoneal drains in the treatment of liver injuries. J. Trauma, 18:393-397, 1978. Review of the relative complication rates of external hepatic drainage in comparison to no drainage in patients with primarily blunt liver injuries.

5.   Flint, L.M. and Polk, H.C.: Selective hepatic artery ligation: Limitations and failures. J. Trauma, 19:319--323, 1979. Discussion of the complications and anatomic reasons for failure of hepatic artery ligation in controlling major liver hemorrhage.

6.   Gottlieb, M.E., Sarfeh, J., et al.: Hepatic perfusion and splanchnic oxygen consumption in patients postinjury. J. Trauma, 23:836-843, 1983. Evaluation of the changes in portal perfusion and oxygen extraction in patients following abdominal trauma. The potential role of hepatic hypoperfusion in causing posttraumatic liver dysfunction is discussed.

7.   Kennedy, P.A., and Madding, G.F.: Surgical anatomy of the liver. Surg. Clin. North Am., 57:233-244, 1977. Excellent review of the pertinent surgical anatomy of the liver and common variations.

8.   Lucas, C.E., and Ledgerwood, A.M.: Prospective evaluation of hemostatic techniques for liver injuries. J. Trauma, 16:442-451, 1976. Detailed review of the results of both conservative and more radical treatment of liver injuries as determined by their anatomic severity.

9.   Mays, E.T.: Vascular occlusion. Surg. Clin. North Am., 57:291-323, 1977. Complete discussion of the experimental and clinical consequences of temporary and permanent hepatic vascular occlusion.

10.   Moore, E.E.: Critical decisions in the management of hepatic trauma. Am. J. Surg., 148:712-716, 1984. Summary of current approach to the management of liver trauma with special emphasis on the utility of the Pringle maneuver and atriocaval shunt in complex injuries.

11.   Pachter, L., and Spencer, F.C.: Recent concepts in the treatment of hepatic trauma. Facts and fallacies. Ann. Surg., 190:423-429, 1979. Review of the technique and results of hepatic inflow occlusion with hepatotomy and individual suture ligation in the treatment of deep liver lacerations.

12.   Sandblom, P., and Mirkovitch, V.: Hemobilia: Some salient features and their causes.
      Surg. Clin. North Am., 57:397-409, 1977. Case review of literature review of the
      clinical hallmarks of hemobilia with emphasis on the pathophysiology of the bile duct
      hemorrhage.
13.   Sclafani, S., Shaftan, G.W., et al.: Interventional radiology in the management of hepatic
      trauma. J. Trauma, 24:256-263, 1984. Case review of the utility and indications for
      angiographic management of intrahepatic vascular lesions and percutaneous liver
      hematoma drainage.
14.   Walt, A.J.: The mythology of hepatic trauma—or Babel revisited. Am. J. Surg.,
      135:12-18, 1978. Critical review of techniques for gaining hemorrhage control and
      preventing septic complications in complex injuries.

21. PANCREATIC AND DUODENAL INJURY
BEN EISEMAN, M.D.

1.   What type of injury may involve the pancreas or the duodenum?
Any type of penetrating injury of the abdomen or lower chest. Lower chest may
mean up to the nipples. These two organs lie retroperitoneally and are therefore
particularly vulnerable to penetration by a stab in the back or a missile that enters
the back. Individuals may be in all sorts of odd positions when shot or stabbed, so
the missile tract may not be a straight line between the wounds of entry and exit
as the patient lies on his or her back on the examining table. Blunt trauma also
may involve the pancreas and the duodenum. Positioned as they are, injury to
them usually involves a severe blow to the upper abdomen. A seat belt injury
commonly involves these two organs, crushing the pancreas against the vertebral
column.

**2.   What are the signs and symptoms of pancreatic and duodenal
injuries?**
Unfortunately there may be very few at first (12 to 18 hours). If duodenal or
pancreatic juice leaks into the peritoneal cavity, the anticipated signs of peritonitis
appear. If the hole is retroperitoneal, there may be no such evidence. Later (18
to 24 hours) there is usually evidence of peritonitis.

3.   What laboratory tests might help in the diagnosis of this injury?
(1) Nasogastric tube to suction return of blood.   (2) Injection of air or a
water-soluble contrast medium is seldom required but if done might demonstrate
a leak from the duodenum. (3) An upright film of the chest or abdomen may show
infradiaphragmatic air or air outside the duodenum, or obliteration of the psoas
shadow. (4) Increased serum amylase is usually present with severe pancreatic or
duodenal injury (sensitive) but is a nonspecific test. All sorts of intraabdominal
injuries can result in hyperamylasemia. (5) Lumbar spine films may show injury of
the vertebrae indicating severe injury to the area and suggesting concomitant
pancreatic or duodenal injury. (6) Peritoneal lavage may or may not be positive. A
retroperitoneal injury will leak behind, not into, the peritoneal cavity.

**4.   If there is any question of pancreatic or duodenal injury, is there
particular harm in watching and waiting?**
Yes, because the best chance to sew up holes in the duodenum with a
reasonable chance for them to heal is when the injury is fresh. After even a few
hours the area becomes enormously edematous and the sutured wound liable to

break down. This is why if there is a high index of suspicion of such an injury, it is best to perform an exploratory laparotomy.

5. **What procedures should be done before operation?**
Prophylactic antibiotics, nasogastric tube to suction, and blood type and match for four units.

6. **What are the main problems the surgeon might anticipate in these injuries?**
(1) Finding a retroperitoneal hole in the duodenum. This requires mobilizing the duodenum and head of the pancreas and getting a direct look at the retroperitoneal duodenum. (2) Deciding whether the bruised and obviously injured pancreas is sufficiently involved to require resection. (3) Associated injuries. These two organs lie surrounded by many other viscera. Seldom are they alone involved.

7. **What procedures is the surgeon apt to perform in repair of the duodenum?**
The surgeon must have a big bag of tricks to fit the various types of injury that may be found. Procedures range from simple suture closure (with or without drain nearby) to actually resecting the duodenum and performing a primary anastomosis.

8. **What procedures might the surgeon perform in the management of a pancreatic injury?**
In general it is advisable to resect the damaged pancreas if it lies to the left of the superior mesenteric artery. If the injury (blunt or penetrating) lies to the right of the superior mesenteric artery, it is wise to be conservative, i.e., stop the bleeding and drain the area, not resect the pancreas.

9. **Why the difference?**
Because resecting the right-hand portion of the pancreas inevitably involves taking out the duodenum as well. This has a very high mortality rate ($\pm 50\%$) when done as an emergency procedure for trauma. It is sometimes better to accept a greater chance of postoperative complications than to risk operative mortality.

10. **What are some of the unique complications that might occur following operation for these two injuries?**
Pancreatic or duodenal fistula, respiratory distress syndrome, pancreatic abscess, duodenal obstruction, and prolonged ileus.

11. **Are there any other procedures that can be done to minimize or treat these complications?**
Yes. A feeding jejunostomy placed at the time of the original operation may save the trouble, risk, and expense of prolonged parenteral feeding.

12. **How much of the pancreas can be resected without causing diabetes?**
Leaving even a thin rim of the head of the pancreas ($\pm 20\%$) will produce sufficient insulin to obviate the need for insulin postoperatively.

BIBLIOGRAPHY

1. Anane-Sefah, J., Norton, L.W., and Eiseman, B.: Operative choice and technique following pancreatic injury. Arch. Surg., 110:161, 1975.

2.   Chambers, R., Norton, L., and Hinchey, E.: Massive right upper quadrant intra-abdominal injury requiring pancreaticoduodenectomy and partial hepatectomy. J. Trauma, 15:714, 1975.
3.   Janson, K.L., and Stockinger, F.: Duodenal hematoma: Critical analysis of recent treatment technics. Am. J. Surg., 129:304, 1975.
4.   Jones, R.C.: Management of pancreatic trauma. Ann. Surg., 187:555, 1978.
5.   Jordan, G.L.: Pancreatic fistula. Am. J. Surg., 119:200, 1970.
6.   Kelly, G., et al.: The continuing challenge of duodenal injuries. J. Trauma, 18:160, 1978.
7.   Lucas, C.E.: Diagnosis and treatment of pancreatic and duodenal injury. Surg. Clin. North Am., 57:49, 1977.
8.   Mahboubi, S., and Kaufmann, H.J.: Intramural duodenal hematoma in children. Gastrointest. Radiol., 1:167, 1976.
9.   Moore, E.E., Dunn, E.L., and Jones, T.N.: Immediate jejunostomy feeding: Its use after major abdominal trauma. Arch. Surg., 116:681, 1981.
10. Morton, J., and Jordan, G.: Traumatic dudenal injuries. J. Trauma, 8:127, 1968.
11. Olsen, W.R.: The serum amylase in blunt abdominal trauma. J. Trauma, 13:200, 1973.
12. Pontius, G., Kilbourne, B., and Paul, E.: Nonpenetrating abdominal trauma. Arch. Surg., 72:800, 1956.
13. Snyder, W., et al.: Surgical management of duodenal trauma. Arch. Surg., 115:422, 1980.
14. Stone, H., and Fabian, T.C.: Management of duodenal wounds. J. Trauma, 19:334, 1979.
15. Stone, H.H., et al.: Experiences in the management of pancreatic trauma. J. Trauma, 21:257, 1981.
16. Vaughan, G., et al.: The use of pyloric exclusion in the management of severe duodenal injuries. Am. J. Surg., 134:785, 1977.

22. PENETRATING NECK INJURIES
JAMES NARROD, M.D., and ERNEST E. MOORE., M.D.

INITIAL GUIDELINES

1.   What tissue plane of the neck must be penetrated to be considered a penetrating neck wound?
The platysma muscle.

2.   Why are penetrating neck injuries worrisome?
In this small area of the body (1% of body surface area) there are many vital structures: pharynx, larynx, esophagus, trachea, thoracic duct, carotid arteries, vertebral and subclavian arteries and veins, external and internal jugular veins, spinal cord, brachial plexus, thyroid gland, etc.

3.   What are level I, II, and III injuries?
Level I injuries are below the top of the sternal notch. Level III injuries are above the angle of the mandible. Level II injuries are between levels I and III. A high carotid injury is the main concern since obtaining vascular control is difficult.

HISTORY AND PHYSICAL EXAMINATION

4.   What questions in the history are critical?
Dysphagia, dysphonia, hoarseness, hemoptysis, hematemesis, and large blood loss at the scene of the accident all suggest a serious injury.

5.   What signs in the physical examination are critical?

Persistent bleeding, enlarging hematoma, crepitus and neurologic deficits all suggest a vital structure was injured.

6. **How often do patients with crepitus have an aerodigestive injury?**
    One third of the time the pharynx, larynx, esophagus, or trachea is injured. Two thirds of the time the air was introduced through the entrance wound and there is no injury.

7. **Are gunshot wounds and knife wounds more likely to cause a significant injury?**
    Yes. However, at least 30% of gunshot wounds entail no significant injury.

8. **Which side of the neck is more likely to be injured?**
    The left side, since the majority of people are right-handed and thus injure their victims who are facing them on the opposite side.

MANAGEMENT

9. **Should arteriograms be performed?**
    Preoperative angiography is generally accepted in level I and III injuries. Its value in a level I wound is to identify injury to the thoracic outlet vessels. Such a lesion necessitates thoracotomy for proximal vascular control before the neck is explored. The primary indication for level III injuries is to exclude internal carotid arterial disruption at the base of the skull.

10. **Are barium swallow study, esophagoscopy, laryngoscopy, and bronchoscopy reliable?**
    No. All the above tests may miss injuries.

11. **In the emergency room, how should bleeding be controlled?**
    Direct pressure should be used; never use blind clamping.

12. **What is the most important problem in the emergency room?**
    The airway must be protected.

13. **Should all penetrating neck injuries be explored?**
    No. Exploring all neck wounds will yield 50% negative explorations.

14. **What is selective management of penetrating neck wounds?**
    All wounds that exhibit signs or symptoms of an injury are explored. Additionally, if the patient cannot be observed owing to intoxication or neurologic deficit, the wound is explored.

15. **What are the advantages of selective management?**
    Negative explorations are reduced and significant injuries are rarely missed.

16. **Should an asymptomatic patient be sent home from the emergency room?**
    No. The patient must be observed for 24 hours to watch for the development of signs and symptoms of a significant injury.

BIBLIOGRAPHY

1. Elerding, S.C., Manart, F.D., and Moore, E.E.: A reappraisal of penetrating neck injury management. J. Trauma, 20:695-697, 1980.

2.   Narrod, J.A., and Moore, E.E.: Initial management of penetrating neck wounds–A
      selective approach. J. Emerg. Med., 2:17-22, 1984.
3.   Narrod, J.A., and Moore, E.E.: Selective management of penetrating neck injuries.
      Arch. Surg., 119:574-578, 1984.
4.   Suryanarayanan, S., and Walt, A.J.: Penetrating wounds of the neck: Principles
      and some controversies. Surg. Clin. North Am., 57:239-250, 1977.

---

23. FACIAL LACERATIONS
R.C.A. WEATHERLEY-WHITE, M.D.

---

1.   What distinguishes facial from other lacerations?
When repairing a facial laceration, it must always be kept in mind that it will "show,"
and that the success of the result will depend largely on technical skill and on the
attention paid to the fine details of wound healing applied to the repair itself.
Debridement of ragged edges, the use of fine suture material in both skin and
subcutaneous tissue, and the early removal of the sutures are paramount to
ensure the optimal results.

2.   What factors influence how the wound is treated?
The principal factors derive from how the injury was sustained. Clean lacerations,
contaminated wounds, crush injuries, animal and human bites are all treated
differently.

3.   How are clean lacerations repaired?
Clean lacerations should be washed and, assuming no loss of tissue, should be
repaired in layers, if necessary, with fine absorbable sutures in the deep tissue
and fine interrupted nylon sutures in the skin. The wound should ideally be
inspected within 24 hours (to check for hematoma or infection), and the skin
sutures removed within 3 or 4 days.

4.   How are dirty lacerations repaired?
In addition to usual skin preparation, dirty lacerations should be thoroughly
irrigated and scrubbed out, after local anesthesia is achieved, to remove all
foreign debris before closing the defect.

5.   Should eyebrows be shaved when repairing facial lacerations?
No. They do not always grow back.

6.   How do you repair crush injuries with associated skin loss?
"Bursting" lacerations, where the skin has been crushed, usually result in ragged
edges and devitalized tissue. These edges must be debrided, as dead tissue
enclosed within the repair will act as a foreign body and predispose to infection. If
there is doubt concerning the viability of tissue, the wound may be cleaned
thoroughly and left open with continuous wet dressings. A delayed primary
closure can be accomplished, usually within 48 hours, when the viability of the
tissue will be more obvious.

7.   How should dog bites be treated?
Dog bites and other animal bites are highly prone to infection. In addition to the
measures outlined above for dirty or crushed wounds (the dog bite having
elements of both), the repair should be done with loose and widely separated
sutures to allow drainage between them. The use of a broad-spectrum antibiotic

and continuous wet dressings is essential. Nonetheless, about 10 to15% of dog bites will become infected. For this reason the wound should be inspected daily; if it is infected, the sutures should be removed to allow adequate drainage.

8. How are human bites treated?
Almost all human bites become infected. For this reason they should never be closed primarily, but left open with wet dressings, and the patient treated with intravenous antibiotics. The wound should be allowed to heal secondarily, although small wounds can be very loosely approximated after a few days without evidence of infection.

9. Should you primarily graft or transfer tissue?
Ordinarily the temptation to use tissue transfer techniques in order to achieve a good cosmetic end result should be resisted. It is better, if possible, to achieve closure in the simplest way and defer reconstruction until the scar is settled and mature. Occasionally when tissue loss is such that direct closure is impossible, it will be necessary to use a skin graft to obtain coverage.

10. Should you use antibiotics?
Attention to the fine points of mechanical wound care–irrigation, debridement, and appropriate handling of tissue–is more germane to the prevention of infection than is the use of antibiotics. However, most surgeons will employ antibiotic coverage when viability is dubious, and bites of all kinds will demand their use.

11. Should victims of bites be admitted to the hospital?
Patients with uncomplicated facial lacerations rarely require admission. Small children with dog bites, for which it would be hard to maintain continuous soaks, may need to be admitted, as should all victims of human bites. Occasionally the treating physician may make the judgment that the home situation is not one in which the appropriate and necessary care will be given.

12. When should scars be revised?
If the result of the repair is less than satisfactory, and if the patient seeks revision, there will be some pressure to "tidy up" the scar. This should be deferred for several months in order to allow maturation and softening of the tissue. Premature scars are a common mistake, and the final result is usually disappointing.

CONTROVERSIES

Fortunately, there are few controversies concerning the management of facial lacerations. Attention to the details of factors known to affect wound healing as outlined above will usually ensure a satisfactory result.

---

24. FROSTBITE
R.C.A. WEATHERLEY-WHITE, M.D.

---

1. What is frostbite and how is it sustained?
Frostbite is a low-temperature thermal injury that may lead to tissue necrosis and even loss of an extremity. It occurs when a part is exposed to low ambient temperatures, either below freezing for a moderately short time, or to a very cool

temperature for longer periods. The severity of the injury will depend on two factors: time and temperature.

2. **Which factors place patients at higher risk for loss of tissue?**
A very rapid loss of heat will overcome the protective "self warming" circulatory shift of warm blood to the exposed part. This occurs when protective clothing is removed (gloves, for example, to effect repairs on a stalled automobile), or if the skin or clothing is wet. Systemic factors that can affect the outcome include alcohol or drug use, diabetes, and other vascular conditions.

3. **What are the stages of frostbite?**
Initially the injured part is white, cold, hard, and lacking in sensation. As circulation returns, it becomes swollen and cyanotic. Later, blisters form with serous or purulent drainage. Ultimately there is demarcation between what is viable and what is destined to slough.

4. **Can the "degree" of frostbite be recognized initially?**
Frostbite is not like a burn, and it is difficult, if not impossible, to predict the outcome based on the physical appearance of the injured part when first examined. A knowledge of the circumstances of injury, particularly the ambient temperature and the length of time exposed, will afford some degree of prognosis.

5. **How is frostbite treated?**
If the part is frozen when first seen, immediate rewarming should be started. This will reduce the length of time that the tissue is exposed to low temperature, and should be carried out in a water bath at a temperature of 40°C. Treatment of severe pain may be necessary during rewarming. If the part has already thawed when first encountered, rewarming will not be helpful. A sterile dressing should be applied, and the decision made whether to admit to hospital. Low molecular weight dextran should be started intravenously during rewarming to diminish the tendency of the blood to "sludge." Neither heparin nor sympathectomy plays any useful role in the acute treatment of frostbite.

6. **When should you operate?**
Surgical treatment should be delayed as long as possible; optimally the necrotic part should separate spontaneously. Premature surgery usually results in the needless loss of tissue that could have survived if left alone. The only urgent surgical situation is for the drainage or debridement of infected tissue.

7. **Which patients should be admitted to the hospital?**
This depends on the severity of the injury. Many can be treated as outpatients quite well, but a judgment must be made as to the patient's reliability. Acutely intoxicated patients should be admitted as well as *all patients with central hypothermia*. These patients must be totally rewarmed and attention paid to both acidosis and cardiac arrhythmias.

CONTROVERSY

The principal controversy still raging deals with the pathophysiology of the injury. Does frostbite result from cellular death at the time of insult, or is it more a vascular injury, which progresses in a finite time-span, and can therefore be treated by supporting the microcirculation?

25. PELVIC FRACTURES

RICHARD C. FISHER, M.D.

DIAGNOSIS

1. **What are the major clinical tipoffs that a patient may have a pelvic fracture?**
    1. History: crush injury, motor vehicle accidents, fall from height
    2. Pain with pelvic compression
    3. Signs and symptoms of severe blood loss

2. **How is the diagnosis of pelvic fracture confirmed?**
    1. Routine x-rays (anteroposterior pelvic) with or without oblique views are usually diagnostic.
    2. For small occult fractures, especially involving the sacral area, technetium bone scans 3 days after the injury sometimes are necessary for confirmation.
    3. CT scans are useful in understanding the fracture geometry.

3. **What are the other commonly associated injuries?**
    1. Hemorrhage
    2. Intraabdominal injuries
    3. Lower urinary tract injuries

4. **Which pelvic fractures should raise your index of suspicion for these complicating associated injuries?**
    There are many classifications of pelvic fractures but the system devised by Conolly and Hedberg seems to be the most functional.
    Major:
    A. Involves a line of weight-bearing transmission from the spine to the acetabulum
    B. Rami on both sides of the symphysis pubis (these include acetabular fractures, hemipelvic fractures (Malgaigne), bilateral pubic rami, acetabular and sacral fractures)
    Minor:
    A. Unilateral pubic rami, isolated iliac fractures, avulsion fractures
    B. Most of the major associated injuries occur with fractures in the major classification

5. **Who was Malgaigne?**
    Joseph François Malgaigne was a French surgeon, scholar, and author who described the unstable pelvic fracture in 1847 in a treatise on fractures and subluxations.

6. **How significant is blood loss in pelvic fractures?**
    In a large series, about 85% of the patients receive some blood replacement. The average transfusion is about 6 units per patient (8 units with intraabdominal injury).

7. **What is the mortality rate?**
    Reported between 9 and 30% (50% with open fractures) occurring in the first 24 hours attributed to hemorrhage. In a large series, all of the patients dying received more than 10 units of blood replacement.

8. **What initial resuscitative measures should be considered?**
    (1) Routine cardiopulmonary resuscitation, (2) fluid and blood replacement, and (3) MAST trousers.

INTRAABDOMINAL AND INTRAPELVIC INJURIES

9. **What percentage of major pelvic fractures are associated with abdominal injuries?**
    22 to 47%

10. **What is the reliability of peritoneal lavage in patients with pelvic fracture?**
    1. Negative taps are usually accurate and do not require laparotomy.
    2. Positive taps should be viewed with suspicion as there is a 12 to 28% reported false-positive rate. (See chapter 17 on Blunt Abdominal Trauma.)
    3. The false-positive taps create a problem, as laparotomy on these patients has a high mortality and complication rate (50% in one reported series). This can be clarified by arteriography.

11. **When is arteriography indicated?**
    As above, in positive peritoneal lavage the arteriogram has been found to be 92% accurate in diagnosing intraabdominal bleeding. With a positive lavage and a negative arteriogram, the patient can probably be watched without immediate laparotomy. Pelvic arteriography is useful for determining large bleeding vessels associated with the fracture in the pelvic area. In addition, arterial embolization has been successful in controlling hemorrhage (see Controversies).

URINARY TRACT INJURIES

12. **What percentage of these patients have urinary tract problems?**
    About 50% with major fractures. These are divided into urethral problems and bladder ruptures.

13. **What urinary work-up should be done?**
    1. Observation. Urethral injuries are often associated with blood in the meatus. More proximal injuries in the bladder area are associated with hematuria.
    2. Urethrograms are diagnostic for urethral injuries. IVP is often necessary to evaluate the remaining urinary tract.

14. **What are the late sequelae of urinary tract injuries?**
    Stricture, impotence, incontinence, fistula, and abscess.

CONTROVERSIES

15. **Repair of urethral injuries: immediate suprapubic cystostomy followed by later reconstruction or immediate urethral repair?**
    Advantages of delayed repair:
    1. Simpler treatment during the acute management phase.
    2. Reported decrease in incidences of stricture, impotence, and incontinence.
    3. Immediate repair often leads to severe blood loss upon disruption of the pelvic hematoma.
    Disadvantages of delayed repair:
    1. Probably not applicable to penetrating injuries.
    2. Requires prolonged use of a suprapubic catheter and additional surgery.

16. Bladder rupture: operative or nonoperative management?
Advantages of nonoperative management:
1. Avoids an extensive surgical procedure in a patient with severe trauma.
Disadvantages of nonoperative management:
1. May require late repair.
2. Requires prolonged indwelling catheters.

Advantages of operative management:
1. Fewer late complications.
2. Can be done at the same time as intraabdominal surgery if that is indicated.
Disadvantages of operative management:
1. Difficult surgery and increased bleeding in an acutely injured patient with massive pelvic hematomas.
Discussion:
Bladder ruptures may be very small puncture type injuries or very large disruptions of the bladder wall and may be intraperitoneal or extraperitoneal. A controversy of operative and nonoperative treatment seems to apply to both intra- and extraperitoneal injuries. Minimal extravasations, on the other hand, may be managed nonoperatively with few of the disadvantages mentioned above.

17. Management of hemorrhage?
Controversy surrounds the treatment of severe hemorrhage associated with pelvic fractures. Initial treatment probably should consist of cardiopulmonary resuscitation and, if necessary, MAST trousers. If bleeding is not controlled, external fixation can be employed. Likewise, if that is not successful, arterial macroembolization and microembolization techniques can be used. Laparotomy to control intraabdominal bleeding is, of course, indicated and is discussed elsewhere. Open arterial ligation has resulted in both a high complication rate and a high rate of continued bleeding.

18. Management of pelvic fractures.
Advantages of bed rest with skeletal traction or pelvic sling:
1. Nonoperative technique with no additional blood loss.
2. Skeletal traction is the best means of controlling proximal migration in hemipelvic injuries.
Disadvantages of bed rest with skeletal traction or pelvic sling:
1. Requires prolonged hospitalization and bed rest.
2. Associated thromboembolism and decubitus ulcers.
3. Poor reduction of fractures.

Advantages of internal fixation:
1. Better anatomic reduction is possible.
2. Early mobilization of the patient.
Disadvantages of internal fixation:
1. A significantly difficult operation with increased risk of blood loss.
2. Often difficult to obtain adequate stable fracture.
3. Many fractures are not amenable to internal fixation.

Advantages of external fixation:
1. Effectively relieves pain, helps to control blood loss, allows early mobilization, and is somewhat effective in maintaining a fracture position.
Disadvantages of external fixation:
1. Infections of the pin tract.
2. Will not always control proximal migration and hemipelvic fractures (Malgaigne).

BIBLIOGRAPHY

1. Brotman, S., Soderstrom, C., Oster-Granite, M., et al.: Management of severe bleeding in fractures of the pelvis. Surg. Gynecol. Obstet., 153:823-826, 1981. Describes the complex vascular anatomy of the pelvic region and explains why any single method of hemorrhage control is not universally successful.

2. Bucholz, R.: The pathological anatomy of Malgaigne fracture-dislocations of the pelvis. J. Bone Joint Surg., 63A:400-404, 1981. Provides an updated classification of pelvic fractures including the importance of posterior ring injuries. A rationale for closed manipulation and external fixation is included.

3. Cass,A., Behrens, F., Comfort, T., et al.: Bladder problems in pelvic injuries treated with external fixation and direct urethral drainage. J. Trauma, 23:50-53, 1983. Describes three cases illustrating urinary tract complications secondary to external fixation of pelvic fractures.

4. Dove, A., Poon, W., and Weston, A.: Haemorrhage from pelvic fractures: Dangers and treatment. Injury, 13:375-381, 1982. Describes the method of management of hemorrhage from pelvic fractures but concentrates on the effective use of MAST trousers.

5. Gilliland, M., Ward, R., Barton, R., et al.: Factors affecting mortality in pelvic fractures. J. Trauma, 22:691-693, 1982. Conditions affecting mortality in pelvic fractures are described from a consecutive series of 100 patients. Mortality was increased by the presence of head injuries, low admitting blood pressure and hemoglobin level, requirements for blood transfusion, and the presence of posterior ring fractures.

6. Gilliland, M., Ward, R., Flynn, T., et al.: Peritoneal lavage and angiography in the management of patients with pelvic fractures. Am. J. Surg., 144:744-746, 1982. Describes the role of peritoneal lavage and the danger of the false-positive result. It emphasizes angiographic correlation and its role in delineating the need for laparotomy.

7. Hawkins, L., Pomerantz, M., and Eiseman, B.: Laparotomy at the time of pelvic fracture. J. Trauma, 10:619-622, 1970. One of the earlier studies on the combination of pelvic fractures and intraabdominal bleeding done at Denver General Hospital. It emphasizes the high mortality and complications associated with this procedure.

8. Hurt, A., Ochsner, J., and Schiller, W.: Prolonged ileus after severe pelvic fracture. Am. J. Surg., 146:755-757, 1983. Describes several cases of prolonged ileus after pelvic fractures and suggests the need for early parenteral nutrition under those circumstances.

9. Kinzl, L., Burri, C., and Coldewey, J.: Fractures of the pelvis and associated intrapelvic injuries. Injury, 14:63-69, 1982. This paper provides controversy by suggesting open treatment for hemostasis and repair of urinary injuries as well as internal fixation of the osseous lesions.

10. Lazarus, H., and Nelson, J.: Technique for peritoneal lavage when a pelvic fracture and suspected hematoma are present. Surg. Gynecol. Obstet., 153:403-404, 1981. A short monograph describes the technique of peritoneal lavage necessary to avoid entering the hematoma from the fractured pelvis.

11. McAninch, J.: Traumatic injuries to the urethra. J. Trauma, 21:291-292, 1981. Reviews management of urethral injuries from blunt trauma with discussion of the controversy of late versus early surgical repair. It stresses the advantages of delayed repair including low incidence of stricture, impotence, and incontinence.

12. Melton, L., Sampson, J., Morrey, B., et al.: Epidemiologic features of pelvic fractures. Clin. Orthop., 155:43-47, 1981. Discusses the incidence of pelvic fractures correlated with age, degree of trauma, and osteoporosis.

13. Peltier, L.: Joseph François Malgaigne and Malgaigne's fracture. Surgery, 44:777-784, 1958. Superb article summarizing the life and works of Joseph Francois Malgaigne.

14. Rafii, M., Firooznia, H., Golimbu, C., et al.: The impact of CT in clinical management of pelvic and acetabular fractures. Clin. Orthop., 178:228-235, 1983. Describes the value of CT examination in better delineating fracture patterns as well as detecting occult fractures and soft tissue injuries following pelvic fractures.

15. Richardson, J., Harty, J., Amin, M., et al.: Open pelvic fractures. J. Trauma, 22:533-537, 1982. A series of 35 patients with open pelvic fractures is discussed, and increased severity of open versus closed fractures is emphasized.

16. Riska, E., and Myllynen, P.: Fat embolism in patients with multiple injuries. J. Trauma, 22:891-894, 1982. The diagnostic criteria for fat embolism syndrome are reviewed as well as the reminder that multiply injured patients are at high risk for this problem.
17. Sandler, C., Harris, J., Corriere, J., et al.: Posterior urethral injuries after pelvic fracture. Am. J. Radiol., 137:1233-1237, 1981. Describes a series of patients with posterior urethral injuries with the extravasation both above and below the urogenital diaphragm. The early management of these lesions is considered.
18. Sclafani, S., and Becker, J.: Traumatic presacral hemorrhage: Angiographic diagnosis and therapy. A.J.R., 138:123-125, 1982. The radiologic diagnosis of pelvic bleeding by angiography is outlined along with its control by small particle embolotherapy.
19. Semba, R., Yasukawa, K., and Gustilo, R.: Critical analysis of results of 53 Malgaigne fractures of the pelvis. J. Trauma, 23:535-537, 1983. The long-term follow-up of patients with Malgaigne fractures is described. Delayed complications include paresthesias of the lower extremity, gait disturbance, low back pain, and incontinence. Adequacy of the reduction correlated with late development of pain.
20. deVries, J., and van der Slikke, W.: False positive peritoneal lavage due to retroperitoneal haematoma. Injury, 12:191-193, 1981. Emphasizes the danger of the false-positive peritoneal lavage resulting in unnecessary laparotomies.
21. Wild, J., Hanson, G., and Tullos, H.: Unstable fractures of the pelvis treated by external fixation. J. Bone Joint Surg., 64A:1010-1020, 1982. The use of external fixation is described in this series of 45 patients. The control of proximal migration of unilateral shear fractures is discussed in relation to the external fixation device.

26. BURNS
EDWARD BARTLE, M.D.

1. **What is the etiology of burns?**
    Burns are caused by excess heat (flame, steam, hot water, hot tar, etc.), chemical contact to skin, and electricity. Scalds, flash flames, or brief contact with tar or grease cause partial thickness burns. Immersions, propane or gas explosion, chemicals, and electricity usually cause full thickness burns.

2. **What determines the depth of a burn?**
    Superficial (first degree) burns are similar to a severe sunburn, with only the epidermis being involved. Partial thickness (second degree) burns histologically injure the epidermis and dermis down to the dermal-subcutaneous tissue level. Full thickness (third degree) burns destroy the entire skin and involve the subcutaneous fat. Hair follicles, sweat glands, and sebaceous glands are located in the deep dermal and subcutaneous layer and can be totally destroyed by deep partial and full thickness burns.

3. **How is the depth of a burn determined clinically?**
    Although there are a number of more sophisticated tests, the simplest way to determine burn depth is by the color of the skin and skin sensation. Sensitivity to pinprick is fairly reliable; insensate skin usually predicts a full thickness burn. Deeply charred or ghostly white skin usually indicates full thickness burns, whereas skin that is pink or has bullous lesions usually signals a partial thickness injury.
    Another way to evaluate is to pull on the hair. If it falls out with resistance or pain, it is likely to be a full thickness or deep partial burn.

4.   **What should be done initially for a burn?**
Scalds, flammable liquids, and explosions constitute the majority of burn injuries. Removing the victim from the inciting agent is important, keeping in mind that patients involved in explosions may have multiple injuries. Stable patients with small burns can be transported by private vehicle with the burns wrapped in sterile dry dressings. If possible, patients with large burns should be transported by ambulance where fluid resuscitation can be initiated.

5.   **How do you get tar off a burn wound?**
Apply neomycin or mineral oil.

6.   **How should the patient be managed initially in the hospital?**
If the patient is stable, the wounds should be debrided, cleansed, and covered with topical antibiotic solution followed by a sterile dressing. Fluid intake should be by predetermined formula (see Controversies), but the important aspect is to keep the urine output at 30 to 50 ml/hr for the first 24 hours and at least 30 ml/hr thereafter. Large burns may require a Foley catheter, an arterial line, and possibly a CVP or a Swan-Ganz catheter. If applicable, tetanus immunization should be administered. Prophylactic antibiotics are not used in adults but penicillin is occasionally used in children because of the high incidence of upper respiratory tract infections at the time of presentation.
Another early problem may be neurovascular compression in an extremity due to increased extracellular fluid trapped in an eschar. Neurovascular monitoring of extremities (especially with a circumferential burn) may uncover problems requiring an escharotomy to relieve pressure.

7.   **What are the essentials of care for burns?**
Early debridement of the burned tissue and coverage are important. This should be done sterilely in the operating room and the burn tissue should be removed by 3 to 5 days post burn (i.e., as soon as a major burn is stable). Minor full thickness burns can be grafted with an autograft soon after presentation. In patients with major burns in whom donor sites are limited, homograft provides good coverage. Major debridements should be limited to 20% of body surface area at one time.

8.   **What needs to be done for patients with inhalation burns?**
Carbonaceous sputum or oropharyngeal char should alert one to the possibility of an inhalation injury. High carboxyhemoglobin levels may confirm this. Although bronchoscopy is not essential, it may help to signal impending airway obstruction. Either way, early "prophylactic" intubation may be necessary. Prophylactic antibiotics and steroids are contraindicated; however, routine culture of sputum every 12 to 24 hours may reveal early pneumonia.

9.   **Are there special considerations for chemical and electrical burns?**
Chemical burns should be decontaminated as soon as possible. The depth of burn is determined by the agent and the duration of contact; otherwise, care is standard. Electrical burns, usually caused by contact with high voltage wires or outlet or wire contact by children, have "entrance" and "exit" sites; thus, a full examination is necessary. Treatment is directed at the areas of injury that tend to be involved, such as muscle, and urine must be checked for myoglobin. If urine myoglobin is high, urine output should exceed 50% ml/hr, and alkalinization of the urine may be necessary.

10. **What is the prognosis for a burn victim?**
Prognosis in mostly based on the extent of burn and age. A 20% burn in a 75-year-old patient carries a 70-80% mortality whereas the same burn in a 25-year-old has a 5% mortality.

11. **What part does nutrition play in care of patients with burns?**
Patients with burns are severely hypercatabolic, with over 200% of normal resting energy expenditure. In patients with large burns, early nutritional support is essential. Whether nutrition should be delivered enterally or parenterally is controversial.

12. **What is important in the treatment of patients with burns after they leave the hospital?**
The end of hospitalization does not end the care, physical or psychological, of patients with burns. A multidisciplinary approach is still essential on an outpatient basis. This includes application of a Jobst garment or burn wound compression, medications for itch (topical lotions and systemic therapy), and psychological support.

CONTROVERSIES

13. **What type of fluid therapy should be used in burn resuscitation?**
A commonly used formula is Parkland's (4 ml/kg/% burn for first 24 hours) using lactated Ringer's crystalloid. Other formulas (Evans and Park) use colloid and crystalloid. There is minimal benefit of the colloid formula over a crystalloid formula and colloid is more expensive. Recently there has been some experience with a concentrated sodium chloride solution, which may be beneficial in that it decreases the amount of total fluid necessary.

14. **Nutrition for burns: enteral or parenteral?**
Enteral: For
Less expensive, more physiologic.
Enteral: Against
Problem delivering enough calories, diarrhea, contamination.
Parenteral: For
Easier to deliver calories, more reliable for caloric delivery, not interrupted for surgery.
Parenteral: Against
Central line complications including sepsis (Candida), necessity of changing lines every 3 days, expensive.

---

27. HEAD INJURY
CORDELL GROSS, M.D.

---

1. **What takes first priority in head injury, to attend to severe hypotension or brain oozing from the ear?**
Hemodynamic support.

2. **What is the first priority in evaluating the injured head?**
Identify major mass lesions or significantly elevated intracranial pressure. This allows herniation syndromes to be minimized and sometimes reversed.

3. **So what?**
    There is a significant negative impact if herniation syndromes evolve.

4. **What is the most effective way to immediately assess the urgency of the situation?**
    Test the ability of the patient to follow simple single-stage commands.

5. **Are oculocephalic reflex tests necessary in the conscious patient? Unconscious patient?**
    No. Yes.

6. **Why?**
    It is important to determine the level of neurologic dysfunction.

7. **Before testing oculocephalic reflexes, what is your obligation?**
    To ascertain the condition of the cervical spine with anteroposterior and lateral x-rays.

8. **Can you evaluate a chemically paralyzed and intubated patient?**
    Not effectively.

9. **Without a pulmonary reason, should a responsive but lethargic patient be intubated?**
    No.

10. **What is the significance of a blown pupil in an unconscious patient?**
    Signifies uncal herniation until proved otherwise.

11. **What is your best response?**
    Hyperosmolar agents.

12. **What drug, what dose, and what rate of administration?**
    Mannitol or urea at 1 gm/kg over 10 to 15 minutes.

13. **What must the patient have when hyperosmolar agents are used?**
    Foley catheter (because of profound diuresis, bladders have been ruptured).

14. **Should shrinkers be used in the face of hypotension?**
    If indicated, yes, and support the intravascular volume as needed with blood or colloid.

15. **What should be your mental priorities in evaluating the unconscious patient?**
    Determine first, level and degree of rostrocaudal dysfunction (i.e., hemispheres, brain stem, cord), and second, in which direction the dysfunction is moving (i.e., toward improvement or deterioration).

16. **What is the utility of the Glasgow coma scale?**
    For those not trained in neurologic evaluation to (1) chart a trend, and (2) communicate to physicians while a neurologically injured patient is in transport or other situations.

17. **What is the true significance of posturing in a patient?**
    The patient is on the brink of disaster and needs diagnostic evaluation acutely and monitoring of intracranial pressure chronically if no surgical lesion is found.

18. **Should every patient with a head injury be given a CT scan?**
No.

19. **Should every unconscious patient with a head injury be given a CT scan?**
Yes.

20. **What if the scanner is down?**
The CT scan is so central to good neurosurgical trauma care and evaluation that it is better to divert the partient to a center with a functional CT scanner.

21. **What if that is not an option?**
Anteroposterior and lateral skull x-ray films can be obtained to inspect for fractures and pineal shifts, and angiography can be considered if the diagnosis is in question.

22. **What if the patient progressively lateralizes and/or otherwise deteriorates from a CNS standpoint?**
Exploratory burr holes are in order, preferably in the operating room.

23. **In the acute situation, what do upgoing toes and brisk deep tendon reflexes indicate?**
Cerebral and/or brain stem injury.

24. **Why not injury of the cord and long tracts?**
Spinal shock. These injuries tend to leave patients paretic and flaccid.

25. **What is the significance of linear nondisplaced skull fractures?**
They suggest a significant smack on the head and, depending on which vascular channels are traversed, they may portend sources of epidural or subdural bleeds.

26. **Of these vascular channels, which channel is of acute interest?**
Middle meningeal artery groove.

27. **What is the channel of delayed interest?**
Venus sinus grooves and posterior middle meningeal artery groove.

28. **What is the best diagnostic study for suspected depressed skull fracture?**
CT scan. Close second: oblique skull films, with the obliquity tangential to the fracture.

29. **Do you need to elevate all compound depressed fractures?**
Probably a good idea. Most neurosurgeons will.

30. **When is something done about a closed depressed skull fracture?**
Usually if it is displaced the full thickness of the skull, i.e., the outer table is even with or deeper than the inner table.

31. **How do you best handle dirty (road rash and hair) scalp lacerations?**
Clean thoroughly, debride, and close with monofilament nylon in one layer (be sure to include the galea).

32. **Should all missile wounds be debrided?**

Yes, but debride only the entrance side (concentrate on the bony fragments) and close the dura. Do not chase the missile any farther than is necessary for bony debridement or significant clot removal.

33. **Why shouldn't nasogastric tubes be placed in patients with obvious facial injuries?**
The tubes can be passed intracranially through basal skull fractures.

34. **What is the most common finding on the lateral x-ray film of patients with basal skull fractures?**
An air-fluid level in the sphenoid sinus.

35. **What is the significance of pneumocephalus?**
Usually indicates a basal skull fracture; antibiotics are probably a good idea, although their efficacy has not been proved.

36. **What is the quickest and safest way to monitor intracranial pressure?**
A transdural bolt.

37. **What is the most widely available bolt?**
A stopcock in a 6/32-inch twist drill hole. The male end of a stopcock that is non-Luer-Lok will pressure fit very nicely into a hole of this size.

38. **How do you get though the dura?**
Gentle but thorough slashing with an 18-gauge needle.

39. **What is the best ongoing indicator that the intracranial pressure monitor is working?**
A saw-tooth waveform on the monitor coincident with the arterial pulse wave.

40. **What is the quickest and easiest way to lower intracranial pressure?**
Hyperventilate to reduce the $PaCO2$, which reduces cerebral blood flow.

41. **Aren't we afraid of dropping the cerebral blood flow too low?**
No. The response to $CO2$ is seen only in vasoreactive areas and this is manifested only in normal, i.e., nonischemic, areas of the brain.

BIBLIOGRAPHY

1.   Plum, F., and Posner, J.B.: The Diagnosis of Stupor and Coma. Contemporary Neurology Series 19, Edition 3. Philadelphia, F.A. Davis, 1980.
2.   Youmans, J. (ed.): Neurological Surgery, Vol. 4. Philadelphia, W. B. Saunders, 1982.

28. SPINAL CORD INJURY
CORDELL GROSS, M.D.

1. **What is the quickest screening examination to rule in spinal cord injury in the unconscious patient?**
Rectal tone. If the patient has a patulous anus, you must proceed as if the cord has been injured.

2. **What is the quickest way to determine spinal cord injury in a conscious patient?**
Ask for extremity movement and response to sensory examination.

3. **What if a patient can move the lower extremities but not the upper extremities?**
Think central cord contusion.

4. **What's that?**
Look it up. It's worth it. It helps to review important cross-sectional anatomy of the cord as well as the vascular supply.

5. **Do you really have to clear C7 to T1 on x-rays?**
Yes. It is so potentially vulnerable since T1 is fixed by ribs and C7 is not.

6. **How do you do it when the patient has wide shoulders?**
Get what is called a swimmer's view, CT scan, or tomography (even though anything beyond a plain x-ray film is difficult to get, it is important enough to establish the stability at the cervicothoracic junction).

7. **How do you look at the odontoid process?**
An open-mouth view and a lateral cervical spine view.

8. **What might be seen on the lateral view?**
A displaced peg or a "fat C2," i.e., the width of the body of C2 which is wider than the body of C3.

9. **What is the lucency usually seen at the base of the odontoid peg on the open-mouth view?**
It is a nutrient channel.

10. **How do you differentiate nutrient channels from fractures?**
With vascular channels, there is usually sclerosis along the border of the lucency. If you do not see this, you have to suspect a fracture.

11. **What do you do if there is dens fracture with displacement?**
Halo stabilization with or without surgery.

12. **If someone comes in completely "out" from a neurologic standpoint from a spinal injury that does not manifest with obvious and profound subluxation displacement, should you watch and wait or obtain a myelogram?**
Get a myelogram. In an acute ruptured disc or hematoma, one has about 6 hours to relieve the pressure if there is going to be any residual function. The sooner the pressure is relieved, the better the chances of improvement.

13. **If there is a gross obvious displacement of the spine with complete myelopathy, what should you do?**
Stabilize with traction and support the vital signs. Be careful with traction in C2 disruption; extraction has, at times, worsened the injury.

14. **Why do people with spinal cord injuries have profound hypotension?**
The transverse myelopathy virtually sympathectomizes the patient below the level of the lesion.

15. **How do you treat it?**
     Volume; since the "problem" with the sympathectomy is relative vasorelaxation and therefore increased intravascular space, adequate filling of the space is the treatment of choice.

16. **What is the significance of a thoracolumbar compression fracture with dislocation and suspected compromise of the canal?**
     There is both peripheral and central nervous system injury by virtue of involvement of the cauda equina and the conus.

17. **So what?**
     Even delayed decompression can result in improved function if the dysfunction is secondary to cauda equina compression in addition to conus injury.

18. **How do you accomplish the necessary reduction of a compression injury in the thoracic or lumbar spine?**
     One of a number of orthopedic internal fixation devices such as extraction rods.

19. **What is a potential source of "blood loss" in thoracolumbar injury?**
     Retroperitoneal hematoma.

20. **How is it diagnosed?**
     A plain film of the abdomen looking for blunting of the psoas shadows or CT scan.

BIBLIOGRAPHY

1.   Haymaker, W. (ed.): Bing's Local Diagnosis in Neurological Disease, Ed. 15. St. Louis, C.V. Mosby, 1969.
2.   Youmans, J. (ed.): Neurological Surgery, Vol. 4. Philadelphia, W. B. Saunders, 1982.

---

29. ACUTE CHOLECYSTITIS
JOYCE A. MAJURE, M.D.

---

1.   **What causes acute cholecystitis?**
     Obstruction of the cystic duct by a gallstone in most cases. Other times (5 to 15%), inspissation of bile by dehydration, or bile stasis during ileus such as may occur after trauma, severe systemic illness, or major surgery. This is known as "acalculous cholecystitis."

2.   **Name six risk factors for cholelithiasis.**
     Female gender, multiparity, > 40 years of age, obesity (traditionally know as the four "F's": female, fertile, forty, and fat), vagotomy, and previous surgical resection of the terminal ileum (such as bypass surgery for obesity).

3.   **What are the classic physical findings? What is pathognomonic?**
     Fever (with or without rigor), tenderness to direct palpation in the right upper quadrant, and positive Murphy's sign (pain in the right upper quadrant upon inspiration, preventing the patient from taking a deep breath). The presence of a tender mass in the right upper quadrant is pathognomonic and occurs in about 20%. The incidence of jaundice is 20 to 30%, with a bilirubin > 1.5 mg/dl in about one third of these.

4. **Which are the best laboratory and x-ray studies to confirm the diagnosis?**
   Laboratory: WBC–leukocytosis; bilirubin and alkaline phosphatase usually only slightly elevated if at all; other liver function tests normal. Amylase may be elevated if there is associated pancreatitis from a common bile duct stone. *X-ray:* plain film of the abdomen or chest film may show radiopaque stones (15 to 20%); if the gallbladder can be visualized, ultrasound is cheap, safe, and accurate (90 to 95% accuracy); technetium (HIDA or PIPIDA) scan using a radioactive isotope which is taken up by the liver and excreted in the bile is also excellent (100% accurate); CT scan is very accurate but more expensive, exposes the patient to more radiation, and is more time-consuming.

5. **What are the most common organisms cultured from the infected gallbladder? What antibiotics are recommended?**
   Escherichia coli, Klebsiella, enterococci, and Aerobacter. Ampicillin, a first- or second-generation cephalosporin, or doxycycline. There is usually no indication for antibiotics in uncomplicated acute cholecystitis. However, they are recommended in the elderly and in diabetic persons.

6. **What is emphysema of the gallbladder?**
   Results from gas-producing organisms infecting the gallbladder, usually Clostridia. Recognized on plain x-ray film as a lucency in the wall or lumen of the gallbladder.

7. **What is empyema of the gallbladder?**
   A gallbladder filled with pus: usually occurs as a result of a delay in surgery, or if treatment of sepsis has occurred for several days without knowing the diagnosis. Often associated with abscesses elsewhere in the abdomen. Has a high association with common bile duct stones and mandates intraoperative cholangiogram.

8. **What does radiographic visualization of air in the bile ducts of the liver signify?**
   Communication with the GI tract, such as gallstone ileus. The gallbladder may become so inflamed and necrotic that it erodes into a loop of adjacent bowel. The stone may then create a mechanical obstruction, usually at the ileocecal valve. The patient reports symptoms of bowel obstruction preceded by symptoms of gallbladder disease. Pneumatobilia may also be present from a surgical anastomosis with the common bile duct, such as a choledochoduodenostomy.

9. **From which artery does the cystic artery usually arise?**
   Right hepatic artery (95%), but anomalies are found in two thirds of cases; the most common anomaly is duplication of the cystic artery, with both branches arising from the right hepatic artery.

10. **Where does the cystic duct usually enter the main biliary tree?**
    Generally at the junction of the middle and upper thirds of the common bile duct. Variations are quite common: spiral insertion, short or absent cystic duct, insertion just proximal to the ampulla of Vater, accompanied by an accessory bile duct.

11. **What are the spiral valves of Heister?**
    A series of folds lining the cystic duct. They may interfere with passage of a probe or catheter for cholangiography.

12. What is biliary dyskinesia?
Functional disorder of the bile ducts with abnormal elevations of pressure and subsequent disorder of bile flow causing biliary symptoms. Diagnosis is difficult, and its existence questionable.

13. What is the difference between acute cholecystitis and biliary colic?
Biliary colic is the result of a stone impacting against or passing through the cystic duct, and will usually subside. It is rarely associated with fever or vomiting, but may have associated transient elevation of alkaline phosphatase. Such patients can be evaluated on an outpatient basis, and surgery performed electively. Cholecystitis is usually accompanied by nausea, vomiting, and fever. These patients need to be admitted, evaluated, given nothing by mouth, and rehydrated. Once the diagnosis is confirmed, cholecystectomy is the treatment of choice.

14. When is the best time to operate for acute cholecystitis?
If the patient responds to initial management, semielective resection of the gallbladder is best done on the third to fifth hospital day. If the patient's condition deteriorates (persistent fever, increased or generalized abdominal tenderness), then cholecystectomy should be performed as soon as possible, as this indicates progression to empyema or necrosis with the potential for perforation.

15. What if the patient has a high operative risk (e.g., severe cardiac or pulmonary disease)?
Cholecystostomy (drainage of the gallbladder with a tube) can be performed under local anesthesia but is indicated in less than 15% of all patients with acute cholecystitis.

16. Should routine intraoperative cholangiograms be performed?
Probably yes. Common duct stones are found in 10 to 25% of patients with acute cholecystitis, and about 15% of patients have concomitant acute pancreatitis demonstrated by an increased amylase level. Unless the inflammation is so severe as to obscure the ductal anatomy and risk common duct injury, cholangiography is recommended.

17. What is white bile?
The mucosa of the gallbladder secretes clear mucus. If a stone completely obstructs the cystic duct, the gallbladder will fill with "white bile."

18. What are the complications of untreated acute cholecystitis?
Perforation with abscess formation or peritonitis, biliary-enteric fistula, sepsis.

BIBLIOGRAPHY

1.   Bennion, L.J., and Grundy, S.M.:   Risk factors for the development of cholelithiasis in man (Part I). N. Engl. J. Med., 229:1161, 1978.
2.   Bennion, L.K., and Grundy, S.M.: Risk factors for the development of cholelithiasis in man (Part II). N. Engl. J. Med., 229:1221, 1978. Review articles on the physiology of gallstone formation (Part I), and risk factors (Part II). Excellent.
3.   Escallon, A., Jr., Rosales, W., and Aldrete, J.S.: Reliability of pre- and intraoperative tests for biliary lithiasis.   Ann. Surg., 201:640, 1985. Discusses OCG, US, HIDA scans as well as intraoperative cholangiography in   both acute and   chronic cholecystitis.

4.   Fry, D.E., Cox, R.A., and Harbrecht, P.J.: Gangrene of the gallbladder: a complication of acute cholecystitis. South. Med. J., 74:666, 1981. Emphasizes high morbidity and mortality of the gangrenous gallbladder. Also notes clinical presentation identical to acute cholecystitis.

5.   Glenn, G., and Dillon, L. D.: Developing trends in acute cholecystitis and choledocholithiasis. Surg. Gynecol. Obstet., 151:528, 1980. Review of 4348 operations for nonmalignant disease of the biliary tract . Gives details of morbidity and mortality and patient profiles over past 46 years, and indicates older, sicker patients and need for prompt surgery.

6.   Jarvinen, H.J., and Hastbacka, J.: Early cholecystectomy for acute cholecystitis: A prospective randomized study. Ann. Surg., 191:501, 1980. Finnish study of 165 patients revealed no increase in morbidity or mortality in early cholecystectomy, while reducing hospital stay, emergency operations, and recurrent attacks.

7.   Jordan, G. L., Jr.:   Choledocholithiasis. Curr. Probl. Surg., 19:721, 1982. Thorough review of diagnosis and management of stones in the common duct, with and without acute cholecystitis.

8.   Laing, F.C.: Diagnostic evaluation of patients with suspected cholecystitis. Surg. Clin. North Am., 64:3, 1984.   Detailed review of radiologic modalities available.

9.   Norrby, S., Herlin, P., Holmin, T., et al.:   Early or delayed cholecystectomy in acute cholecystitis? A clinical trial. Br. J. Surg., 70:163, 1983. Swedish prospective study of 192 patients supporting early surgery for acute cholecystitis for both medical and economic reasons.

10. Stryker, S.J., and Beal, J.M.: Acute cholecystitis and common-duct calculi. Arch. Surg., 118:1063, 1983.   Importance of intraoperative cholangiograms with acute cholecystitis, demonstrating 12.5% incidence of choledocholithiasis.

30. CHRONIC CHOLECYSTITIS
JAMES NARROD, M.D.

1.   What is the most common type of gallstone?
Mixed cholesterol stones account for 80% of gallstones in patients in the U.S.

2.   Who gets pigment stones?
Pigment stones are green or black and occur in patients with hemolytic anemia. In the Orient they occur commonly with *Ascaris lumbricoides* or *Escherchia coli* infections.

3.   Are men or women more likely to get gallstones?
Women.

HISTORY AND PHYSICAL EXAMINATION

4.   Where is the pain of cholecystitis?
The pain is located in the right upper quadrant or epigastrium with radiation to the tip of the scapula or infrascapular area.

5.   What symptoms suggest stones in the common bile duct?
A history of jaundice, dark urine, pruritus, and clay-colored stools all suggest an episode of choledocholithiasis.

6.   What is Murphy's sign?
The patient inspires while the examiner is palpating under the liver; inspiration stops in mid-cycle by painful contact of the gallbladder with the palpating hand. This is more common in acute than in chronic cholecystitis.

7. **What is Courvoisier's law?**
    Dilatation of the gallbladder does not occur in obstructive jaundice due to a stone in the common bile duct because of previous scarring of the gallbladder wall; in obstruction from carcinoma of the head of the pancreas, there is no scarring and a dilated gallbladder results. This law is not always true.

DIAGNOSTIC TESTS

8. **What percentage of gallstones are visualized on a plain abdominal radiograph?**
    Only 10 to 15% of gallstones are radiopaque.

9. **What are the two important findings of oral cholecystography (OCG)?**
    Radiolucent shadows in the opaque dye are gallstones. Nonvisualization of the gallbladder would indicate obstruction of the cystic duct or chronic cholecystitis such that the gallbladder is unable to concentrate the dye. The test is 95% accurate.

10. **What else can cause a nonvisualized gallbladder?**
    Serum bilirubin greater than 1.8 mg/dl, emesis of or interstitial malabsorption of the dye, inadequate hepatic excretion due to liver disease, or failure of the patient to take the pills can give a false-positive OCG.

11. **What are the advantages of ultrasonography?**
    It can be used in pregnancy. Additionally, jaundice and liver failure as well as emesis and malabsorption do not affect the test. Enlargement of the common bile duct can also be detected. It is highly accurate if the gallbladder can be visualized.

TREATMENT

12. **Should a patient with gallstones have surgery?**
    Once symptoms of gallstones develop, the patient will continue to have problems and is at risk for acute cholecystitis. Cholecystectomy has a mortality rate of less than 0.1% in patients under 50 years of age and 0.8% in patients over 50. The risk of surgery increases by a factor of 2 to 3 if the surgery is performed on an emergency basis.

13. **What about dissolving the gallstones?**
    Chenodeoxycholic acid taken for 2 years can dissolve radiolucent gallstones in up to one third of patients. The stones recur if the medication is stopped. Side effects include liver toxicity and diarrhea.

OPERATIVE CONSIDERATIONS

14. **Should a drain be placed during cholecystectomy?**
    In general, a drain is not required following cholecystectomy for chronic cholecystitis (see Controversies).

15. **What is the triangle of Calot?**
    This is a space bounded by the liver, the common hepatic duct, and the cystic duct. The cystic artery is usually found in the triangle of Calot.

16. **What are the ducts of Luschka?**

These are the hepatocholecystic ducts that drain bile from the liver directly into the gallbladder.

CONTROVERSIES

17. During cholecystectomy, should a drain be placed?
Elective cholecystectomies without common bile duct explorations do not need to be drained if the field is dry at the time of closure. Drains have been shown to increase the incidence of wound infection and postoperative fever. By using a closed drainage system instead of Penrose drains, the incidence of infection can be reduced. Theoretically, a drain will allow a bile leak to be adequately decompressed. Randomized prospective studies have favored no drains.

18. Should intraoperative cholangiograms always be done?
If there are signs of common duct stones (jaundice, hyperamylasemia, multiple small stones, dilated common bile duct), duct exploration is positive in only 20 to 30%. Intraoperative cholangiograms will reduce negative duct explorations to less than 20%. If there are no indications for duct exploration, doing intraoperative cholangiograms is controversial and probably not indicated.

BIBLIOGRAPHY

1. Farha, G.J., Frederic, C.C., and Matthews, E.H.: Drainage in elective cholecystectomy. Am. J. Surg., 142:678-680, 1981.
2. Ferrucci, J.T., Fordtran, J.S., Cooperberg, P.L., et al.: The radiological diagnosis of gallbladder disease. Radiology, 141:49-56, 1980.
3. Gracie, W.A., and Ransohoff, D.F.: The innocent gallstone is not a myth. N. Engl. J. Med., 307:798-799, 1982.
4. Isselbacher, K.J.: Chenodiol for gallstones: Dissolution or disillusion? Ann. Intern. Med., 95:377-378, 1981.

---

31. JAUNDICE*
G. RICHARD NEELEY, M.D.

---

1. What clinical features suggest a benign etiology for jaundice?
A short, acute course associated with pain and fever in an otherwise healthy patient.

2. How is the diagnosis of gallstones usually made?
By ultrasound, which has a high rate of accuracy (90 to 95%), provides an immediate answer, and may also show a dilated duct.

3. If a jaundiced patient has gallstones and an obstructive pattern on liver function tests, what operation should be performed, and what preoperative measures are necessary?
Cholecystectomy and common duct exploration. Preoperative tests should ensure that clotting is normal (vitamin K may be required for prolonged protime), and antibiotics should be given to cover for cholangitis. An acutely ill patient may require urgent decompression.

Note: Questions pertaining to jaundice may also be found in Chapter 33, Pancreatic Cancer.

4. **What is the goal of surgery?**
    To relieve obstruction of the liver, and ideally to remove all stones or other causes of obstruction (e.g., strictures).

5. **How is the operation carried out?**
    The gallbladder is removed, unless needed for bypass, if the obstruction proves to be malignant. Operative cholangiogram via the cystic duct documents the level and often the cause of obstruction. The duct is opened and the stones are removed either directly or with biliary Fogarty catheters. A choledochoscope is increasingly applied to visualize the duct directly. Bakes dilators are passed into the duodenum through the sphincter. At the completion of exploration, a T-tube is placed in the common duct and a radiograph is taken to confirm that the duct is clear and that the channel into the duodenum is patent.

6. **What if the duct is empty and can pass dilators but dye does not go into the duodenum?**
    This is probably caused by spasm of the sphincter as a result of manipulation. It is usually better to place a T-tube in the duct and repeat the cholangiogram post-operatively. If residual stones are present, they can usually be removed by the radiologist via the T-tube tract, or by an endoscopist by endoscopic retrograde cholangiopancreatography (ERCP).

7. **When is sphincterotomy indicated?   How is it done?**
    It is indicated for recurrent common duct stones, or impacted stones, which cannot be removed by usual means. It is performed through a duodenotomy under direct vision with care being taken to avoid damage to the pancreatic duct orifice. Bypass of the obstruction via choledochoduodenostomy or choledo-chojejunostomy (usually a Roux-en-Y) is preferred by some surgeons in this situation. Disadvantages include the potential of leaving the pancreatic duct obstructed and leaving a so-called distal stump.

8. **When is the T-tube removed?**
    Usually 1 to 3 weeks postoperatively, after a normal cholangiogram has been obtained.

9. **What are the most common symptoms of malignant jaundice?**
    Major weight loss (more than 10%); unexplained upper abdominal or back pain (about 50% of patients); and painless obstructive jaundice (about 20% of presenting patients). Less common presentations include steatorrhea, diabetes, and thrombophlebitis (Trousseau's sign).

10. **Which drugs should be considered as producing cholestatic jaundice?**
    Chlorpromazine derivatives, isoniazid, and anabolic steroids.

11. **What is the best initial test in a patient thought to have pancreatic carcinoma?**
    Ultrasound. Sensitivity is 82%; specificity is 84%.

12. **What are the sensitivity and specificity of CT?   ERCP?**
    77% and 82%.   86% and 90%.

13. **What are the chief advantages and disadvantages of ERCP?**
    Advantage: tissue diagnosis possible. Disadvantage: technical failure rate is about 20%.

14. **What is the major problem in improving the miserable results in the treatment of pancreatic carcinoma?**
The tumor is usually advanced and unresectable by the time symptoms appear.

15. **What is Courvoisier's law?**
The gallbladder is distended and is sometimes palpable in malignant jaundice but may not distend if there are stones and chronic thickening of the wall.

16. **What are the intraoperative dilemmas when malignant jaundice is suspected?**
Making the diagnosis. This may be done by lymph node biopsy if enlarged nodes are present. The problem is similar findings of a hard mass in the head of the pancreas and the question as to whether this represents a malignant tumor or an area of pancreatitis.

17. **How is the pancreas biopsied?**
Some surgeons believe that the pancreas should not be biopsied because of the risk of precipitating pancreatitis. Others argue that the pancreas should not be resected without positive tissue diagnosis. Biopsy may be incisional or carried out with a needle (either direct or transduodenal in the hope of decreasing the risk of fistula). Fine needle biopsy is gaining increasing application owing to its safety and demonstrated accuracy. (See Chapter 33, Pancreatic Cancer.)

18. **What is the chance of obtaining a positive biopsy of pancreatic cancer at the time of surgery?**
18 of 55 proven cases were false negatives.

19. **What is the accuracy of clinical impression at operation?**
It is incorrect about 4 to 9% of the time.

20. **What are the complications of pancreatic biopsy?**
Hemorrhage, fistula, pancreatitis, and subphrenic abscess.

21. **How often do these complications occur?**
Isaacson (Mayo Clinic): 527 biopsies, 6% complications, none fatal. Lightwood: 177 biopsies, 4.7% complications, 1.7% fatal.

22. **What are the arguments in favor of biopsy?**
   1.   Clinical impression carries a false-positive rate of 7 to 18%.
   2.   Biopsy is accurate. Pathology has false-positive and false-negative rate of 3 to 4%.
   3.   The complication rate is acceptably low, only 5 to 10%, and less when only those not resected are counted.

23. **What is currently the best technique for intraoperative biopsy?**
Fine needle aspiration. Positive in 87% of proven cases.

24. **What is the differential diagnosis of obstructive jaundice?**
Benign: (1) common duct stone, (2) stricture secondary to previous surgery, (3) obstruction in intrapancreatic portion of common duct secondary to chronic pancreatitis.
Malignant: (1) pancreaticoduodenal carcinoma, (2) tumor of distal common duct (cholangio-carcinoma), (3) obstruction at hilum (Klatskin tumor), carcinoma of gallbladder invading ducts.

25. **What is PTC?**
Percutaneous transhepatic cholangiography.

26. **How is it done?**
By radiologists. The needle is placed in the dilated bile duct, the guide wire is passed through the needle; then the catheter is passed over the guide wire (Seldinger technique).

27. **What are the risks of PTC?**
Inability to cannulate ducts, bleeding from the liver, and bile leak.

28. **What is percutaneous biliary drainage?**
Following PTC, a catheter is left in place to decompress an obstructed biliary tree.

29. **What are the most common complications of percutaneous biliary drainage?**
Dislodgement and bleeding; sepsis secondary to cholangitis.

30. **Is preoperative external biliary drainage worthwhile?**
Probably not. Initial enthusiasm has waned as additional studies have documented complications and a lack of significant benefit.

31. **What are the mortalities and prognoses of various operations for pancreatic carcinoma?**

	Mortality (%)	Survival (months)
Biopsy only	44	3.6
Biliary bypass	16	6.2
Biliary and GI bypass	26	4.8
Partial pancreatectomy (Whipple)	12	16.2
With gross tumor out		20.3
With tumor left in		12.9
Palliative Whipple		6.8
Total pancreatectomy	17	26.0

32. **What are the corresponding mortalities and survival for peri-ampullary carcinoma?**

	Mortality (%)	Survival (months) (av.)	Survival (months) (5 yr.)
Ampullary	14	46	24
Bile duct carcinoma	13	58	25
Duodenal carcinoma	0	27	0

(Reference: Forrest et al.: Ann. Surg., 189:129-138, 1979.)

33. **What is the overall 5-year survival following Whipple resection for pancreatic carcinoma?**
5%

34. **What is a "Whipple operation" ?**
A pancreaticoduodenal resection (see Figure on opposite page).

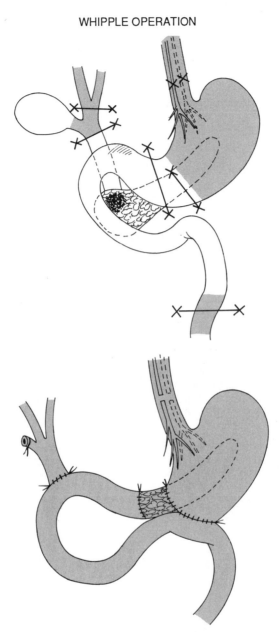

(Adapted from Reber, H.A., and Way, L.W.: Pancreas. In Way, L.W. (ed.): Current Surgical Diagnosis and Treatment, 6th ed. Los Altos, Lange, 1983, p. 553.)

35. What is the rationale for total pancreatectomy versus Whipple?
(1) Removes potential for recurrence due to multifocal disease. (2) Avoids pancreaticojejunostomy with attendant risk of leak.

36. What is the rationale for vagotomy in association with pancreatic resections?
The high incidence of stomal ulceration and bleeding if vagotomy is not done; for example, 50% of 14 patients without vagotomy bled in Scott's series.

37. **Should gastroenterostomy be done in addition to biliary bypass?**
This is controversial. About 15% of patients with biliary bypasses will have an obstructed duodenum and require subsequent operation.

38. **What is the overall resectability rate in pancreatic carcinoma?**
10 to 15%

39. **What is the role of adjuvant therapy for unresectable pancreatic carcinoma?**
It is only palliative. There is some evidence that multiple drug chemotherapy and chemotherapy combined with radiation may provide some objective palliation.

BIBLIOGRAPHY

1.   Bodner, E., Schwamberger, K., and Mikuz, G.:   Cytological diagnosis of pancreatic tumors. World J. Surg., 6:103-106,1982.
2.   Brooks, J.R.: Operative approach to pancreatic carcinoma. Sem.Oncol., 6:357-367,1979.
3.   Forrest, J.F., and Longmire, W.P.: Carcinoma of the pancreas and periampullary region. A study of 279 patients. Ann. Surg., 189:129-138, 1979.
4.   Hatfield, A.R.W., Tobias, R., Terblanche, J., et al.: Preoperative external biliary drainage in obstructive jaundice. A prospective controlled clinical trial. Lancet, 896-899, 1982.
5.   Ihse, I., Toregard, B.M., and Akerman, M.: Intraoperative fine needle aspiration cytology in pancreatic lesions. Ann. Surg., 190:732-734, 1979.
6.   Lee, Y.-T. N.:   Tissue diagnosis for cancer of pancreas and periampullary structures. Cancer, 49:1035-1039, 1982.
7.   Moossa, A.R., and Levin, B.: Collaborative studies in the diagnosis of pancreatic cancer. Sem. Oncol., 6:298-308, 1979.
8.   Mueller, P., Van Sonnenberg, E., and Ferrucci, J.T.:   Percutaneous biliary drainage: Technical and catheter-related problems in 200 procedures. A.J.R., 138:17-23,1982.
9.   Osteen, R.T., Brooks, D.C., Gray, E.B., et al.: Evaluation of palliative procedures for pancreatic cancer. Am. J. Surg., 141:430-433, 1981.
10. Sarr, M.G., Gladen, H.E., Beart, R.W., et al.: Role of gastroenterostomy in patients with unresectablecarcinoma of the pancreas. Surg. Gynecol. Obstet.,152:597-600,1981.
11. Scott, H.W., Dean, R.H., Parker, R.H., et al.: The role of vagotomy in pancreaticoduodenectomy. Ann. Surg., 191:688-696,1980.
12. Smith, F.P., and Schein, P.S.: Chemotherapy of pancreatic cancer. Sem. Oncol., 6: 368-376, 1979.

---

32. ACUTE PANCREATITIS
LAWRENCE W. NORTON, M.D.

---

1.   **What are common causes of acute pancreatitis?**
Alcoholism (40%) and biliary tract disease (40%).

2.   **What are uncommon causes?**
Idiopathic (1 to 2%), postoperative (1 to 2%), hereditary (1 to 2%), hypercalcemia (1 to 2%), and drugs such as isoniazid, estrogens, and thiazides (10%).

3.   **Does hyperamylasemia in a patient with abdominal pain confirm pancreatitis?**
No. Amylase levels can be elevated as a result of perforated peptic ulcer, bowel obstruction, salpingitis, and other disease states.

4.   **How can hyperamylasemia due to pancreatitis be identified?**
By measurement of the pancreas-specific isoenzyme. The amylase/creatinine clearance ratio is a less reliable means of differentiation.

5. **What are the frequency and mortality of severe (fulminant) pancreatitis?**
    Frequency < 10%; mortality > 50%

6. **By what means can severe pancreatitis be predicted?**
    When three or more Ranson indices are positive at 48 hours, severe disease is likely in 65 to 85% of patients. Other means of determining severe disease are diagnostic peritoneal lavage, measurement of serum methemalbumin, and CT scanning.

7. **What are Ranson indices?**
    Eleven physiologic measurements or blood chemistries that are useful in predicting the occurrence of severe pancreatitis. (See reference.)

8. **What is the best drug to relieve pain in mild pancreatitis?**
    Meperidine (Demerol) may have some advantage over morphine because it causes less constriction of the sphincter of Oddi. The difference in effectiveness of the two analgesics is slight.

9. **Should antibiotics be given to patients with mild pancreatitis?**
    No. Antibiotics neither improve the course of early pancreatitis nor prevent later septic complications.

10. **Is nasogastric suction effective treatment for mild pancreatitis?**
    No. Controlled, prospective studies show no advantage of nasogastric suction in patients with mild disease.

11. **What are possible *local* complications of severe pancreatitis?**
    Hemorrhage from adjacent vessels, colonic perforation, fistula or obstruction, lesser sac abscesses, pancreatic phlegmon, or pancreatic fistula.

12. **What is the significance of hypoxemia early in the course of pancreatitis?**
    Atelectasis caused by severe pancreatitis results in hypoxemia that occurs early in the disease. The respiratory distress syndrome occurs frequently thereafter. Mechanical ventilation, if instituted when PaO2 falls below 60 mm Hg, is useful treatment.

13. **What is the cause of hypocalcemia in severe disease?**
    No single explanation of hypocalcemia is accepted. Possible causative factors include: (1) "soap" formation in the lesser sac, (2) calcitonin release stimulated by glucagon, (3) hypomagnesemia, (4) hypoalbuminemia, (5) decreased levels of parathormone, and (6) hypovolemia.

14. **Why does shock occur in severe pancreatitis?**
    Hypotension is less often due to hypovolemia than to hemodynamic changes resembling sepsis. Cardiac output is usually increased despite evidence of impaired ventricular function, and peripheral vascular resistance is decreased.

CONTROVERSIES

15. **Cimetidine.**
    Blockade of H2 receptors to decrease acid stimulation of secretion in the duodenum would seem to be reasonable treatment for early pancreatitis. Animal studies showed that cimetidine either failed to alleviate disease or made it worse. Clinical use of cimetidine shows neither harm nor apparent benefit.

16. **Peritoneal lavage.**
Dilution of vasoactive peptides and enzymes elaborated by the severely inflamed pancreas is the rationale for therapeutic peritoneal lavage. Results of lavage in patients with severe pancreatitis were encouraging initially. Recent reports suggest no improvement with peritoneal lavage.

17. **Pancreatic resection.**
Removal of necrotic pancreas seems reasonable. Unfortunately, the presence and degree of necrosis cannot be determined accurately by operative inspection. Results of resection of all or nearly all of the pancreas in the presence of life-threatening disease are variable. The procedure is performed rarely in the United States but commonly in Finland and France.

BIBLIOGRAPHY

1. Acosta, J.M., Pellegrini, C.A., and Skinner, D.B.: Etiology and pathogenesis of acute biliary pancreatitis. Surgery, 83:367, 1978.
2. Howes, R., Zuidema, G., and Cameron, J.L.: Evaluation of prophylactic antibiotics in acute pancreatitis. J. Surg. Res., 18:197, 1975.
3. Norton, L.W., and Eiseman, B.: Near total pancreatectomy for hemorrhagic pancreatitis. Am. J. Surg., 127:191, 1974.
4. Ranson, J.H.C., Rifkind, K.M., and Turner, J.W.: Prognostic signs and nonoperative peritoneal lavage in acute pancreatitis. Surg. Gynecol. Obstet., 143:209, 1976.
5. Stone, H.H., Fabian, T.C.: Peritoneal dialysis in the treatment of acute alcoholic pancreatitis. Surg. Gynecol. Obstet., 150:878, 1980.

33. PANCREATIC CANCER[*]
NATHAN PEARLMAN, M.D.

1. **What are the presenting signs of pancreatic cancer?**
(1) Painless jaundice in 30% of patients, (2) pain alone (epigastric, right upper quadrant, back) in 20%, (3) pain with jaundice in 30 to 40%, and (4) signs of metastases (hepatomegaly, ascites, lung nodules, supraclavicular nodes) in 10 to 20%.

2. **A patient presents with jaundice and a markedly elevated alkaline phosphatase level, but other liver functions and clotting studies are relatively normal. There is no history of similar episodes in the past, no fever, and no pain. What is the next best test to determine what is going on?**
The next best test to obtain is ultrasound or CT scan. The accuracy of either depends on the machine being used and/or expertise of the radiologist or ultrasonographer carrying out the test. Ultrasound, in our experience, is accurate in diagnosing extrahepatic biliary obstruction in 90+% of cases and, if the pancreas can be seen (more than two thirds of patients), will also demonstrate a mass, if present. Similar accuracy exists with modern CT equipment. Fine needle aspiration and/or ERCP with cytologic examination of pancreatic duct aspirate may

[*]Note: Questions pertaining to pancreatic cancer may also be found in the chapter on Jaundice. The following discourse represents personal experience with pancreatic cancer and may not parallel all surgeons' experience with this problem.

also provide a diagnosis in upwards of 90% of cases; but these techniques are relatively expensive, depend on the presence of experienced pathologists and endoscopists, and are no more accurate than ultrasound and/or CT scan.

3. **The ultrasound or CT scan scan shows dilated bile ducts and, perhaps, a mass in the region of the head of the pancreas. Why not proceed directly to the operating room?**
    Because not all such patients have cancer of the pancreas. Some have impacted stones in the distal common bile duct, some have pancreatitis, and some have proximal bile duct cancer. Also, the patient's family is not always understanding when surprised by the information that the surgeon unexpectedly found cancer and is proceeding with an operation that has a 10 to 20% mortality rate.

4. **How can we avoid getting into such a predicament?**
    If the ultrasound and/or CT scan show dilated intrahepatic or extrahepatic bile ducts, ERCP or transhepatic cholangiography should be performed. This will provide more information as to whether the obstruction is due to tumor or stones, and at what level it is. The surgeon, patient, and family will be more prepared (mentally and physically) for a major operation, should that prove necessary.

5. **With information from ERCP and/or transhepatic cholangiography in hand, why not proceed to the operating room now?**
    Depending on the level of jaundice and nutritional status of the patient, one might want to delay surgery for 7 to 10 days to carry out biliary decompression (in the hope of improving liver function) and nutritional replenishment. The benefits of such preoperative measures are unclear at the present time, however.

6. **Okay. We finally made it to the operating room, have entered the abdomen, and there is a discrete, rock-hard mass in the head of the pancreas, no liver metastases, and no ascites. What next?**
    Try to determine if the mass is cancerous with a transduodenal or direct needle biopsy and frozen section of the mass. Alternatively, a wedge biopsy can be carried out, with closure. These biopsy attempts should not be overly aggressive, because the morbidity or mortality may outweigh any benefits of the information obtained.
    Then, while the pathologist is trying to decide between cancer and pancreatitis (it is often quite difficult), try to determine whether the tumor is resectable for cure should a diagnosis of cancer be reported. Grab the mass and gently rock it up and down to see if it is free of retroperitoneal structures. Check for suspicious nodes and/or suspicious induration around the celiac axis, in the root of the mesentery (where the middle colic artery originates), and in the hilum of the liver. If suspicious nodes or induration is found in one or all of these locations, do not presume that cancer is present and forego resection. Send the biopsy specimen for pathologic confirmation.

7. **Suppose biopsy of nodes in the celiac axis, root of the mesentery, or hilum of the liver shows cancer on frozen section. Is the tumor resectable for cure? How about for palliation?**
    No, and no.

8. **Suppose, however, that biopsy of these nodes shows no cancer on frozen section but the pathologist finds pancreatitis only in the needle biopsies sent down earlier. Is it justified to proceed with resection on the basis of clinical judgment alone?**

For many experienced pancreatic surgeons, the answer is "yes." Others, however, demand proof of malignancy before proceeding to remove the tumor. The reason for this is that most pancreatic tumors are surrounded by a rim of pancreatitis, and this often feels almost as hard as the tumor. It is relatively easy, therefore, to biopsy this area of pancreatitis and miss the tumor, which may be only millimeters away.

9. **The pathologist calls back to inquire if you are going to carry out a Whipple procedure; if so, he wants to alert the blood bank to call in donors (he remembers the last time you tried one). What's a "Whipple"?**
En bloc removal of the gallbladder, common bile duct, duodenum, head of the pancreas over to the portal vein and, generally, the antrum of the stomach, with or without an accompanying vagotomy. See Figure on page 93.

10. **If this is a Whipple procedure, what is a "total" pancreatectomy?**
Removal of all of these structures as well as the body and tail of the pancreas and spleen.

11. **Why do some surgeons champion the Whipple procedure, whereas others always seem to carry out total pancreatectomies?**
Theoretically, there is about a 20% incidence of multifocal, or residual, disease left behind in the body and tail of the pancreas with a Whipple procedure. In addition, a major source of morbidity and mortality after the latter operation historically has been leaks from the anastomosis of the pancreatic remnant to the small bowel. Both of these problems are avoided if a total pancreatectomy is performed. On the other hand, a total pancreatectomy commits the patient to lifelong diabetes, which is often difficult to manage. Furthermore, survival figures for pancreatic cancer are no better with total pancreatectomies than with Whipple procedures. We believe that the morbidity associated with total pancreatectomy generally outweighs any theoretical benefit it might achieve, and therefore we carry out Whipple procedures whenever possible.

12. **Why take out the gallbladder, duodenum, and stomach if the tumor is in the pancreas?**
Once the ampulla of Vater is removed, the gallbladder does not function well and forms stones. The duodenum shares a common blood supply with the head of the pancreas; because of this, it usually is devascularized when the latter is removed. The gastric antrum has, historically, been removed to achieve a better margin around the tumor. A vagotomy is often added to removal of the antrum to prevent marginal ulceration where the gastric remnant is anastomosed to small bowel. Recently, however, there has been evidence that the antrum and pylorus may not always require resection to obtain reasonable margins and, in that case, the need for vagotomy is less compelling.

13. **We decide to proceed with a standard Whipple procedure, since the tumor seems mobile and node biopsies are negative. Besides knowing how to remove the structures already listed, is there anything else we should know at this point?**
Whether the superior mesenteric vein or portal vein is free of invasion where it passes behind the neck of the pancreas.

14. **Suppose that the portal vein seems stuck to the tumor in this location. Does that mean that the tumor is unresectable?**

Most pancreatic surgeons would say "yes." A few would remove this short portion of the portal vein, if that were the only finding of "unresectability," and either replace the defect with a vein graft or prosthesis, or mobilize the two ends for a direct anastomosis.

15. **Well, we decide that adherence to the portal vein does mean incurability. Should anything be done before closing the abdomen?**
At a minimum, a biliary-enteric bypass (cholecystojejunostomy or choledochojejunostomy). The duodenum should not be used for this purpose, since the tumor tends to grow upward toward the liver and will gradually obstruct a choledochoduodenostomy. To prevent gastric outlet obstruction at a later date, some authors routinely recommend a gastroenterostomy as well; however, there is little evidence this benefits most patients. Some authors also believe that alcohol injection of the celiac ganglion is useful in controlling pain from cancer of the pancreas; however, we have not found this to be helpful.

16. **The patient recovers nicely from these bypass procedures and wants to know if anything else can be done. What is available for locally unresectable pancreatic cancer at this time?**
Both radiotherapy and chemotherapy (5-fluorouracil, or a combination of 5-fluorouracil, Adriamycin, and mitomycin-C). There is some evidence of a modest prolongation of survival (3 to 4 months) with the use of such modalities, either alone or in combination.

17. **What is the chance of survival if a resection has been possible?**
50 to 60% at one year; 25 to 39% at 2 years; and 5 to 25% at 5 years.

18. **With such dismal survival figures, why are surgeons always so eager to resect pancreatic cancer?**
Because these survival figures are better than can be achieved with either radiotherapy or chemotherapy, or both in combination. Median survival when the tumor cannot be removed is only about 6 to 8 months.

BIBLIOGRAPHY

1. Cubilla, A.L., Fitzgerald, P.J.: Cancer of the exocrine pancreas: The pathologic aspects. CA, 35:2-18, 1985.
2. Fortner, J.G.: Regional, total and subtotal pancreatectomy. Cancer, 47:1712-1718,1981.
3. Hansson, J.A., Hoevels, J., et al.: Clinical aspects of nonsurgical percutaneous transhepatic bile drainage in obstructive lesions of the extrahepatic bile ducts. Ann. Surg., 189:58-61, 1979.
4. Haslam, J.B., Cavanaugh, P.J., Strapp, S.L.: Radiation therapy in the treatment of unresectable adenocarcinoma of the pancreas. Cancer, 32:1341-1345, 1973.
5. Mackie, C.R., Cooper, M.J., et al.: Non-operative differentiation between pancreatic cancer and chronic pancreatitis. Ann. Surg., 189:480-487, 1979.
6. Moertel, C.G., Childs, D.S., et al.: Combined 5-fluorouracil and supervoltage radiation therapy of locally unresectable gastrointestinal cancer. Lancet, 2:865-867, 1969.
7. Pliam, M.B., ReMine, W.H.: Further evaluation of total pancreatectomy. Arch. Surg., 110: 506-512, 1975.
8. Traverso, L.W., Longmire, W.P.: Preservation of the pylorus in pancreaticoduodenectomy. A follow-up evaluation. Ann. Surg., 192:306-309, 1980.
9. Warren, K.W., Choe, D.S., et al.: Results of radical resection for periampullary cancer. Ann. Surg., 182:534-538, 1975.

34. CHRONIC PANCREATITIS
LAWRENCE W. NORTON, M.D.

1. **What is chronic pancreatitis?**
   The classic syndrome consists of abdominal pain, diabetes, steatorrhea, and pancreatic calcifications. Frequently one or more of the latter three are absent.

2. **How does chronic pancreatitis differ from chronic relapsing pancreatitis?**
   The pain of chronic pancreatitis is severe and unremitting, usually causing drug addiction for analgesia. Chronic relapsing pancreatitis is characterized by intermittent pain without endocrine or exocrine insufficiency and calcification.

3. **Is chronic pancreatitis the result of acute pancreatitis?**
   Many patients have not had acute pancreatitis, although alcoholism is common to both.

4. **What are the signs and symptoms of steatorrhea?**
   Diarrhea is frequently but not invariably associated with pancreatogenous steatorrhea. Stools typically are soft, greasy, and foul-smelling. An oily ring is left in the toilet bowl.

5. **What test confirms steatorrhea?**
   Increased neutral fat (triglyceride) in the stool can be detected microscopically or biochemically. A fecal fat concentration in excess of 10% is characteristic of pancreatogenous steatorrhea.

6. **What tests might differentiate various causes of steatorrhea?**
   The *D-xylose* test is positive in the presence of small bowel disease and usually is normal in patients with pancreatic exocrine insufficiency. The Schilling test for vitamin B12 absorption shows decreased urinary secretion of labeled cyanocobalamin in 40% of patients with chronic pancreatitis but may also be positive in the presence of pernicious anemia, bacterial overgrowth, or ileal disease.

7. **In a patient with abdominal pain due to chronic pancreatitis but no steatorrhea, is there any means of detecting pancreatic insufficiency?**
   The secretion stimulation test becomes abnormal when more than 75% of pancreatic function is lost. Normally, the peak concentration of bicarbonate in pancreatic juice is greater than 80 mEq/L. Patients with abdominal pain secondary to chronic pancreatitis who do not have steatorrhea have concentrations in the range of 60 to 80 mEq/L.

8. **Is serum amylase elevated in chronic pancreatitis?**
   No. Serum pancreatic isoamylase is usually normal or decreased.

9. **What is the treatment of steatorrhea?**
   Most patients respond to replacement of pancreatic enzymes. If this fails to reduce fecal fat excretion to less than 15 to 20 gm/day, fat content in the diet is decreased. If steatorrhea persists, aluminum-containing antacids, and finally, cimetidine are introduced.

10. How is pain relieved?
Alcohol and narcotics are withdrawn (under cover of clonidine) if possible. The narcotic bowel syndrome may contribute to pain. Medically intractable pain suggests the need for operation.

11. What information is essential before operating upon a patient with chronic pancreatitis?
A radiographic contrast study of the pancreatic duct. The best approach is by ERCP. During operation, the duct can be visualized by: (1) direct needle injection of a contrast material into the enlarged duct, (2) duct cannulation via duodenotomy, or (3) cannulation of the distal duct after amputation of the tail of the gland.

12. What procedures might relieve pain if the pancreatic duct is obstructed only at the ampulla of Vater?
Sphincteroplasty is the procedure of choice. Distal pancreatectomy with Roux-en-Y pancreaticojejunostomy (Duval) is an alternative.

13. What procedure is indicated for multiple duct obstructions resulting in the "chain-of-lakes" appearance?
The Puestow operation opens the obstructed duct system longitudinally and provides drainage from the head to the tail via a Roux-en-Y pancreatico-jejunostomy.

14. What procedures may be useful for patients with a normal pancreatic duct?
Near-total (95%) pancreatectomy (Child) preserves the duodenum while eliminating virtually all of the pancreas. Diabetes, if not already present, is inevitable after this operation. Total pancreatectomy is a more radical procedure and is no more effective.

15. What is the usual result of these operations?
Pain relief in 70% of patients by the end of one year; 50% by the end of five years.

CONTROVERSIES

16. Visceral ganglionectomy.
Neurectomy of sympathetic fibers supplying the pancreas performed at the level of the celiac axis is sometimes recommended for pain relief in patients failing resection or as an alternative to pancreatic operations. Pain relief is variable (50 to 90%).

17. Ligation of pancreatic duct.
Ligating the ducts of both Wirsung and Santorini as they penetrate the wall of the duodenum causes atrophy of acini and ducts but preserves islet cell function. Results of this procedure for pain relief are not encouraging.

BIBLIOGRAPHY

1. Ammann, R.W., Akovbiantz, A., Largiades, F., et al.: Course and outcome of chronic pancreatitis. Gastroenterology, 86:820, 1984.
2. Cooperman, A.: Chronic pancreatitis. Surg. Clin. North Am., 61:71, 1981.
3. Frey, C.F.: Role of subtotal pancreatectomy and pancreaticojejunostomy in chronic pancreatitis. J. Surg. Res., 31:361, 1981.

4.   Moore, D. C., Bush, W.H., and Burnett, L.L.: Celiac plexus block: A roentgenographic
      anatomic study of technique and spread of solution in patients and corpses. Anesth.
      Analg., 60:369, 1981.
5.   Warshaw, A.L., Popp, J.W., and Schapiro, R.H.: Long-term patency, pancreatic function
      and pain relief after lateral pancreaticojejunostomy for chronic pancreatitis.
      Gastroenterology, 79:289, 1980.

35. ESOPHAGEAL VARICES AND PORTAL HYPERTENSION

A.L. CAMBRE, M.D., and G. VAN STIEGMANN, M.D.

1.   **What is portal hypertension?**
      Portal hypertension is an elevation in pressure of the portal venous circulation.
      Normal portal venous pressure ranges from 7 to 10 mm Hg, while average portal
      pressure in portal hypertension is 20 mm Hg with a range of 15 to 60 mm Hg.

2.   **What are the causes of portal hypertension?**
      Portal hypertension may be caused by increased resistance to portal blood flow
      or increased portal blood flow. Increased resistance to flow is divided into three
      main categories: (1) prehepatic (portal vein thrombosis, extrinsic compression
      [tumors]); (2) hepatic (cirrhosis, congenital hepatic fibrosis, schistosomiasis); and
      (3) posthepatic (Budd-Chiari syndrome, constrictive pericarditis). Increased portal
      blood flow may be caused by arterial-portal venous fistulas or increased splenic
      flow, as seen in various forms of splenomegaly.

3.   **Which veins join to form the portal vein?**
      The portal vein is 8 to 9 cm in length and is formed by the confluence of the
      splenic and superior mesenteric veins. The portal vein lies dorsal and medial to
      the common bile duct and hepatic artery in the hepatoduodenal ligament. There
      are no valves in the portal circulation.

4.   **Characterize the blood flow to the liver.**
      Total hepatic blood flow is approximately 1500 ml/min, or roughly 25% of cardiac
      output. Approximately three fourths of the total blood flow and one fourth of the
      oxygen supply are derived from the portal vein, and one fourth of total blood flow
      and three fourths of the oxygen supply are provided by the hepatic artery.

5.   **Describe the venous drainage from the liver.**
      There are three major hepatic veins: the right, middle, and left. There are no
      valves in the hepatic venous system. The segmental anatomy of the liver is
      defined by the hepatic venous drainage. Two main hepatic veins empty into the
      inferior vena cava, one from the left and middle hepatic lobe, and one from the
      right hepatic lobe.

6.   **How long can portal vein and hepatic arterial flow to the liver be
      interrupted?   What is the Pringle maneuver?**
      In the normothermic liver, blood flow can be interrupted for 15 minutes without
      hepatocellular damage. If prolonged control of hepatic blood flow is necessary,
      the occlusion can be briefly released, then reapplied every 10 to 15 minutes.
      The Pringle maneuver consists of occlusion of the portal triad (portal vein, hepatic
      artery, common bile duct) by placement of a vascular clamp across the
      hepatoduodenal ligament.

7. **What is the most common cause of portal hypertension in in adults? In children?**
   Cirrhosis of the liver, most frequently caused by chronic alcoholism, is th. common cause of portal hypertension in Western countries. Alcoholic cir. causes obstruction of portal venous blood flow on the hepatic vein side ot sinusoid (*post*sinusoidal). Laennec's cirrhosis accounts for 85% of cases of portal hypertension in the U.S. Extrahepatic portal venous occlusion is the second most common cause of portal hypertension and is the most common cause of portal hypertension in children. This is most commonly a consequence of cavernomatous malformation of the portal vein.

8. **Describe the collateral vessels that become functional in cases of portal hypertension in order of their clinical importance.**
   1. The coronary vein joins the portal vein and the esophageal mesenteric plexus, which subsequently empties into the azygous and hemiazygous veins (esophageal varices).
   2. The superior hemorrhoidal vein, a branch of the inferior mesenteric vein, communicates via a submucosal plexus with the middle and inferior hemorrhoidal veins, subsequently entering the systemic circulation via the inferior vena cava (hemorrhoids).
   3. The umbilical vein communicates the increased pressures in the portal tree to superficial veins of the abdominal wall, which ultimately drain via the superior and inferior epigastric veins into the systemic circulation (caput medusae associated with Cruveilhier-Baumgarten syndrome).
   4. The veins of Retzius form a collateral circuit between the mesenteric and peritoneal veins, then empty into the inferior vena cava.

9. **Where in the GI tract may varices occur? From which site is bleeding most likely?**
   Varices have been demonstrated in the GI tract from the esophagus to the rectum. Most commonly, however, the esophagus and cardia of the stomach are involved, with the lesser curvature of the stomach involved less frequently. Varices of the esophagus are most likely to bleed. Ninety-five percent of variceal hemorrhage occurs in the area of the gastroesophageal junction.

10. **What percentage of patients with hepatic cirrhosis will bleed from esophageal varices?**
    Approximately 30% of cirrhotic patients will experience a bleeding episode. Variceal hemorrhage can be anticipated within 2 years of the diagnosis of esophageal varices in most cases.

11. **What percentage of patients will have a second variceal hemorrhage? Is the mortality risk increased?**
    Forty to sixty percent of cirrhotic patients who have bled once from esophageal varices will rebleed within 1 year of the first episode. Risk of fatal hemorrhage is 50% for the initial episode and is not increased by subsequent episodes of variceal bleeding.

12. **How is the diagnosis of esophageal varices made?**
    Flexible fiberoptic endoscopy has assumed the primary role in diagnosis of variceal hemorrhage. Not only does the procedure allow visualization of actively bleeding varices, but it also allows a thorough examination of the stomach and duodenum to rule out gastritis, peptic ulcer disease, or extraesophageal varices. Barium swallow can detect varices in 85 to 90% of patients but provides no information regarding the site of bleeding.

13. **If a patient with known varices experiences upper GI bleeding, what is the likelihood that varices are the source?**
Twenty-five percent or more of patients in the above circumstances will have bleeding from another source (peptic ulcer, Mallory Weiss tear, gastritis). Endoscopic evaluation is mandatory to guide proper treatment.

14. **What is the initial treatment of a patient with suspected esophageal varices?**
Initial resuscitation should include placement of multiple large-bore intravenous lines and crossmatching of blood. Gastric lavage should be performed with a large-bore tube (Ewald). Endoscopy is then performed when the patient has become hemodynamically stable. If esophageal varices are identified as the source of bleeding, vasopressin, 0.4 to 0.8 units/minute, is administered by constant intravenous infusion. Since rates of rebleeding approach 80 to 90% following cessation of vasopressin, semiemergent endoscopic sclerotherapy is usually employed.
Patients who do not repond to vasopressin treatment require placement of the Sengstaken-Blakemore tube. Balloon tamponade will control variceal hemorrhage in most patients, but is also associated with a substantial (50 to 60%) rate of rebleeding once the balloons are deflated. We believe that injection sclerotherapy should be performed within 12 hours of insertion of the Sengstaken-Blakemore tube.

15. **What is a Sengstaken-Blakemore tube?**
The Sengstaken-Blakemore tube consists of two balloons, one of which is inflated in the stomach, the other in the esophagus. Once the gastric balloon is inflated (250 cc of air), the tube is drawn up tight against the gastroesophageal junction by placing it on traction. If bleeding is not controlled by inflation of the gastric balloon alone, the esophageal balloon may be inflated to a sphygmomanometer-controlled pressure of 20 mm Hg. Risks of balloon tamponade include perforation of the esophagus, necrosis of esophageal mucosa, and suffocation from migration of the balloon into the hypopharynx. Balloon tamponade is a temporary measure for control of bleeding, with up to 50 to 60% of patients rebleeding following balloon deflation.

16. **What is injection sclerotherapy?**
Injection sclerotherapy involves the injection of a sclerosing substance into or around a varix, creating fibrosis and thickening of the variceal wall and paravariceal mucosa. This may be performed through flexible or rigid endoscopes.

17. **What are the results of injection sclerotherapy?**
Acute variceal hemorrhage may be controlled with a single injection in 70 to 80% of patients. It may be controlled with 1 to 3 injection sessions in up to 95% of patients. Chronic injection therapy at weekly or monthly intervals is capable of obliterating esophageal varices. About half of patients treated by injection sclerotherapy, however, will rebleed at some time. These repeated bleeds tend to be of decreased severity and occur with less frequency than those in patients who are untreated. Injection sclerotherapy probably does not increase overall survival in patients with bleeding esophageal varices. It does, however, provide a relatively safe and inexpensive method of controlling bleeding.

18. **What complications are associated with injection sclerotherapy?**
Esophageal perforation (either mechanical, due to the endoscope itself, or chemical, due to the sclerosing substance), esophageal stenosis, fever, pleural effusion, and precipitation of hemorrhage are potential complications. Fever is

most common, usually resolving within 24 to 36 hours after injection. Superficial mucosal slough may occur in up to one fourth of patients. Overall, complications of treatment during acute bleeding episodes occur in up to 50% of patients. Most, however, are of little clinical significance.

19. **What if bleeding cannot be controlled by injection sclerotherapy?**
Five to ten percent of patients treated with injection sclerotherapy will continue to bleed. Mortality in this group approximates 70 to 100%. An active decision must be made as to whether to withhold further therapy, to attempt percutaneous transhepatic variceal or coronary vein embolization, or to perform an emergency operation.

20. **Should a patient with documented esophageal varices, who has *never* bled, undergo prophylactic treatment to prevent bleeding?**
Injection sclerotherapy may be performed on an elective basis for the prevention of variceal hemorrhage. Efficacy is unproven, however. Prophylactic shunt operations are contraindicated. One cannot predict which patients will bleed, and there is no documented improvement in survival.

21. **What is the operative mortality for a patient with acute bleeding (*emergency* shunt)?**
Emergency operations for variceal bleeding are associated with a mortality of 30 to 50%. The variability in these mortality figures can be accounted for by the differences in prehemorrhage patient risk characteristics as well as the presence or absence of shock and massive transfusion prior to emergent operative therapy. Hepatic failure is the cause of death in two thirds of those who die after emergency shunt.

22. **What operations are available to treat bleeding from esophageal varices?**
A host of operations have been devised for preventing recurrent or treating acute variceal hemorrhage. These operations may be divided into two broad categories: (1) portosystemic shunting operations, and (2) devascularization operations:

Shunting Operations	Devascularization Operations
Portocaval shunt	Esophageal transection
Mesocaval shunt	Direct ligation of esophageal varices
Splenorenal shunt	Splenectomy
Selective splenorenal shunt	Esophageal devascularization + splenectomy

23. **What is the difference between selective and nonselective shunts?**
Selective shunts are designed to decompress esophageal varices while allowing prograde portal blood flow to the liver. The selective splenorenal shunt currently in use involves anastomosis of the proximal (splenic side) splenic vein to the left renal vein. The coronary vein (left gastric) and other large periesophageal collateral veins are also ligated. This allows decompression of the esophageal varices via the short gastric veins to the spleen, and hence from the newly anastomosed splenic vein to the systemic circulation at the left renal vein. High pressures are maintained in the portal vein, which continues to perfuse the liver. Nonselective shunts decompress the entire portal system, reducing portal pressure throughout, and often result in stagnation or reversal of the portal hepatic flow. This reduction in prograde hepatic blood flow may result in hepatic encephalopathy.

24. **What is hepatic encephalopathy?**
Hepatic encephalopathy is a constellation of central nervous system symptoms occurring in patients with chronic liver disease and in some patients who undergo portosystemic shunting. Symptoms may range from minor personality changes to frank psychosis, with most patients demonstrating lethargy, asterixis, and confusion. Factors responsible for hepatic encephalopathy include increased systemic ammonia levels resulting from breakdown of blood by colonic bacteria in conjunction with depressed liver function and increased sensitivity of the central nervous system.

25. **What is the treatment of encephalopathy?**
Acute encephalopathy is treated by diminishing dietary protein intake, purgation of the colon, and administration of lactulose (30 ml every 6 hours) and neomycin (1 gm every 6 hours) by mouth. Patients with chronic encephalopathy who fail to respond to this medical regimen may require ileostomy, colectomy, or colonic exclusion.

26. **What criteria are used to select patients for elective shunt operations?**
Most patients who survive an episode of documented variceal hemorrhage should be considered for an elective operation designed to prevent rebleeding. Prime candidates are patients under the age of 60 with good hepatic and nutritional function according to Child's classification. The venous phase of selective splenic and superior mesenteric arteriograms and preoperative measurements of portal and caval venous pressures are required preoperatively.

27. **What is Child's classification?**

CHILD'S CLASSIFICATION

	A	B	C
Serum bilirubin (mg/dl)	Below 2.0	2.0-3.0	Over 3.0
Serum albumin (mg/dl)	Over 3.5	3.0-3.5	Under 3.0
Ascites	None	Easily controlled	Poorly controlled
Neurologic disorder	None	Minimal	Advanced
Nutrition	Excellent	Good	Poor

Child's classification is based on an assessment of hepatic function and nutrition. Patients who are Child's class A are good-risk patients and have low operative mortality. Those in Child's class C are high-risk patients with correspondingly higher operative mortality.

28. **What is the operative mortality for elective portosystemic shunts? What percentage of patients rebleed? What is the cause of rebleeding?**
The operative mortality in elective portosystemic shunts is 5% for Child's A, 10% for Child's B, and 20 to 40% for Child's C patients. Rebleeding occurs in approximately 5% of patients, usually due to thrombosis of the shunt.

29. **What operations are used for emergency treatment of variceal hemorrhage?**

The goal of emergency operation for variceal hemorrhage is control of bleeding. Less concern is placed on postoperative sequelae (encephalopathy) when exsanguination is the alternative. A form of central (nonselective) portosystemic shunt is usually employed in the emergency setting. The most expeditious shunt is performed by placing a graft between the proximal superior mesenteric vein and the vena cava (mesocaval shunt). Other emergent operations including direct esophageal varix ligation, splenectomy, or esophageal transection are often only temporarily effective in controlling bleeding.

30. What management options are available for patients who are at risk of repeat variceal hemorrhage (elective treatment)?
Elective operations for high-risk patients (Child's C) are probably not warranted. Survival in this group is limited regardless of treatment and most are best managed with chronic injection sclerotherapy. Better risk patients (Child's A and B) are best treated with some form of portosystemic shunt. In patients with favorable anatomy (patent splenic vein, normal left renal vein), a selective splenorenal shunt is preferred because of the lower incidence of hepatic encephalopathy.

BIBLIOGRAPHY

1. Burnett, D.A., and Sorrell, M.F.: Alcoholic cirrhosis. Clin. Gastroenterol.,10:443, 1981.
2. Cello, J.P. et al.: Endoscopic sclerotherapy versus portocaval shunt in patients with severe cirrhosis and variceal hemorrhage. N. Engl. J. Med.,311:1589-1593, 1984.
3. Chojkier, M., and Conn, H.O.: Esophageal tamponade in the treatment of bleeding varices: A decadal progress report. Dig. Dis. Sci., 25:267, 1980.
4. The Copenhagen Esophageal Varices Sclerotherapy Project: Sclerotherapy after first variceal hemorrhage in cirrhosis. A randomized multicenter trial. N. Engl. J. Med., 311:1574-1600, 1984.
5. Sivak, M.V.: Endoscopic sclerotherapy of esophageal varices. Gastroenterology Series, Vol. 1. New York, Praeger Publishers, 1984.
6. Warren, W.D., et al.: Ten years of portal hypertensive surgery at Emory: Results and new perspectives. Ann. Surg., 195:530-542, 1982.

36. DYSPHAGIA
RICHARD K. PARKER, M.D.

1. What is dysphagia?
Dysphagia is difficulty swallowing or inability to swallow. It is usually a subjective type of complaint, and it is rather difficult to date the exact time of onset as well as the cause. Often, however, the patient will provide a general idea of the area of difficulty, such as upper, middle, or lower section of the esophagus.

2. What causes dysphagia?
In general, dysphagia can be broken down into several different categories or etiologies: (1) anatomic disorders such as congenital abnormalities or atresias, as well as webs, cysts, and rings that may conform to the contour of the esophagus;

(2) congenital neurologic problems, such as chalasia or achalasia, or acquired neurologic problems such as strokes or other degenerative diseases; (3) inflammatory changes in the esophagus resulting from the presence of foreign bodies, infections, or reflux; and (4) benign tumors such as myomas, and malignant tumors, which are usually primary squamous cell carcinomas of the mid and upper esophagus, as well as adenocarcinomas at the gastroesophageal junction or extending from the stomach itself.

3. **Does the etiology differ according to the age of the patient?**
Certainly the pediatric age group has problems entirely different from those of adult or elderly populations. Newborn infants with dysphagia usually present with atresias (versus esophageal webs), vascular rings, or congenital neurologic problems. However, toddlers may present with chalasia, vascular rings, foreign bodies, cysts, or strictures. Adolescents usually have neurologic problems, duplication cysts, or strictures caused by reflux. In adults, strictures resulting from reflux esophagitis, cysts, acquired neurologic problems, or tumors are likely. In elderly patients, neurologic problems, diverticula, neoplasms, foreign bodies, and strictures may cause dysphagia.

4. **How is a newborn infant with dysphagia evaluated?**
The first and easiest test is to pass a nasogastric tube into the stomach to verify patent versus atretic esophageal anatomy. Also, radiographs of the chest and abdomen should be obtained.

5. **In a child, what would be the next step?**
After a history is taken and a physical examination performed, one should proceed directly to a barium swallow study; endoscopy should also be considered.

6. **In evaluating an adult, would you proceed differently?**
Once again, the history and physical examination will usually provide information about the problem. Following a barium swallow study, the patient should also be given an endoscopic examination with biopsy. Manometric studies should be considered to evaluate the neurologic function of the esophagus.

7. **What thought process is involved after you have obtained the studies mentioned above?**
Generally the first step is to differentiate physiologic or motor disorders from anatomic disorders.

8. **What can be done for motor disorders?**
The treatment for motor disorders is to try to establish the primary problem and to treat the primary disease process. If primary treatment fails, one may have to resort to a feeding gastrostomy with or without a spit fistula in the neck.

9. **What is the difference between chalasia and achalasia?**
In chalasia, there is inability of muscle to tighten, and therefore the esophagus remains wide open throughout. This permits a conduit from the mouth to the stomach; however, there is minimal or no motility seen. The greatest problem this creates is free reflux from the cardioesophageal junction back into the esophagus. Achalasia is the inability of the esophagus to relax, creating a persistent stricture that does not allow the upper esophagus to empty totally. On examination the abnormal muscular area is that of the small tight esophagus, not of the dilated esophagus above this level.

10. What are the common anatomic abnormalities found in the esophagus?
Stricture, neoplasm (both benign and malignant), foreign bodies, dupication cysts, and diverticula.

11. What type of cysts are usually seen in the esophagus?
The cysts found alongside the esophagus are usually duplication cysts, which result from congenital remnants. These may present at an early age, or may not present until adolescence or adulthood.

12. What causes diverticula of the esophagus?
In the upper esophagus, the diverticula are usually Zenker's, which results from a hypertensive cricopharyngeal muscle and may or may not be associated with a stroke. Traction diverticula usually occur in the midesophagus as a result of inflammatory changes of the subcarinal lymph nodes and are usually associated with tuberculosis or other granulomatous diseases. The distal esophagus may be affected by an epiphrenic hernia which is also the result of chronic inflammatory disease.

13. When should one consider dilatation versus direct repair of esophageal strictures?
All strictures should be evaluated by endoscopy and biopsy. If the biopsy confirms a benign process, the treatment of choice is repeated esophageal dilatations. Failure of the esophagus to remain open following repeated dilatation is indication for open repair combined with an antireflux procedure.

14. Which types of tumors occur in the esophagus?
Benign tumors are usually myomas or occasionally other types of small duplication cysts along the esophageal wall. However, the most common malignant tumor is carcinoma of the esophagus; sarcomas also occur occasionally. Metastatic tumors rarely involve the esophagus with the exception of direct extension of the lung carcinoma.

15. Do different types of tumors occur at various levels of the esophagus?
Primary squamous cell carcinomas usually occur in the upper and midesophagus, and are more prevalent in persons with a history of significant alcohol intake and in smokers. Tumors in the distal third of the esophagus are more likely to be adenocarcinomas occurring at the gastroesophageal junction or in the location of a Barrett's esophagus. An adenocarcinoma of the stomach may extend directly from the fundus into the esophagus.

---

37. REFLUX ESOPHAGITIS
LAWRENCE W. NORTON, M.D.

---

1. What symptoms suggest reflux esophagitis?
Frequent substernal burning discomfort after meals or at night associated occasionally with regurgitation of gastric juice is typical. Pain is relieved by sitting up. Severe disease can cause dysphagia because of stricture.

2. **What is the difference between heartburn and reflux esophagitis?**
    The lay term "heartburn" can describe the discomfort of reflux esophagitis but, generally, it refers to mild intermittent reflux without esophagitis.

3. **Is an upper GI series a useful first step in diagnosing esophageal reflux?**
    No. Barium studies cannot confirm reflux and do not establish esophagitis.

4. **Is hiatal hernia an essential finding in the diagnosis of reflux esophagitis?**
    No. Hiatal hernia is associated with reflux esophagitis in only 80% of patients.

5. **What is the initial treatment of patients with symptoms of reflux esophagitis?**
    (1) Diet management (avoid overeating; avoid foods that relax the lower esophageal sphincter such as chocolate); (2) avoidance of tight clothing, which increases intraabdominal pressure; (3) elevation of head of bed on 6-inch blocks; and (4) antacid therapy.

6. **What steps should be taken if initial treatment fails to relieve symptoms within 4 to 6 weeks?**
    Endoscopy is indicated to confirm the presence of esophagitis. Cimetidine and metoclopramide may be added to the treatment regimen.

7. **If esophagitis cannot be identified by endoscopy, can symptomatic reflux be confirmed?**
    The Bernstein acid test determines whether acid dripped onto the distal esophageal mucosa reproduces the patient's pain and suggests that reflux is responsible for the symptom.

8. **When should an operation be recommended for symptomatic reflux esophagitis?**
    Failure of nonoperative treatment should be demonstrated over several months (perhaps a year) before operation is recommended. Exceptions are patients with stricture or ulceration in the distal esophagus.

9. **What is the goal of operation?**
    The primary objective of an operative procedure is to stop gastroesophageal reflux by mechanically improving the competency of the lower esophageal sphincter. Secondary goals are to preserve esophagogastric motility and to return the stomach to the abdomen.

10. **What procedures are available to prevent reflux?**
    One transthoracic and three transabdominal operations are used currently. The Belsey IV operation, performed through the chest, and the Nissen fundoplication each provide an "ink-well"-type valve at the cardia by wrapping the stomach around the esophagus. The Hill gastropexy secures the cardia to preaortic fascia. The Angelchik prosthesis, an experimental device, restores competence by increasing the acuteness of the cardia angle. See figures on pages 111 and 112.

11. **Which operation is best?**
    Difference in results after the Belsey IV, Nissen, and Hill operations is slight. The Angelchik prosthesis appears to be at least as effective as the other procedures in preventing reflux.

The following three figures were redrawn from Nardi, G.L., and Zuidema, G. D. (eds.): Surgery: Essentials of Clinical Practice. Boston, Little, Brown, 1982, pp. 404-405, with permission.

BELSEY IV OPERATION

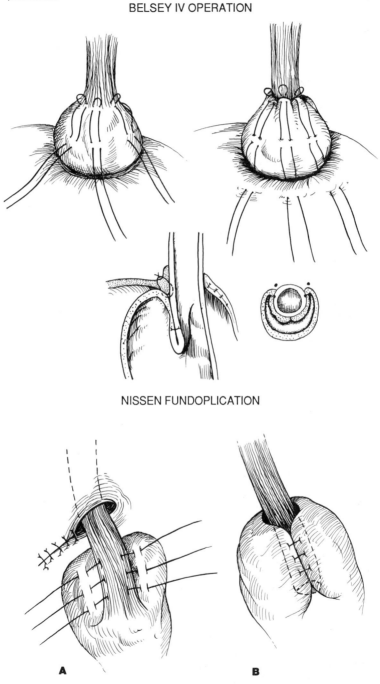

NISSEN FUNDOPLICATION

A   B

HILL GASTROPEXY

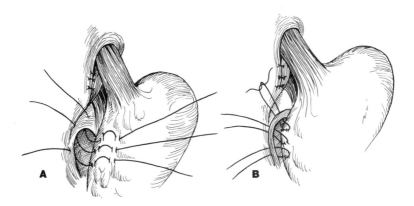

12. **Can these operations cause problems or fail?**
Yes. The Nissen fundoplication can cause the "gas-bloat" syndrome. The Nissen fails (10 to 20%) because of loss of wrap or "slippage." Rarely, the wrapped stomach perforates. The Belsey and Hill procedures fail slightly more often but cause fewer complications. The Angelchik prosthesis may dislodge, disrupt, or erode into an adjacent viscus.

13. **How can stricture from reflux esophagitis be managed?**
Pliable (unfixed) strictures can be dilated. Fixed strictures require surgical repair. One such operation is to patch the narrowed esophagus with stomach wall (Thal).

CONTROVERSY

14. **Is the Angelchik prosthesis effective?**
Despite widespread use and popularity because of ease of insertion, this prosthesis is condemned by many surgeons for its high rate of complications. Two studies show it to be more effective than Nissen fundoplication.

BIBLIOGRAPHY

1.   Brand, D.L., Eastwood, J.R., Martin, D., et al.: Esophageal symptoms, manometry and histology before and after antireflux surgery: A long-term study. Gastroenterology, 76:1398, 1979.
2.   Johnson, L.F., and DeMeester, T.R.: Evaluation of elevation of the head of the bed, bethanechol and antacid foam tablets on gastroesophageal reflux. Dig. Dis. Sci., 26:673, 1981.
3.   Richter, J.E., and Castell, D.O.: Gastroesophageal reflux. Ann. Intern. Med., 97:93, 1982.
4.   Starling, J.R., Reichelderfer, M.O., Pellett, J.R., et al.: Treatment of symptomatic gastro-esophageal reflux using the Angelchik prosthesis. Ann. Surg., 195:686, 1982.
5.   Winnan, G.R., Meyer, C.T., and McCallum, R.W.: Interpretation of the Berstein test: A reappraisal of criteria. Ann. Intern. Med., 96:320, 1982.

38. ESOPHAGEAL CARCINOMA
MICHAEL R. JOHNSTON, M.D.

1. **Esophageal carcinoma accounts for only 1 to 3% of all cancers in the U.S. In what three countries is this disease a major cause of death from cancer?**
Iran, China, and South Africa.

2. **Which population group In the U.S. is most at risk for the development of esophageal carcinoma?**
Elderly black males in the southeast section of the country.

3. **What benign disorders of the esophagus are considered to be "premalignant"?**
Barrett's esophagus, leukoplakia, achalasia, Plummer-Vinson syndrome, caustic injuries to the esophagus, and probably scleroderma.

4. **What is Barrett's esophagus?**
A glandular metaplasia of the esophageal mucosa, usually secondary to chronic reflux esophagitis.

5. **Dysphagia and weight loss are common findings in a patient presenting with esophageal carcinoma. What pulmonary findings will these patients often exhibit?**
Aspiration pneumonia secondary to esophageal obstruction.

6. **Mass screening has been used successfully to diagnose esophageal carcinoma in some Oriental countries. What technique is most often used?**
Exfoliative cytology using a mesh-covered balloon catheter.

7. **What findings on the preoperative work-up militate against a "curative" resection?**
A totally obstructing lesion; acute angulation or cavitation of the esophageal lumen demonstrated by barium swallow study; a lesion longer than 5 cm; constant, boring back pain; tracheoesophageal fistula; and vocal cord paralysis.

8. **Which sites are most commonly involved with distant metastatic esophageal carcinoma?**
Liver, lung, and bone.

9. **In treating a patient with esophageal carcinoma, what is the overriding consideration no matter what treatment modality is chosen? Why?**
Palliation, i.e., the ability to swallow oral secretions and maintain reasonable oral alimentation, is of primary importance. Although aggressive attempts at curative therapy should be made in good-risk patients, results are so poor that durable palliation should be the major consideration.

10. **With the thoracic esophagus being a left-sided structure, why is the surgical approach to the mid and upper esophagus through a right thoracotomy?**

The esophagus passes behind the aortic arch as the aorta passes from an anterior to a left posterior mediastinal structure. This effectively shields the upper portion of the esophagus from easy accessibility through a left-sided approach. On the right side, the only intervening structure is the azygous vein, which can be sacrificed with impunity.

CONTROVERSIES

11. **In the good-risk patient with a small localized carcinoma of the distal esophagus, what is considered the primary treatment?**
    Most clinicians believe that lesions at or below the level of the aortic arch should be surgically resected while those above the arch should have primary radiation therapy. Others believe that since the surgical cure rate is low (10 to 30% 5-year survival) and the risk from surgery substantial (5 to 20%), all patients should be irradiated. Combined modality therapy, most recently with chemotherapy followed by surgery, may be advantageous, but as yet is unproved.

12. **Other than surgical resection, what options are available to a patient with an obstructing esophageal carcinoma?**
    There are many approaches other than surgical resection for the patient with an obstructing carcinoma; however, there is no unanimity as to the best approach. Radiation therapy is effective in relieving the obstruction if the tumor is not invading contiguous structures. However, tracheoesophageal, bronchoesophageal, or aortoesophageal fistulas may occur when invasive tumors are irradiated. Also, even though radiation therapy will usually open an obstructing lesion, the palliation is not durable and at least 50% of patients will have reobstruction before they die. Another option is to place an endoesophageal prosthetic tube to maintain patency of the esophagus. Placement of these tubes is difficult and, even in experienced hands, carries a 5 to 25% mortality. Dislodgement and impaction of the tubes are frequent occurrences and most patients can swallow only liquids. Esophageal diversion by performing a cervical esophagostomy and a gastrostomy for feeding is considered by most experienced clinicians as unacceptably poor palliation. The esophagostomy is difficult to manage and patients generally find long-term maintenance of nutrition by gastrostomy feedings intolerable. Laser recanalization of the esophageal lumen has recently been successful in relieving esophageal obstruction. More experience and longer follow-up is needed with this appealing approach. Basically, there are multiple methods available to relieve a malignant esophageal obstruction because none is ideal. An individualized approach to each patient and the experience of the clinician are the key ingredients for successful palliation.

BIBLIOGRAPHY

1. Ellis, F.H., and Gibb, S.P.: Esophagogastrectomy for carcinoma. Ann. Surg., 190:699, 1979.
2. Franklin, R., Steiger, Z., Vaishampayan, G., et al.:   Combined modality therapy for esophageal squamous cell carcinoma. Cancer, 51:1062, 1983.
3. Murray, G.F., Benson, R.W., and Starek, P.J.K.:   The assessment of operability of esophageal carcinoma. Ann. Thorac. Surg., 23:393, 1977.
4. Naef, A.P., Savary, M., and Ozzello, L.: Columnar-lined lower esophagus: An acquired lesion with malignant predisposition. J. Thorac. Cardiovasc. Surg., 70:826, 1975.
5. Pearson, J.G.: The value of radiotherapy in the management of squamous oesophageal cancer. Br. J. Surg., 58:794, 1971.
6. Postlethwait, R.W.:   Squamous cell carcinoma of the esophagus.   In Surgery of the Esophagus. New York, Appleton-Century-Crofts, 1979.

39. UPPER GASTROINTESTINAL BLEEDING
MICHAEL MILL, M.D.

1. **What is upper gastrointestinal bleeding?**
Upper gastrointestinal bleeding occurs from lesions of the gastrointestinal tract proximal to the ligament of Treitz. The usual presentation is that of hematemesis and/or melena.

2. **How much blood loss is necessary to cause melena?**
As little as 50 ml of blood can cause clinically obvious melena. With a bleed of 1000 ml, melena can persist for 5 days, and stool can remain Hemoccult-positive for 3 weeks.

3. **What salient features of a patient's history must always be obtained?**
(1) Prior history of symptoms or diagnosis of peptic ulcer disease; (2) a history of cirrhosis or alcohol abuse; (3) history of retching; and (4) an accurate history of drug abuse, including ethyl alcohol, salicylates, steroids, nonsteroidal anti-inflammatory agents, etc. (i.e., any "barrier breakers").

4. **List the differential diagnosis for an upper gastrointestinal hemorrhage and the relative frequencies of each.**
(1) Peptic ulcer disease, 50 to 52% (duodenal ulcers occur 4 times more frequently than gastric ulcers, although they have an equal propensity for bleeding); (2) acute mucosal lesions, 13 to 18%, which include esophagitis, gastritis, "stress ulcers," etc.; (3) esophagogastric varices, 8 to 14%; (4) Mallory-Weiss tears, 7 to 8%; (5) gastric neoplasms, 2 to 4%, which include carcinomas, leiomyomas, leiomyosarcomas, and lymphomas; (6) diaphragmatic hernias, 2% (reflux esophagitis from hiatal hernias, hemorrhagic gastritis in paraesophageal hernias); (7) hemobilia, 1%; and (8) miscellaneous: arteriovenous malformations, duodenal diverticula, polyps, aortic, hepatic artery, splenic artery aneurysms with fistulas, and aortoduodenal fistulas after aneurysm surgery.

5. **How often is upper gastrointestinal bleeding the first symptom of peptic ulcer disease?**
Sixteen percent of patients with bleeding ulcers will present with melena as the first symptom of peptic ulcer disease.

6. **In patients with hemorrhage secondary to peptic ulcer disease, which vessel is the culprit in duodenal ulcers? In gastric ulcers?**
Duodenal ulcers, gastroduodenal artery. Gastric ulcers, left or right gastric artery.

7. **What is the anatomic location of acute mucosal lesions in the stomach?**
Erosions are generally multiple rather than single and typically occur in the body and fundus, sparing the antrum, and involve the lesser and greater curvatures with equal frequency.

8. **What are the most common causes of upper gastrointestinal hemorrhage in cirrhotic patients?**
(1) Esophagogastric varices, 53%, of which 70% will be massive bleeds; (2) gastritis, 22%, of which 84% will be mild to moderate bleeds; and (3) peptic ulcer disease, 20%.

9. **Which diagnosis is responsible for the majority of deaths from upper gastrointestinal bleeding?**
    Esophagogastric varices.

10. **Define Cushing's ulcers and Curling's ulcers.**
    Cushing's ulcers: acute gastroduodenal lesions following intracranial operations or severe head injuries. Described in 1932. *Curling's ulcers*: acute gastroduodenal lesions associated with major burn injuries occur in 12% of hospitalized patients with burns. Incidence increases with size of burn. Described in 1842.

11. **What is the most common cause of upper gastrointestinal bleeding in children?**
    Esophagogastric varices secondary to extrahepatic portal vein obstruction.

12. **What are the symptoms of hemobilia?**
    Intermittent colicky pain, jaundice, and hematemesis.

13. **What initial steps should be taken in the work-up and management of a patient with upper gastrointestinal bleeding?**
    (1) Establishment of intravenous access. Preferably a central line and 1 or 2 large-bore peripheral lines for volume replacement and monitoring of fluid status. (2) Nasogastric or Ewald tube to confirm diagnosis and to clear the stomach of blood and to gauge continued bleeding. (3) Foley catheter to monitor urine output. (4) Laboratory values: (a) hematocrit may be unreliable initially because equilibration takes 4 to 8 hours, but should be monitored every 4 to 6 hours, (b) PT/PTT and platelet count to rule out coagulopathy, (c) BUN will be elevated owing to blood absorption in the GI tract, and (d) liver function tests to rule out underlying liver disease. (5) Blood transfusion and replacement of blood components (FFP, platelets).

14. **What are the best methods for diagnosing upper gastrointestinal hemorrhage?**
    (1) Esophagogastroduodenoscopy is the most reliable method (85 to 95% accuracy). (2) Technetium sulfur scans may be helpful in patients with intermittent bleeding, but are compromised by liver and spleen uptake, which may obscure the exact location of bleeding. (3) Selective angiography of the celiac axis and superior mesenteric artery is 90% accurate if blood loss is at least 3 to 5 ml/minute and is 20% accurate for varices with venous phase film. (4) Upper gastrointestinal contrast series is 56% accurate for ulcers, 50% accurate for varices, 25% accurate for acute mucosal lesions, and has a false-negative rate of 24%. (5) Laparotomy for emergent situations in which other studies have been inconclusive.

15. **What are the nonsurgical options for the management of upper gastrointestinal bleeding?**
    Iced-saline gastric lavage, antacids for peptic ulcer disease and acute mucosal lesions, intraarterial or intravenous vasopressin (0.2 to 0.4 units/minute), and Sengstaken-Blakemore tube for variceal hemorrhage. Note that H2 blockers, though widely used, have not been demonstrated to be effective in controlling acute upper gastrointestinal bleeding.

16. **What are the indications for operative intervention?**
    (1) Blood loss of 2000 to 2500 ml during the first 24 hours, or 1500 ml during the second 24 hours; (2) hematocrit < 25; (3) recurrent bleeding during the initial hospitalization; (4) significant history of peptic ulcer disease or recurrent bleeding from peptic ulcer disease; and (5) associated illnesses or advanced age, which make patients poor risks for tolerating shock or stress from significant or recurrent hemorrhage.

17. What are the surgical options for treatment of upper gastrointestinal bleeding?

(1) Duodenal ulcers: ligation of the bleeding vessel, and definitive ulcer operation (vagotomy) and pyloroplasty, vagotomy and antrectomy, highly selective vagotomy). (2) Gastric ulcer: vagotomy and pyloroplasty or hemigastrectomy with or without vagotomy. All ulcers must be biopsied to rule out malignant disease, and preferably wedged out if not included in a standard gastric resection. (3) Acute mucosal lesions: vagotomy and pyloroplasty or vagotomy and antrectomy. Total gastrectomy is no longer advocated. (4)Varices: endoscopic sclerosis, esophagogastric devascularization (Sugiura procedure), and emergency portocaval shunt. (5) Mallory-Weiss tears, oversewing of tears. (6) Cancer: of distal stomach, hemigastrectomy; of proximal stomach, total gastrectomy. (7) Diaphragmatic hernias: hiatal hernia, antireflux procedure; paraesophageal hernia, reduction of hernia and plication of diaphragm. (8) Hemobilia: intrahepatic, hepatic resection; extrahepatic, arterial ligation or repair.

CONTROVERSIES

18. Should all patients with massive upper gastrointestinal bleeding undergo immediate endoscopy?

For: In the hands of experienced endoscopists, endoscopy is a relatively safe (complication rate 0.25%), rapid, and accurate (85 to 95%) means of diagnosing the etiology of upper gastrointestinal bleeding. Early knowledge of the exact location and type of bleeding lesion can facilitate further resuscitative efforts and aid in choosing the appropriate operation should early operative intervention be indicated.

Against: Special expertise is required, and massive bleeding may make accurate diagnosis technically difficult, if not impossible. Emergency endoscopy in critically ill patients does carry increased risks of aspiration and respiratory compromise. More accurate and useful information may be obtained after initial resuscitation and stabilization, followed by endoscopy on a nonemergent basis.

19. Should vasopressin be administered intraarterially?

For: Intraarterial infusion allows maximal concentration of the vasoconstrictive drug at the actual bleeding site. It can be used as an adjunct to angiography in those patients requiring angiograms to localize the source of gastrointestinal bleeding. Intraarterial vasopressin has been shown to be effective in controlling bleeding, especially from esophagogastric varices and acute mucosal lesions.

Against: Intraaterial vasopressin administration requires invasive angiographic procedures and maintenance of accurate catheter position to prevent inadvertent infusion into other vascular regions or the liver. Excessive local administration may lead to local bowel ischemia and infarction. The overall complication rate has been reported as high as 35%. Recently, intravenous vasopressin infusion has been demonstrated to be as efficacious, and safer and easier to administer than by the intraarterial route.

20. Should gastric lavage be performed with iced saline?

For: Iced saline theoretically produces local mucosal hypothermia and vasoconstriction, which may reduce or stop bleeding, especially from acute mucosal lesions.

Against: Studies have not clearly demonstrated any benefit to the use of iced saline. Rather it appears that the mechanical action of the lavage in removing blood clots from the gastric lumen and in preventing gastric distention is responsible for any beneficial results from gastric lavage.

BIBLIOGRAPHY

1. Atkenson, R.J., and Nyhus, L.M.: Gastric lavage for hemorrhage in the upper part of the gastrointestinal tract. Surg. Gynecol. Obstest., 146:797, 1978.
2. Chojkier, M., Broszmann, R.J., et al.: Controlled comparison of continuous intraarterial and intravenous infusions of vasopressin in hemorrhage from esophageal varices. Gastroenterology, 77:540, 1979.
3. Conn, H.O., Ramsby, G.R., Storer, E.H., et al.: Intraarterial vasopressin in the treatment of upper gastrointestinal hemorrhage: A prospective, controlled clinical trial. Gastroenterology, 68:211, 1975.
4. Dronfield, M.W., Langman, M.J.S., Atkinson, M., et al.: Outcome of endoscopy and barium radiography for acute upper gastrointestinal bleeding: Controlled trial in 1037 patients. Br. J. Med., 248:545, 1981.
5. Himal, H.S., Perrault, C., and Mzabi, R.: Upper gastrointestinal hemorrhaage: Aggressive management decreases mortality. Surgery, 84:448, 1978.
6. Peterson, W.L., Barnett, C.C., Smith, H.J., et al.: Routine early endoscopy in upper gastrointestinal bleeding: A randomized, controlled trial. N. Engl. J. Med., 304:925, 1981.
7. Villar, H.V., Fender, H.R., Watson, L.C., et al.: Emergency diagnosis of upper gastrointestinal bleeding by fiberoptic endoscopy. Ann. Surg., 185:367, 1977.

---

40. DUODENAL ULCER DISEASE
M.A. AMMONS, M.D., and G. VAN STIEGMANN, M.D.

---

1. Who gets duodenal ulcers?

Five percent of the United States' population has active peptic ulcer disease. Men have an incidence 3 to 4 times higher than that of women. Duodenal ulcers are 10 times more common than gastric ulcers in the young population, but the incidence equalizes with increasing age. The overall incidence of duodenal ulcers has been declining for unknown reasons and is now about half that of 20 years ago.

2. What causes duodenal ulcers?

Duodenal ulcers tend to occur in patients who have hypersecretion of gastric acid. They may, however, also occur in those with normal acid secretion. Back-diffusion of gastric acid through a "leaky" mucosal barrier may play a role in the development of duodenal ulcers but is probably more important in gastric ulcers.

3. What are the stimuli for gastric acid secretion?

1. Cephalic phase: sight, smell, taste, or thought of food increases gastric acid secretion via vagal stimulation.

2. Gastric phase: distention of the gastric antrum and products of protein digestion stimulate gastrin release.

3. Intestinal phase: food in the small bowel releases a hormone (enteroxyntin) that increases acid release.

4. What inhibits gastric acid secretion?

An antral pH less than 2.5 inhibits gastrin release. Somatostatin may also serve as an inhibitor of gastrin release. Secretin and CCK-PZ block acid secretion experimentally but may not be physiologically important.

5. What physiologic abnormalities have been observed in patients with duodenal ulcer?

(1) Increased numbers of parietal and chief cells, (2) increased sensitivity of parietal cells to gastrin stimulation, (3) increased gastrin response to a meal, (4) decreased inhibition of gastrin release in response to acidification of gastric contents, and (5) increased rates of gastric emptying. Not all of the above abnormalities are present in every patient with duodenal ulcers.

6. **Are there any physiologic markers for patients at high risk for developing duodenal ulcers?**
    Blood group O is associated with a higher incidence of duodenal ulcer. Twenty-five percent of people do not secrete blood group antigens (H, A, B) in gastric juice and are also at high risk for developing duodenal ulcer.

7. **What other groups are at high risk?**
    Patients with multiple endocrine adenopathy, type I, have a 50 to 85% incidence of gastrinoma with severe ulcer diathesis. Patients with chronic liver or lung disease and those with chronic pancreatitis may also be at higher risk.

8. **What are the symptoms of a duodenal ulcer?**
    1. Pain is the most common presenting symptom of duodenal ulcer. Usually burning or gnawing and located in the midepigastrium, the pain is well localized. Radiation to the back is a sign of pancreatic penetration. Pain often occurs before meals or at night (early morning) and is relieved by ingestion of food or antacids. Pain may also be episodic with long periods of remission. Nausea and vomiting may also occur, even in the absence of obstruction.
    2. Bleeding (see chapter on Upper Gastrointestinal Bleeding).
    3. Obstruction may occur as a result of inflammatory mass, pyloric spasm, or secondary to repeated episodes of duodenal scarring and fibrosis. Obstruction usually results in nausea, vomiting, and anorexia, which may lead to severe metabolic debilitation.
    4. Perforation constitutes a surgical emergency and has an associated mortality rate of 5 to 10%. Ulcers located on the anterior surface of the duodenum are prone to perforation and may perforate without a significant prior history of duodenal ulcer disease. Free air is present on upright chest x-ray films in about 80% of patients.

9. **What medical treatment is appropriate for treatment of duodenal ulcers?**
    1. Diet: barrier breakers (aspirin, nonsteroidal anti-inflammatory agents) should be avoided. Although increased frequency of meals may be useful in symptomatic treatment, there is no evidence that dietary restrictions are beneficial to healing.
    2. Antacids are useful in neutralizing gastric pH and are prescribed 1 to 3 hours after meals.
    3. H2 antagonists, cimetidine or ranitidine, decrease acid secretion.
    4. Sucralfate adheres to the ulcer base, providing a resistant coating to the actions of pepsin and acid digestion.
    5. Bismuth compounds also provide a coating action and are used widely for gastric ulcers.

10. **What is the success rate of medical treatment?**
    With the above treatment schemes, approximately 75 to 95% of duodenal ulcers will heal in 4 to 6 weeks. Recurrence is common, however, and 70% will recur within 1 year of cessation of treatment.

11. **What complications are associated with medical treatment?**

Magnesium-containing antacids may cause diarrhea and calcium-containing agents may cause constipation. H2 receptor blockers may induce changes in mental status, gynecomastia, interference with cytochrome oxidase-metabolized drugs (anticoagulants, diazepam, propranolol, and lidocaine), and others. Potential for developing gastric cancer, once thought to be a possible complication of H2 blockers, does not appear likely.

12. **How is gastric analysis performed and when should it be employed?**
Gastric analysis may be useful when severe ulcer diathesis leads to suspicion of Zollinger-Ellison syndrome. Basal acid output (BAO) is measured in milliequivalents per hour under fasting conditions, and maximal acid output (MAO) is measured after histamine, pentagastrin, or betazole (Histalog) stimulation. Normal BAO is 1.5 to 2.5 and in patients with duodenal ulcers averages 3 to 5.5. MAO is normally 20 to 30 but averages 30 to 40 in patients with duodenal ulcers. Gastric analysis is infrequently used today because of availability of serum gastrin analysis. There is great overlap in values of normal and abnormal acid secretion, and neither proclivity for ulcer development nor rationale for type of operative treatment can be based accurately on gastric analysis.

13. **When should serum gastrin levels be obtained?**
Serum gastrin levels should be obtained in patients who present with recurrent ulcers after operation, multiple ulcers, or ulcers in unusual locations, and in all patients with evidence of endocrine adenomatosis syndromes. Normal serum gastrin levels are 50 to 100 pg/ml. Patients with G-cell hyperplasia may exhibit values up to 400 to 500, whereas those with Zollinger-Ellison syndrome are generally above 500.

14. **How is the diagnosis of duodenal ulcer made?**
Barium study of the upper gastrointestinal tract may have a false-negative rate of up to 50%, particularly if superficial mucosal ulcerations are present. Flexible upper gastrointestinal endoscopy in experienced hands has a 95% sensitivity with corresponding specificity and allows complete visualization of the entire upper gastrointestinal tract.

15. **What are the indications for operative treatment of duodenal ulcers?**
Failure of medical management to control bleeding, obstruction, and intractability are common indications. Perforation of the duodenal ulcer is nearly an absolute indication unless the patient is seen 24 to 48 hours following the event and Gastrografin in the upper gastrointestinal series confirms that perforation is well sealed.

16. **What operations are used to treat duodenal ulcer?**
(1) Truncal vagotomy and pyloroplasty or gastrojejunostomy, (2) vagotomy and antrectomy with B1 or B2 anastomosis (without vagotomy), (3) subtotal gastrectomy with B1 or B2 anastomosis (without vagotomy), (4) highly selective vagotomy, and (5) total gastrectomy.

17. **What is the rate of recurrence of ulcer following surgical treatment?**
Vagotomy and pyloroplasty, 10%
Vagotomy and antrectomy, 1 to 2%
Subtotal gastrectomy, 1 to 2%
Highly selective vagotomy, 10 to 15%
Total gastrectomy, less than 1%

18. **What is the mortality of these operations when performed electively?**
Vagotomy and pyloroplasty, 1%; vagotomy and antrectomy, 1–3%; subtotal gastrectomy, 1–3%; highly selective vagotomy, 0.1%; total gastrectomy, 2–5%.

19. **What is the treatment for perforated duodenal ulcer?**
Graham closure is commonly used and consists of closing the defect with an omental patch secured by several seromuscular sutures placed on either side of the perforation. An acid-reducing operation (highly selective vagotomy, vagotomy and pyloroplasty) may be used in addition but only in very fit patients with a longstanding history of ulcers. Definitive operations such as these should not be performed for perforations that have gone untreated for more than 6 to 12 hours.

20. **What is the long-term result following Graham closure of a perforated ulcer?**
One third will remain asymptomatic, one third will have symptoms controlled by medical treatment, and one third will require definitive ulcer operation.

21. **What are Billroth I and Billroth II anastomoses?**
Billroth I anastomosis refers to an anastomosis between the duodenum and the gastric remnant (gastroduodenostomy). Billroth II is constructed by sewing the jejunum to the gastric remnant (gastrojejunostomy). Billroth I is generally preferred to Billroth II, but objective superiority of one over the other is difficult to measure. See figure below. (Adapted from Nardi, G.L., and Zuidema, G.D. (eds.): Surgery: Essentials of Clinical Practice. Boston, Little, Brown, 1982, p. 493.)

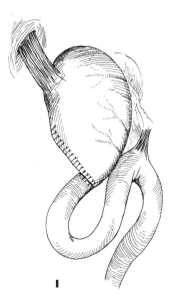

I

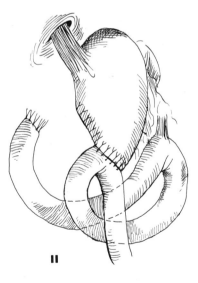

II

22. Who was Billroth?
Christian Albert Theodor Billroth (1829 to1894) was an Austrian surgeon credited with performing the first gastric resection in 1881.

23. What are the early complications of operation for duodenal ulcer disease?
1.   Duodenal stump leakage may occur following a Billroth II anastomosis. Three to six days postoperatively, the patient may experience severe upper abdominal pain and appear toxic and febrile. Treatment consists of prompt reoperation and controlled drainage of the leaking duodenal closure.
2.   Gastric retention may occur because of edema at the anastomosis or atony of the stomach following vagotomy. Gastric retention usually resolves spontaneously, although 3 to 4 weeks may be required in some cases.
3.   Bleeding may occur from a suture line, a missed ulcer, or from other gastic mucosal lesions. Most postgastrectomy bleeding ceases spontaneously; however, endoscopy and electrocoagulation or laser treatment may be necessary in some cases.

24. Where do ulcers recur following operation?
Ulcers usually recur adjacent to the gastric anastomosis on the intestinal side (jejunum, duodenum).

25. What factors may account for recurrent ulceration?
Recurrent ulcers may occur because of inadequate gastric resection, incomplete vagotomy, inadequate drainage of the gastric remnant (stasis of gastric contents proximal to the anastomosis), or from retained gastric antrum (Billroth II anastomosis).

26. What is a Roux-en-Y operation?
A Roux-en-Y anastomosis is created to prevent reflux of bile and pancreatic secretions into the stomach. Such reflux may produce troublesome symptoms referred to as a "bile reflux gastritis." See figure below. (Redrawn from Keen, G.: Operative Surgery and Management. Bristol, Wright/PSG, 1981, p. 47.)

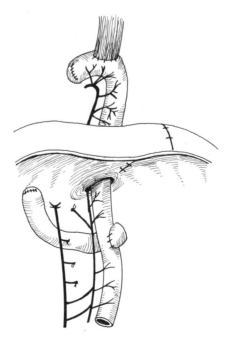

27. What is the dumping syndrome?
The dumping syndrome is a collection of symptoms occurring after gastric resection and is experienced by 10 to 20% of patients in the early postoperative period, but remains a long-term problem in only 1 to 3%. Following ingestion of food, patients experience nausea, vomiting, crampy abdominal pain, diaphoresis, flushing, diarrhea, and, occasionally, syncope. The rapid entry of a hypertonic bolus of food into the small bowel is responsible for the osmotic and glucose shifts which produce these symptoms. Dietary manipulation (low carbohydrate and high fat and protein content), in addition to anticholinergic drugs, usually alleviates the symptoms. Rarely, further corrective operations may be needed to reverse severe cases.

28. What is the afferent loop syndrome? How may it be prevented?
Afferent loop syndrome refers to postprandial abdominal pain which is often relieved by bilious vomiting. The mechanism consists of a narrowing at the junction of the stomach and duodenal side of a Billroth anastomosis. Biliary and pancreatic secretions build up within this afferent limb, causing pain. Relief of pain occurs when the contents are discharged into the stomach, often resulting in vomiting or severe bile reflux. Prevention requires avoidance of a long or twisted afferent limb and construction of a patent anastomosis.

BIBLIOGRAPHY

1.   Carter, D.C. (ed.):   Clinical Surgery International, Vol. 7:   Peptic Ulcer. New York, Churchill Livingstone, 1983.
2.   Bunte, H., and Langhans, P.: A Century of Ulcer Surgery: Medical and Surgical Therapy Today. Baltimore, Urban & Schwarzenburg, 1984.
3.   Goligher, J.C., et al.: Several standard elective operations for duodenal ulcer: Ten to 16 year clinical results. Ann. Surg., 198:18, 1979.
4.   Korman, M.G., et al.: Relapse rate of duodenal ulcer after cessation of long-term cimetidine treatment: A double-blind controlled study. Dig. Dis. Sci., 25:88,1980.
5.   Schirmer, B.D., et al.: Marginal ulcer: A difficult surgical problem. Ann. Surg., 195:653, 1982.
6.   Fiore, A.C., et al.: Surgical management of alkaline reflux gastritis. Arch. Surg., 117:689, 1982.
7.   Kennedy, T.: The failure of gastric surgery. Br. J. Surg., 68:677, 1981.

41. GASTRIC ULCERS AND GASTRIC CANCER

GEORGE MOORE, M.D., and CHARLES ABERNATHY, M.D.

BENIGN GASTRIC ULCERS

1. What is the key concept in the initial management of gastric ulcers?

That they may be either benign *or* malignant (as opposed to duodenal ulcers).

2. What are the techniques for evaluating a gastric ulcer?

Gastroscopy and biopsy are the most direct. An upper gastrointestinal series can be helpful but is not diagnostic; it will differentiate duodenal from gastric ulcers.

3. How do benign gastric ulcers differ from duodenal ulcers?

Benign ulcers are difficult to treat and have a high incidence of recurrence and complications. It is estimated that benign gastric ulcers are responsible for 50% of the deaths caused by peptic ulcer disease.

4. What is a "trial of healing"?

A trial of therapy (antacids, H2 antagonist) for 6 weeks to see if ulcer heals 90%. Few experienced surgeons bypass this "trial" and proceed directly to operation (primarily because of the high incidence of recurrence of benign ulcers and the small but definite false-negative rate on endoscopic biopsy).

5. Can a malignant gastric ulcer show healing?

Yes. Some gastric ulcers with foci of malignant disease heal completely on a medical regimen.

6. Do H2 antagonists help to heal benign gastric ulcers?

The efficacy of H2 antagonists in benign ulcers has yet to be established. The mainstay of therapy continues to be antacids.

7. Which operation is done for benign gastric ulcer?

Operation usually is a hemigastrectomy or subtotal gastrectomy without vagotomy. The ulcer is removed with the specimen if possible.

8. What if the ulcer is so high (proximal) in the stomach that it cannot be removed with a subtotal gastrectomy?

Usually the ulcer is "wedged" out. A supplementary acid-reducing operation is optional. The age of the patient and the cause or causes of the ulcer are important factors.

9. Do patients with gastric ulcers have hyperacidity?

Usually not (fewer than 5%). The etiology of benign gastric ulcers is thought to be mucosal injury (by "barrier breaker" medications such as aspirin or bile salts or corticoid-like substances). (See the chapter on Duodenal Ulcer.)

10. How do malignant ulcers differ from benign ones?

Clinically impossible to distinguish. Very large ulcers in the elderly and those on "barrier breaker" medications are usually benign. Endoscopy and biopsy is the only sure way to differentiate. Very large shallow ulcers are usually benign.

11. How important is gastric cancer?

About 15,000 persons die from gastric cancer yearly; it is the seventh most common cause of death from malignant disease.

12.   The epidemiology of gastric ulcers and gastric cancers varies enormously between countries.   Are there any clues as to etiologic factors?
There are many fascinating statistics, such as the high incidences in Japan, Chile, the Pacific islands, and in the Scandinavian countries. The incidence of gastric cancer has fallen rapidly over the last 30 years. The age-adjusted death rate in the United States has fallen from 30 to 5 deaths per 100,000 affected. Even in Japan there is some decrease in occurrence of gastric ulcers. The hypothesis for the pandemicity of gastric cancer and its subsequent decline have included dietary changes, the use of refrigeration, the influenza of 1918 to 1920 (viral origin), and many others. It is ironic that specific factors have not been identified in this most significant decrease of all lethal cancers.

13.   How is atrophic gastritis related to gastric cancer?
Studies from several countries have suggested that atrophic gastritis and intestinal metaplasia are precancerous alterations of the gastric mucosa and that the risk of subsequent cancer in 10 to 20 years is related to the extent of the gastritis.

14.   Is pernicious anemia a causal factor in gastric cancer?
It is estimated that 5 to 10% of such patients develop gastric cancer even if treated adequately.

15.   There are over 2000 reported cases of gastric cancer developing after gastric resections for duodenal ulcer. Is this coincidental?
Gastric cancer has developed after various operations of the stomach. The median time to development is about 20 years; however, the incidence of gastric cancer can be expected to be higher in all patients who are 20 years older. The thesis may be correct, but it is a very weak carcinogenic factor.   Perhaps such operations promote atrophic gastritis.

16.   When should one operate upon gastric cancer and what should be done?
1. Curative gastrectomy. Whenever possible, partial gastrectomy is performed since multiple primary cancers are rare. Usually 80 to 90% of the stomach is resected with inclusion of the nodes along the major vessels. Radical resection of the stomach including a more extensive dissection and excision of the body and tail of the pancreas and the spleen is associated with a higher mortality rate and no greater number of cures.
2. A patient with metastases. Patients with distant and liver metastases or ascites rarely benefit from palliative bypass operations. The median survival is about 3 months. The diagnosis can be established by gastroscopy. Both enteral catheters and intravenous hyperalimentation may be used for nutritional support.
3. A patient in whom the adjacent organs are involved. The resection of gastric cancer that has directly infiltrated into the left lateral lobe of the liver, the mesocolon, or the pancreas is reasonable because there is a slight chance (5%) of cure, and there is a modest palliation (3.9 months).
4. Total gastrectomy is required for some diffuse lesions, especially if located along the lesser curvature. The operation may also be required for large malignant lymphomas. The mortality and morbidity associated with this operation are much higher and it should rarely be used for palliation.

17.   Is radiation therapy or chemotherapy of therapeutic value for gastric cancer?

Radiation therapy as an adjuvant to resection of gastric lymphomas may cure 40% of patients. It is of little value against the epithelial malignant diseases. Chemotherapy is relatively useless even for palliation. Combinations of drugs with 5-fluorouracil or cisplatin have provided a few extra months of survival but at the cost of toxicity and a risk of prolonged and expensive hospitalization. Adjuvant chemotherapy is ineffective. Second-look operations and resections of multiple metastases are ineffective.

18. **What is the outcome of performing subtotal and total gastrectomies?**
The immediate mortality rates are about 3% and 10%, respectively, and 15% if extended resections of the distal pancreas and spleen are done.

19. **What is the survival expectancy for patients in the United States with resected lesions without and with metastases?**
About 15% and 5% at 5 years. There are no effective adjuvant therapies except curative radiation therapy for gastric lymphomas. The Japanese report much higher survival figures because of a difference in tumor biology.

20. **What postoperative instructions are helpful to patients who undergo partial or total gastrectomies?**
A majority of patients will suffer some degree of dumping syndrome, which consists of faintness, lowered blood pressure, and nausea after eating. This can be reduced by eating more meals (6 per day) with smaller volumes of food. Liquids should be taken separately from meals. Patients often develop a distaste for sweets, milk, and meats, but will eat cheeses and tart foods. Patients should lie down for 15 to 30 minutes after eating whenever possible. The head should be slightly elevated to minimize regurgitation. A permanent 15% weight loss can be expected.

21. **What is Sister Mary Joseph's sign?**
Dr. William Mayo's long-time surgical assistant, Sister Mary Joseph, noted that patients with a hard nodule at the umbilicus and an intraabdominal malignancy (particularly gastric cancer) did not do well, thus making the association of metastases to the umbilicus with intraabdominal cancer.

BIBLIOGRAPHY

1. Au, F.C., et al.: The role of cytology in the diagnosis of carcinoma of the stomach. Surg. Gynecol., 151:601, 1980.
2. Bizer, L.S.: Adenocarcinoma of the stomach: Current results of treatment. Cancer, 51:743, 1983. In a review of 171 patients, only 10% lived for 5 years.
3. Boddle, A.W., Jr., et al.: Palliative total gastrectomy and esophagogastrectomy: A reevaluation. Cancer, 51:1195, 1983.
4. Dupont, J.B., Jr.: Adenocarcinoma of the stomach: Review of 1497 cases. Cancer, 41:941, 1978. Of 84 patients who had total gastrectomy, only 6 survived 5 years.
5. Gastrointestinal Tumor Study Group: A comparative clinical assessment of combination chemotherapy in the management of advanced gastric carcinoma.Cancer, 49:1362, 1982.
6. Kaibara, N., et al.: Significance of mass survey for gastric cancer from the standpoint of surgery. Am. J. Surg., 142:543, 1981. In Japan, 20 to 25% of all cases of gastric cancer are detected by mass survey.
7. Lawrence, W.T., and Lawrence, W., Jr.: Gastric cancer: The surgeon's viewpoint. Semin. Oncol., 7:400, 1980.
8. Ochsner, A., Weed, T.E., and Neussle, W.R.: Cancer of the stomach. Am. J. Surg., 141:10, 1981. Endoscopy should be used liberally.

42. SMALL BOWEL OBSTRUCTION

MICHAEL MILL, M.D.

1. **Name the three mechanisms for the development of small bowel obstructions and give an example of each one.**
   (1) Obturation of the bowel lumen: e.g., gallstone ileus, bezoars, foreign bodies, and worms; (2) mural disease with encroachment of the lumen: e.g., inflammatory conditions (regional enteritis, tuberculosis, eosinophilic granulomas), carcinoma, traumatic or radiation strictures, and hematomas; and (3) extrinsic lesion: e.g., adhesions, hernias, carcinomatosis, and intraperitoneal abscesses.

2. **What are the most common causes of small bowel obstructions today?**
   (1) Adhesions from prior abdominal procedures; (2) incarcerated or strangulated hernias (in order of frequency): inguinal, femoral, umbilical, and ventral hernias; and (3) neoplasms. These three, listed in order of frequency, account for 80% of all cases of small bowel obstruction.

3. **What are the most common presenting symptoms?**
   Abdominal pain begins as a diffuse, poorly localized, cramping pain that coincides with the waves of peristalsis as the bowel tries to force its contents past the obstruction. Vomiting is more frequent and profuse with proximal obstructions and is bilious in nature; it is less frequent and "feculent" in nature in distal obstructions. There is failure to pass flatus and feces. Note that abdominal distention is a late symptom.

4. **What are the most common physical findings on presentation?**
   Mild, diffuse abdominal tenderness (severe, localized tenderness or signs of peritoneal irritation are indicative of complications, and may also indicate the cause of the obstruction); high-pitched, "tinkling" bowel sounds; an old abdominal scar; and abdominal distention, generally a late finding.

5. **What systemic manifestations are often present?**
   Dehydration, low urine output, and low-grade fever.

6. **What is the single best diagnostic test to establish the diagnosis?**
   Three-way view of the abdomen, or "obstruction series," which includes a posteroanterior chest film and upright and supine abdominal films.

7. **What are the characteristic findings on the three-way series?**
   (1) Distended loops of small bowel with air and fluid levels arranged in a "step-ladder" or "inverted J" pattern; (2) absence of rectal gas; (3) elevated hemidiaphragms due to bowel distention; (4) a "ground-glass" appearance suggests ascites secondary to peritoneal extravasation of fluid from the congested, edematous bowel wall; and (5) free air, if present, is an ominous sign of bowel perforation.

8. **What laboratory abnormalities are usually present?**
   (1) Increased BUN secondary to dehydration and decreased urine output. (2) Increased urine specific gravity. (3) Mild metabolic acidosis. (4) WBC may be normal or slightly elevated. If > 15,000, this suggests strangulated bowel; if > 40,000, a mesenteric vascular occlusion should be suspected. (5) Severe electrolyte abnormalities (increased Na^+, decreased Cl^-, decreased HCO_3^-)

127

suggest severe, longstanding obstruction. (6) Hyperamylasemia suggests strangulated or dead bowel.

9. **Name the three types of obstruction based upon bowel viability.**
Simple obstruction: the lumen is obstructed, but the blood supply is not compromised. *Strangulated obstruction:* twisting of the mesentery has resulted in vascular compromise of the involved bowel. *Closed loop obstruction:* both limbs of the involved segment are obstructed; the vascularity is compromised, and the involved loop cannot decompress itself proximally, resulting in massive distention and a high risk of rupture or perforation.

10. **What steps should be taken in the initial treatment of small bowel obstructions?**
(1) Intravenous fluid resuscitation to correct dehydration, fluid and electrolyte abnormalities, and establish adequate urine output. (2) Nasogastric suction to decompress proximal distention. In some patients, this may prevent a partial obstruction from becoming a complete obstruction, and avoid an operation (see Controversies). (3) Timed surgical intervention.

11. **How can a partial obstruction be differentiated from a complete obstruction?**
The most important clinical finding is the continued passage of flatus or feces. An upper GI contrast series (see Controversies).

12. **List the differential diagnosis for a patient with a presumed mechanical small bowel obstruction.**
　　1. Paralytic ileus
　　History: recent operation with prolonged return of bowel function, or associated illness, e.g., pneumonia, sepsis, renal failure, and retroperitoneal hematoma.
　　Physical examination: absence of bowel sounds.
　　Laboratory tests: three-way series shows both small and large bowel gas without differential air/fluid levels.
　　2. Mesenteric vascular occlusion
　　History: elderly patient with recent MI or atrial fibrillation; sudden, severe abdominal pain.
　　Physical examination: abdominal tenderness out of proportion to physical findings.
　　Laboratory tests: markedly elevated WBC count, hyperamylasemia, unexplained, persistent metabolic acidosis.
　　3. Large bowel obstruction
　　History and physical examination: marked abdominal distention before significant symptoms appear.
　　Laboratory tests: three-way series shows distended gas-filled colon.

13. **What factors must be considered in the timing of surgical intervention?**
　　1. Duration of obstruction, especially the severity of fluid and electrolyte abnormalities. Prolonged obstructions should forego a trial of "conservative" therapy (IV hydration/nasogastric suction), and proceed to more urgent surgery.
　　2. Development of signs of peritoneal irritation, markedly elevated WBC count, or hyperamylasemia suggests strangulated and/or dead bowel.
　　3. Improvement of vital organ function: cardiovascular stability, and adequate renal and pulmonary function must be assured in order for a patient to tolerate a general anesthesia and laparotomy.

4.   In general, the old adage "never let the sun rise or set on a bowel obstruction" still holds. The above factors can be adequately evaluated and corrected within 6 to 8 hours.

14.   Who performed the first recorded surgical procedure for an intestinal obstruction?
Praxagoras created an enterocutaneous fistula to relieve an obstruction in 350 B.C.

15.   List the surgical options at the time of laparotomy.
    1.   Lysis of adhesions.
    2.   Reduction and repair of hernias.
    3.   Bypass of obstructing lesions.
    4.   Enterocutaneous fistula proximal to the obstruction, especially for perforation and/or significant peritoneal contamination.
    5.   Resection of obstructing lesions with primary anastomosis.
    6.   Resection of compromised or dead bowel with exteriorization or primary anastomosis.
    7.   Placement of long intestinal tube to minimize risk of recurrent obstruction (see Controversies).

16.   What are the best gross criteria of bowel viability at laparotomy?
Color, peristalsis, and arterial pulsations. Other methods used include fluorescein dye, Doppler studies, "nicking" the serosa to gauge bleeding, all with variable accuracy reported.

17.   What is the mortality of surgical treatment of small bowel obstructions?
Modern, timely treatment has reduced the mortality from 50% three decades ago, to <1% in patients operated upon with 24 hours of presentation. The mortality for strangulated hernias still remains ~ 25%.

18.   What is the risk of recurrent obstruction after laparotomy?
Many authors estimate the lifetime risk of developing an obstruction secondary to adhesions after laparotomy to be about 20%. However, which patients will be affected cannot be accurately predicted by any specific criteria, although some individuals have a tendency to form adhesions.

19.   Can adhesion formation be prevented?
No. Although adhesions can be demonstrated to be caused by intraperitoneal sepsis, blood in the peritoneal cavity, and foreign bodies (including talc from surgical gloves, and lint from gowns, drapes, laparotomy pads, etc.), nothing has been shown to significantly prevent or reduce adhesion formation. Novel treatments attempted include instillation of saline or heparin into the peritoneal cavity, the use of long intestinal tubes, and the closing, or not closing , of surgical incisions of the peritoneum (see Controversies).

CONTROVERSIES

20.   Nasogastric versus long tube decompression (Miller-Abbott or Cantor tubes).
Although long tubes (passed transpylorically to just above the obstruction) may decompress the obstructed bowel more efficiently than nasogastric tubes, they require more time and effort for proper placement, and may lead to unneccessary delays in definitive treatment. Their use has been gradually abandoned in favor of nasogastric suction and appropriately timed surgery.

21. **Upper gastrointestinal contrast x-rays.**
Water-soluble or thin barium contrast material given orally or via a nasogastric tube may be of use in differentiating partial from complete obstruction and in pinpointing the location and occasionally the cause of an obstruction. If a complete obstruction is identified, then nasogastric suction must be promptly resumed, and the surgeon prepared for expeditious surgical intervention to prevent aspiration or perforation from the fluid added to the already distended bowel.

22. **Long tubes to prevent recurrent obstruction secondary to adhesions.**
Baker tubes placed nasogastrically or via gastrostomy or jejunostomy have been used to "stent" the small bowel after laparotomies for recurrent obstructions. Theoretically they allow the bowel to become "plicated" in gentle curves as new adhesions form, although the long-term efficacy of such tubes has not been conclusively demonstated.

23. **Peritoneal intergrity and adhesion formation?**
Although some surgeons contend that closing the peritoneum of incisions covers a "raw" facial surface and prevents adhesions, others have demonstrated that the abdominal cavity reperitonealizes by growth of mesenchymal rests on intraabdominal surfaces and not by ingrowth from the edges of cut peritoneum. They further contend that closing the peritoneum actually promotes adhesion formation by interfering with normal healing in addition to adding foreign bodies (sutures) that may act as a nidus for adhesion formation.

BIBLIOGRAPHY

1. Baker, J.W.: Selective usage of the original and modified Baker intestinal tube. Surg. Gynecol. Obstet., 149:577, 1979.
2. Bizer, L.S., Liebling, R.W., Delaney, H.M., and Gliedman, M.L.: Small bowel obstruction: The role of nonoperative treatment in simple intestinal obstruction and predictive criteria for strangulation obstruction. Surgery, 89:407, 1981.
3. Ellis, H.: Collective review: The cause and prevention of postoperative intraperitoneal adhesions. Surg. Gynecol. Obstet., 133:497, 1971.
4. Hofstetter, S.R.: Acute adhesive obstruction of the small intestine. Surg. Gynecol. Obstet., 152:141, 1981.
5. Stewardson, R.H., Bombeck, C.T., and Nyhus, L.M.: Critical operative management of small bowel obstruction. Ann. Surg., 187:189, 1978.
6. Weigelt, J.A., Snyder, W.H., III, and Norman, J.L.: Complications and results of 160 Baker tube plications. Am. J. Surg., 140:810, 1980.

---

43. INTESTINAL ISCHEMIA
WILLIAM PEARCE, M.D., and MARY MOCKUS, PH.D.

PREOPERATIVE

1. **Will chronic occlusion of one of the three major arteries be sufficient to produce the clinical signs of intestinal ischemia?**
No. The abundant collateral circulation between the celiac artery, superior mesenteric artery, and inferior mesenteric artery will generally provide adequate flow to the gut even when one of these three vessels are occluded.

2.   **What are the causes of intestinal ischemia?**
     Decreased low and/or a redistribution of flow due to hypovolemia, shock, heart failure, mesenteric vasoconstriction, bowel obstruction, vasculitis, or emboli. Preoperatively, arteriography is useful in differentiating between atherosclerotic stenosis or occlusion, embolism, and low flow. Where ischemia is the result of a gradual process, the arteriogram will reveal the development of collaterals. When the ischemia is caused by a more abrupt process (emboli), the block in flow may be visualized as well as the failure to develop a rich collateral blood supply. Low-flow states will be apparent as poor filling throughout the vascular bed.

3.   **What is the pathogenesis of nonocclusive mesenteric ischemia and what is the associated mortality rate?**
     Nonocclusive mesenteric ischemia results from splanchnic vasoconstriction in response to decreased cardiac output, hypovolemia, vasopressors, or hypotension. Predisposing factors include myocardial infarction, congestive heart failure, renal failure, hepatic failure, or major intraabdominal or thoracic surgery. The mortality rate is 90%.

4.   **What is the typical presentation of chronic intestinal ischemia?**
     Food avoidance from recurrent postprandial intestinal angina, nonspecific abdominal pain, and ischemic gut.

5.   **What is the diagnostic triad of acute superior mesenteric artery occlusion?**
     Catastrophic abdominal pain, gut-emptying by vomiting and/or diarrhea, and cardiac disease, often with a past history of emboli.

6.   **How often is abdominal pain absent in intestinal ischemia?**
     Twenty-five percent of patients will not present with the characteristic picture of acute abdominal pain that is out of proportion to physical findings.

7.   **What laboratory findings are suggestive of intestinal ischemia?**
     Early in the course of the disease, there may be no abnormalities in blood chemistry, and in highly suspicious cases, arteriography should be performed. Late in the course of the disease, the following may be observed: increased hematocrit and hemoglobin concentration due to plasma loss into the gut, unexplained metabolic acidosis due to anaerobic metabolism, leukocytosis due to an inflammatory reaction, elevations in serum amylase, LDH and CPK, and Hemoccult-positive stools.

8.   **What drug causes constriction of the superior mesenteric artery?**
     Digitalis.

9.   **What is celiac artery compression syndrome?**
     Compression of the celiac artery by the crus of the diaphragm. The diagnosis can be difficult to make because angiography may reveal a narrowing of the celiac artery in asymptomatic patients. In addition, the narrowing of the celiac artery in symptomatic patients often does not correlate well with the severity of symptoms. Minimal diagnostic criteria include postprandial abdominal pain, weight loss, an abdominal bruit, and a smooth narrowing of the superior portion of the celiac artery by angiogram.

10. **How does the distribution of intestinal ischemia differ in patients with atherosclerotic occlusion *versus* superior mesenteric artery embolus?**

See Figure below. *Left*, the distribution of intestinal ischemia with an embolus to the superior mesenteric artery. Note the sparing of the proximal jejunum and right colon. *Right*, the distribution of intestinal ischemia following thrombosis of the origin of the superior mesenteric artery.

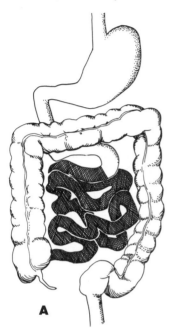 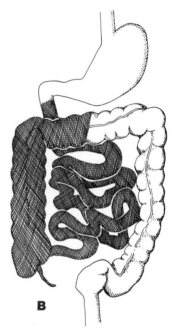

A   B

11. **What conditions are associated with mesenteric venous thrombosis?**

Hypercoagulable states such as polycythemia, venous outflow obstruction, intraabdominal sepsis, and abdominal trauma.

OPERATIVE

12. **What are the collateral arteries between the celiac trunk and the superior mesenteric artery?**

The superior and inferior pancreaticoduodenal arteries via the gastroduodenal artery.

13. **In patients with either atherosclerotic occlusion or embolism and intestinal ischemia, what is the most appropriate management?**

Revascularization and resection. Resection alone is associated with 90% mortality. Revascularization improves the mortality rate to around 50%.

14. **What are the surgical options in the management of ischemic gut?**

Revascularization may be achieved by direct thromboendarterectomy, bypass grafting, or reimplantation.

15. **Intraoperatively, what techniques can be applied to determine bowel viability?**
Palpable mesenteric pulses, Doppler, and fluorescein.

16. **When and on what criteria is a decision made for a second-look operation?**
The decision is made intraoperatively. Thirty to forty-five minutes after revascularization of the bowel, the viability of the intestines is assessed and dead bowel is resected. A decision to reoperate 12 to 24 hours later may then be made to further evaluate the status of the bowel, as clinical signs may not be helpful at this time. Also, fluid and electrolyte status may be improved during the interval betwen the first and second surgery.

17. **How much small intestine is required to sustain adequate nutrition? Is the ileocecal valve important?**
50 to 100 cm. Yes. The ileocecal valve is important, at least in experimental models.

18. **What is the aortoiliac steal syndrome?**
When the aortoiliac circulation is repaired, the increased flow to the extremities leads to decreased flow in the meandering mesenteric artery. If there is significant disease in the celiac and superior mesenteric arteries, the decrease in flow to the meandering mesenteric artery may lead to intestinal ischemia.

19. **What is the long-term prognosis following revascularization for chronic intestinal ischemia?**
Eighty to ninety percent of patients have good pain relief; 75% of patients have relief of malabsorption.

20. **What is the cause of death in most patients with chronic intestinal ischemia?**
Atherosclerotic coronary artery disease.

21. **What are some of the sequelae of revascularization and gut ischemia?**
Poor healing of the anastomosis, stricture formation, and intestinal fistula formation.

BIBLIOGRAPHY

1. Brandt, W. , and Boley, S.J.: Celiac axis compression syndrome: A critical review. Am. J. Dig. Dis., 23:633, 1978.
2. Connolly, J.E., and Kwaan, J.H.M.: Management of chronic visceral ischemia. Surg. Clin. North Am., 62:345, 1982.
3. Hen, F.W., Silen, W., and French, S.W.: Intestinal gangrene without apparent vascular occlusion. Am. J. Surg., 110:231, 1965.
4. Stoney, R.J., Ehrenjeld, W.K., and Wylie, E.J.: Revascularization methods in chronic visceral ischemia caused by atherosclerosis. Ann. Surg., 186:468, 1979.
5. Stoney, R.J., and Olcott, C.: Visceral artery syndromes and reconstructions. Surg. Clin. North Am., 59:637, 1979.
6. Zelenock, G.B., et al.: Splanchnic arteriosclerotic disease and intestinal angina. Arch. Surg., 115:497, 1980.

44. DIVERTICULAR DISEASE OF THE COLON
LAWRENCE W. NORTON, M.D.

1. **What causes colonic diverticula?**
    Two theories are popular . One postulates a weakness of the bowel wall at the site of vessel perforation that allows mucosal extrusion. The other relates diverticula to increased intraluminal pressure as a result of low dietary fiber and chronic constipation (Burkitt).

2. **How can a diverticulum cause pain?**
    Pain is apparently the result of perforation of the diverticulum. The resulting leakage may be scant and contained within pericolic fat or be extensive involving the mesentery, other organs, or peritoneal cavity.

3. **Where are diverticula usually located in the colon?**
    Most are in the left colon but diverticula of the right colon and cecum are not rare.

4. **At what age is diverticulitis most common?**
    After age 50.

5. **What treatment would you recommend to decrease the risk of diverticulitis in a patient with multiple diverticula?**
    A diet high in fiber (bran, cellulose, etc.) appears to reduce the risk of diverticulitis.

6. **What is the best means of diagnosing diverticular disease?**
    Barium enema examination is superior to colonoscopy in detecting and detailing colonic diverticula.

7. **Can diverticular disease cause bleeding?**
    Yes. Bleeding occurs at some time in about 25% of patients with multiple diverticula. The disease accounts for at least half of all instances of colonic bleeding.

8. **How can bleeding be localized to one diverticulum or colon segment?**
    The most accurate means of localization is angiography performed via the inferior mesenteric artery and, if necessary, the superior mesenteric artery. Tagged red blood cell studies are less useful. Colonoscopy is rarely helpful.

9. **If a bleeding site is located in the colon, when should operation be performed?**
    Replacement of 5 to 6 units of blood within 24 hours or rebleeding during hospitalization are indications for emergency resection of a segment of colon containing a bleeding diverticulum.

10. **If bleeding is life-threatening but cannot be localized within the colon, what treatment is required?**
    Subtotal colectomy with ileostomy and closure of the sigmoid colon at the peritoneal reflection (Hartmann's operation).

11. **When perforation of a diverticulum results in an intraabdominal abscess, which of the following causes the lowest operative mortality?**

(1) Diverting colostomy with abscess drainage? (2) Resection of involved colon with proximal colostomy and distal mucous fistula or closure (Hartmanr, pouch)? or (3) Resection with primary anastomosis? (See Controversy). Operative mortality is lowest after resection and proximal colostomy for fecal diversion.

12. **What is the clinical evidence of a vesico- or urethro-colic fistula following diverticular perforation?**
Pneumaturia.

13. **What procedure is required to repair vesico- or urethro-colic fistula?**
If pneumaturia occurs early after diverticulitis, a proximal diverting colostomy is performed. About 3 months later, the involved colon is resected, the colostomy is taken down, and the colon is anastomosed primarily. If pneumaturia occurs late or is longstanding, preliminary diversion by means of colostomy is unnecessary.

CONTROVERSY

14. **Can a primary anastomosis be done for acute perforated diverticulitis?**
Resection and primary anastomosis for acute perforation of a colonic diverticulum in the presence of an intraabdominal abscess causes complications in 30% of patients and death in 5%. Primary anastomosis after acute perforation without an abscess involves less risk but is not recommended despite the advantage of a one-stage operation.

BIBLIOGRAPHY

1. Behringer, G.E., and Albright, N.L.: Diverticular disease of the colon, a frequent cause of massive rectal bleeding. Am. J. Surg., 125:9, 1972.
2. Larson, D.M., Masters, S.S., and Spiro, H.M.: Medical and surgical therapy in diverticular disease: A comparative study. Gastroenterology, 71:723, 1976.
3. Painter, N.S., and Burkitt, D.P.: Diverticular disease of the colon: A deficiency disease of Western civilization. Br. Med. J., 2:450, 1971.
4. Winzelberg, G.G., Froelich, J.W., McKusik, K.A., et al.: Radionuclide localization of lower gastrointestinal hemorrhage. Radiology, 139:465, 1981.
5. Wise, L.: Surgical management of ruptured diverticulitis. Am. J. Surg., 14:122,1981.

45. ACUTE LARGE BOWEL OBSTRUCTION
ROBERT SAWYER, M.D.

1. **How is the diagnosis made?**
Physical examination reveals distention and high-pitched bowel sounds with rushes. A silent abdomen and localized tenderness are serious signs. Plain abdominal films show gas in the dilated colon with haustral markings.

2. **How is the diagnosis confirmed?**
Plain film is usually enough; however, if there is uncertainty, an unprepared barium enema is confirmatory.

3. **What causes large bowel obstruction?**
Cancer, diverticulitis, volvulus, and toxic megacolon.

4. **When do you operate?**
Early in colon obstruction. Danger signs are quiet abdomen, right lower quadrant tenderness, and increasing pain. Preoperative intravenous fluids, nasogastric suction, and antibiotics are necessary to prepare patients for surgery.

5. **Why is tenderness in the right lower quadrant important?**
The cecum is the area most likely to perforate. The larger diameter of the cecum causes more tension on the cecal wall at the same intraluminal pressure.

6. **Which operation should be performed?**
It is important to decompresss the colon before it perforates. Standard procedure is the decompressing colostomy. Adequate resection of a malignant tumor cannot be done satisfactorily under emergency conditions. Diverticulitis can be resected but an anastomosis cannot be done primarily. Volvulus should be reduced or resected; reduction is likely to recur.

7. **Where is the cancer usually located?**
In the left colon. Lesions of the right colon usually do not obstruct; they tend to bleed occultly.

8. **Where is the volvulus located?**
In either the sigmoid or the cecum. Right colon or cecal volvulus is a congenital entity caused by failure of the peritoneal attachments to form during the thirteenth week of gestation. Sigmoid volvulus occurs in the older population because the sigmoid elongates with diet changes in the elderly.

9. **What is toxic megacolon?**
Dilation of the entire colon secondary to acute ulcerative colitis, which may require an emergency colectomy with formation of an ileostomy.

10. **What is Ogilivie's syndrome?**
Ogilvie's syndrome is enormous dilation of the right colon without a mechanical obstructing lesion.

11. **How much can the cecum dilate before it is liable to perforate?**
When the cecum reaches 15 cm in diameter, the tension on the wall is so great that decompression is essential.

---

46. INFLAMMATORY BOWEL DISEASE
GILBERT HERMANN, M.D.

---

1. **What two clinical entities encompass the diagnosis of inflammatory bowel disease?**
Crohn's disease and ulcerative colitis, the latter being either acute or chronic.

2. **While there is often an overlap between these two diseases, they can usually be distinguished by clinical, radiologic, and pathologic criteria. What are some major clinical differences?**

Rectal bleeding is unusual in Crohn's disease but common in chronic ulcerative colitis. The findings of abdominal mass and anal complications (fissure, fistula) are more common in Crohn's disease (15 to 50%).

3. **What are some major radiologic differences?**
Terminal ileal involvement, skip areas, internal fistulas, and thumb printing are all rare or absent in chronic ulcerative colitis but common in Crohn's disease.

4. **What are some major morphologic differences?**
Granulomas in the intestinal wall and adjacent lymph nodes are absent in ulcerative colitis but occur in 60% of patients with Crohn's disease.

5. **Whereas Crohn's disease has been documented to affect the gastrointestinal tract from the pharynx to the anus, what are the most common clinical patterns of gastrointestinal involvement?**
Small-bowel-type only, 28%; both ileum and colon (ileocolitis), 41%; and colon only, 27%. This latter goes by several names, among those being Crohn's colitis and granulomatis colitis.

6. **Crohn's colitis and chronic ulcerative colitis are often difficult to distinguish clinically. What are some major differences that one can note on colonoscopy?**
The colonic appearance of Crohn's disease is that of focal, predominantly right-sided disease. The mucosa is cobblestone in appearance with transverse ulcerations in affected areas. Biopsies reveal transmural disease with focal granulomas. On colonoscopy, chronic ulcerative colitis usually appears as a diffuse disease. However, if only a portion of the colon is involved, it is on the left side and almost always involves the rectum. Pathologic changes involve primarily the mucosa and submucosa.

7. **What are major indications for surgery in Crohn's disease?**
It depends on the site of involvement. Enteroenteral fistulas (controversial), abscess, and intestinal obstruction are the most common indications for small intestinal and ileocolic types. Perianal disease and medical failure as well as ileocolic fistulas and abscess formation are the most common indications for surgery in the colonic type.

8. **How does this contrast with surgical indications in chronic ulcerative colitis?**
Medical intractability including failure to thrive in children, diarrhea, weight loss, and abdominal pain, toxic megacolon with or without perforation, and concern about development of colonic cancer (controversial) are the main indications.

9. **What is the surgical procedure for the treatment of ulcerative colitis?**
Total colectomy with formation of a standard ileostomy, Kock pouch, or ileoanal anastomosis (controversial). Ileorectal anastamosis with preservation of rectum has been advocated by some (controversial).

10. **What are the acceptable surgical procedures for the treatment of complications of Crohn's disease?**
Complications initiating surgery are surgically corrected by removing all areas of bowel involved in the complications, i.e., obstruction, abscess, etc. Grossly clear margins are satisfactory with maximum preservation of intestinal length. Skip areas are left alone, unless they are directly adjacent to resectioned intestine.

11. **What should the patient be told to expect regarding occurrence of the inflammatory bowel disease following surgery?**
With chronic ulcerative colitis, surgery is definitive and curative. With Crohn's disease, however, the aim of surgery is to treat the complications, i.e., obstruction, sepsis, etc. Recurrence can be expected in a high percentage of cases if the patient is followed long enough. The incidence of recurrence following total colectomy for Crohn's colitis is controversial.

CONTROVERSIES

12. **All patients with enteroenteral fistulas secondary to Crohn's disease should have surgery when the fistula is discovered.**
For: These patients do poorly, will develop further intraperitoneal septic complications and will always eventually need surgery.
Against: Studies have indicated that many patients with enteroenteral fistulas do well without operative treatment provided they remain asymptomatic.

13. **All patients with documented chronic ulcerative colitis for over 10 to 15 years, whether active or not, should have a colectomy to avoid the risk of carcinoma of the colon.**
For: The incidence of carcinoma of the colon overall is 3 to 5 %, which is 10 to 15 times higher than that for the general population. In addition, the cancers tend to be multifocal and are at a more advanced stage when diagnosed.
Against: Using biopsy techniques, only those patients whose colons show dysplastic changes need have a colectomy if the disease is quiescent.

14. **Ileorectal anastomosis is an acceptable operation following colectomy for ulcerative colitis.**
For: The patients have reasonable normal bowel habits and avoid the problems and complications associated with other procedures.
Against: At least 50% of these patients need to be reoperated upon for recurrence of disease. Also, the remaining rectum can be a site for the development of cancer.

15. **Standard (Brooke) ileostomy is a good way to handle the terminal ileum following total colectomy for chronic ulcerative colitis.**
For: Complication rate is very low. Over 90%+ of the patients studied lead very satisfactory lives.
Against: There are definite psycho-social-sexual problems associated with the use of external appliances. This is particularly true in the teenage group where chronic ulcerative colitis is quite common.

16. **The Kock pouch is a good procedure to use following colectomy for chronic ulcerative colitis.**
For: It avoids the use of an external appliance and is quite easy to manage.
Against: Approximately 20 to 30% of all patients who have a Kock pouch need to have a revision because of slippage of the valve mechanism allowing the pouch to become incontinent.

17. **An ileoanal anastomosis is a good operation following colectomy for chronic ulcerative colitis.**
For: It allows the patient to avoid any external appliances or ostomies. This is, of course, very well accepted by the patients.
Against: It is more difficult technically to construct, and, thus, the complication rate is higher. The average number of bowel movements is at least four to six a day, and there is sometimes soilage at night.

BIBLIOGRAPHY

1. Allan, R., et al.: Crohn's disease involving the colon: an audit of clinical mangement. Gastroenterology, 73:723, 1977. Followed 204 patients. Despite high morbidity, the long-term prognosis was good with appropriate surgery and limited use of corticosteroids.

2. Beart, R.W., et al.: Surgical management of inflammatory bowel disease. Curr. Probl. Surg., 1980. An excellent review article from the Mayo Clinic Group.

3. Broe, P.J., Bayless, T.M., and Cameron, J.L.: Crohn's disease. Are enteroenteral fistulas an indication for surgery? Surgery, 91:249, 1982. Enteroenteral fistulas, if asymptomatic, are by themselves not an indication for surgery. However, they are usually associated with active disease. If asymptomatic and patients required surgery later, there was no increased morbidity.

4. Buchmann, P., et al.: Natural history of chronic perianal Crohn's disease. Ten year follow-up: A plea for conservatism. Am. J. Surg., 140:642, 1980. Ten-year follow-up of 109 patients with Crohn's and perianal disease. Perianal complications of Crohn's disease pursue a benign course and are rarely an indication for proctectomy.

5. Butt, J.H., and Morson, B.: Dysplasia and cancer in inflammatory bowel disease. Gastroenterology, 80:865, 1981. Excellent editorial with bibliography setting forth the problems associated with detecting cancer prone patients with IBD by precancerous histologic changes on biopsy.

6. Farmer, R.G., Hawk, W.A., and Turnbull, R.B., Jr.: Indications for surgery in Crohn's disease. Analysis of 500 cases. Gastroenterology, 71:245, 1976. This study reveals the significant differences in surgical indications depending on the location of Crohn's disease.

7. Farmer, R.G., Hawk, W.A., and Turnbull, R.B., Jr.: Clinical patterns in Crohn's disease: a statistical study of 615 cases. Gastroenterology, 68:627, 1975. An excellent overview of the clinical aspects of Crohn's disease.

8. Fazio, Y.W.: Regional enteritis (Crohn's disease). Indications for surgery and operative strategy. Surg. Clin North Am., 63:27, 1983. Discusses in some detail the broad experience of the Cleveland Clinic with surgical aspects of regional enteritis.

9. Glotzer, D.J.: Operations in inflammatory bowel disease. Indications and type. Clin. Gastroenterol., 9:371, 1980. Good overview of entire subject by an experienced surgeon.

10. Goligher, J.C.: Procedures conserving continence in the surgical management of ulcerative colitis. Surg. Clin. North Am., 63:49, 1983. Discusses the pros and cons of the Kock pouch, ileoanal anastamosis and ileorectaol anastamosis following colectomy for ulcerative colitis.

11. Greenstein, A.J., et al: Reoperation and recurrence in Crohn's colitis and ileocolitis. N. Engl. J. Med., 293:685, 1975. A good study using actuarial methods. Shows an inexorable tendency of Crohn's ileocolitis to require reoperations, approaching 90% by the 15th year.

12. Johnson, W. R., et al.: Carcinoma of the colon and rectum in inflammatory disease of the intestine. Surg. Gynecol. Obstet., 156(2):193, 1983. Definite increased risk for colonic carcinoma in patients with longstanding ulcerative colitis. Reached 19% after 34 years. No increased risk with Crohn's colitis.13.

    Kewenter, J., Hulten, L., and Ahren, C.: The occurrence of severe epithelial dysplasia and its being on treatment on longstanding ulcerative colitis. Ann. Surg., 195:209, 1982. Another report attempting to determine the role of dysplasia found on biopsy as an indication for prophylactic colectomy in longstanding chronic ulcerative colitis.

14. Kock, N.G., et al.: Continent ileostomy. An account of 314 patients. Acta Chir. Scand., 147:67, 1981. Reviews the personal experience of the leader in this field. Revisional surgery for malfunction of the nipple valve has decreased to 6% in this report.

15. Locke, M.R., et al.: Recurrence and reoperation for Crohn's disease. The role of disease location in prognosis. N. Engl. J. Med., 304:1586, 1981. The initial distribution of disease determines the subsequent clinical course. The ileocolic type had the highest recurrence rates.

16. Meyer, S., Wolfish, J.S., and Sacher, D.B.: Quality of life after surgery for Crohn's disease. A psychosocial survey. Gastroenterology, 78:1, 1980. Study of 51 patients followed 5 to 10 years. Despite recurrence in 27 patients and ileostomy in 14, 47/51 patients were satisfied that surgery had substantially improved their preoperative status.

17. Nugent, F.W., et al.: Prognosis after colonic resection for Crohn's disease of the colon. Gastroenterology, 65:398, 1973. Follow-up of 33 patients over 16 years. Only 1 (3%) developed recurrent disease.

18. Pennington, L., Hamilton, S.R., Bayless, T.M., and Cameron, J.L.: Surgical management of Crohn's disease. Influence of disease at margins of resection. Ann. Surg., 192:311, 1980. The presence or absence of microscopic disease at the anastomosis did not influence anastomotic wound healing or the recurrence rate.

19. Steinberg, D.M., et al.: Sequelae of colectomy and ileostomy: comparison between Crohn's colitis and ulcerative colitis. Gastroenterology, 68:33, 1975. A study of over 500 patients. Patients with ulcerative colitis fared much better.

---

47. APPENDICITIS
BRUCE BARTON, M.D.

---

1. What is characteristically the first symptom of acute appendicitis?
Pain starting in the periumbilical area and moving to the right lower quadrant is classic.

2. Where is McBurney's point?
The junction of the outer one third and inner two thirds of a line joining the anterosuperior iliac spine and the umbilicus.

3. What is the blood supply to the right colon?
The ileocolic, right colic, and middle colic vessels.

4. Which abdominal layers are traversed in the exposure of the appendix through a McBurney incision?
From superficial to deep: aponeurosis of the external oblique, muscle, internal oblique muscle, transversalis fascia and muscle, and peritoneum.

5. What is the mortality of surgery for (a) nonperforated appendicitis? (b) perforated appendicitis?
(a) 0.1% or less. (b) approximately 3.5% (some modern series of perforated appendicitis have reported a < 0.5% mortality).

6. Who first correlated the clinical symptoms with the pathologic findings of inflammation of the appendix?
Fitz in 1886.

7. In what two groups of patients is the incidence of perforation of the appendix *greatest* prior to operation?
Young children (especially < age 5) and the elderly, in whom the incidence of perforation may reach 75%.

8. In children, what two other conditions commonly mimic acute appendicitis?

Gastroenteritis and mesenteric adenitis. Mesenteric lymphadenitis describes the inflammatory condition of the lymph nodes clustered in the mesentery of the terminal ileum, which presents with pain and tenderness of the right lower quadrant. Recently, *Yersinia enterocolitica* has been identified as a possible cause of both the adenopathy and associated enteritis.

9. **In which group of patients will the incidence of false-positive diagnosis of appendicitis be highest?**
    In women between the ages of 20 and 40 years. In common surgical practice it is quite acceptable to remove appendices that are normal (approximately 15% of all operations). Extended observation of patients increases both the associated morbidity and mortality as the number of perforated appendices increases.

10. **In older patients (age > 50 years) what condition may be indistinguishable from acute appendicitis?**
    Acute diverticulitis. Diverticular inflammation of either the cecum or a redundant sigmoid colon may present with right lower quadrant symptoms.

11. **Does fever accompanying pelvic inflammatory disease (PID) tend to be higher or lower than the fever of acute appendicitis?**
    Higher. Other differentiating features of PID include pain with cervical motion (Chandelier sign), bilaterality of pain, and pain related to the onset of menses.

12. **What is the term used to describe the pain accompanying the rupture of an ovarian follicle at mid-menstrual cycle in the female?**
    Mittelschmerz (German for "middlepain").

13. **Gas in the portal venous system accompanied by chills, fever and jaundice suggests what condition associated with appendicitis?**
    Pylephlebitis, or suppurative thrombosis of the portal vein. Because of preoperative antibiotic coverage it is now rarely seen after gangrenous or perforated appendicitis.

14. **A patient explored for right lower quadrant pain appears to have regional enteritis (Crohn's disease). What is the appropriate management of the appendix?**
    If the base of the appendix and surrounding cecum are grossly free of disease, the organ is removed (see Controversies).

15. **If the patient explored for right lower quadrant pain has a carcinoma of the cecum, what should the surgeon do?**
    Right hemicolectomy.

16. **What is the most common tumor of the appendix?**
    The carcinoid. It is found in approximately 0.3% of appendectomies.

17. **What is the best treatment of a 2-cm carcinoid involving the base of the appendix?**
    Right hemicolectomy (see Controversies).

18. **What is "pseudomyxoma peritonei"?**
    This term describes the rare laparotomy finding of massive gelatin-like mucinous ascites associated with an ovarian or appendiceal neoplasm. Pseudomyxoma peritonei is perhaps best characterized as a mucin-secreting adenocarcinoma of the ovary or appendix with peritoneal metastasis. The literature is extremely con-

fusing in the differentiation of this condition from benign mucus-producing tumors of the appendix (mucocele) or ovary (cystadenoma). Clinical presentation includes abdominal pain, distention, and small bowel obstruction. Operative intervention is aimed at reduction of tumor bulk. Appendectomy and oophorectomy is advocated. Adjuvant chemotherapy with 5-fluorouracil and melphalan and radiotherapy are of benefit in the postoperative treatment of these patients. Five-year survival is > 50%.

19. **Should wide peritoneal drainage be done for treatment of diffuse (perforated) appendiceal peritonitis?**
No. Wide drainage of the peritoneum has been studied and shown to be unsuccessful and possibly may be harmful to the patient. It is acceptable therapy, however, to mechanically drain loculated intraperitoneal pus (abscess).

20. **Is simple drainage of an appendiceal abscess without appendectomy acceptable treatment of this complication?**
Yes. In the face of an established abscess with an inaccessible appendix, the abscess is approached and drained mechanically. An appendectomy should be scheduled 6 to 8 weeks later. The incidence of recurrent appendicitis in the unremoved appendix is approximately 20%.

21. **What is the preferred method of drainage of a pelvic abscess that develops after appendectomy?**
Transrectal drainage. This approach avoids the peritoneal contamination incurred with transabdominal drainage and should be used if possible.

22. **What is the most common complication following appendectomy?**
Subcutaneous wound infection.

23. **What is the most common organism of the large bowel in man?**
Bacteroides fragilis is most prevalent, with 10% organisms per gram of wet feces.

24. **Assuming no antibiotic prophylaxis, what is the frequency of postoperative infections in appendicitis without perforation? With perforation?**
Without perforation, approximately 6 to 10%. With perforation, approximately 50%.

25. **Has preoperative antibiotic therapy been shown to be of benefit in the management of appendicitis?**
Yes. In several studies the incidence of infection after appendectomy has been substantially reduced *both* in perforated and nonperforated cases with the administration of a single dose of antibiotic preoperatively.

CONTROVERSIES

26. **Carcinoid tumor of the appendix.**
Most carcinoid tumors of the appendix are small lesions (< 1.5 cm) which are incidental findings at appendectomy. They are commonly located at the tip of the appendix (70% of cases). In these instances, simple appendectomy is adequate therapy. For tumors of the base of the appendix, for limited lymphocyte invasion, and for invasion into the mesoappendix, simple appendectomy has been advocated by some as adequate treatment, and right hemicolectomy by others. It is largely agreed upon, however, that tumors that are 2 cm or larger represent aggressive carcinomas requiring more radical resections (right hemicolectomy).

27. **Crohn's disease of the appendix.**
A commonly held belief is that appendectomy in the face of Crohn's disease is safe only if the appendix and surrounding cecum are grossly free of involvement. It was reasoned that the removal of an appendix from an area of granulomatous inflammation would result in a higher incidence of fecal fistulas. This, in fact, has not been substantiated in the literature, and apprehension concerning appendectomy in this situation is probably unwarranted.

BIBLIOGRAPHY

1.   Conte, J.E., Jr., Jacob, L.S., and Polk, H.C.: Antibiotic Prophylaxis in Surgery. Philadelphia, J.B. Lippincott Co., 1984.
2.   Fernandez, R.N., and Daly, J.M.: Pseudomyxoma peritonei. Arch. Surg., 115:409, 1980.
3.   Fitz, R.H.: Perforating inflammation of the vermiform appendix, with special reference to its early diagnosis and treatment. Trans. Assoc. Am. Phys., 1:107, 1886.
4.   Gottrup, F.: Prophylactic metronidazole in prevention of infection after appendectomy: Report of a double blind trial. Acta Chir. Scand., 146:133, 1980.
5.   Habson, T., and Rosenman, L.D.: Acute appendicitis: When is it right to be wrong? Am. J. Surg., 108:306, 1964.
6.   Haller, J.A., Jr., Shaker, I.J., et al: Peritoneal drainage versus non-drainage for generalized peritonitis from ruptured appendicitis in children. Ann. Surg., 177:595, 1973.
7.   Janik, J.S., and Firor, H.V.: Pediatric appendicitis: A 20-year study of 1640 children at Cook County (Illinois) Hospital. Arch. Surg., 114:717, 1979.
8.   Lewis, F.R., Holcroft, J.W., Boeys, J., et al.: Appendicitis: A critical review of diagnosis and treatment in 1000 cases. Arch. Surg., 110:677, 1975.
9.   Moertal, C.G., Dockerty, M.B., and Judd, E.S.: Carcinoid tumors of the vermiform appendix. Cancer, 21:270, 1968.
10.   Nugent, F.W.: Crohn's disease of the appendix. Am. J. Gastroenterol., 65:83, 1976.
11.   Yang, S.S., Gibson, P., et al.: Primary Crohn's disease of the appendix: A report of 14 cases and review of the literature. Ann. Surg., 189:334, 1979.

---

48. LOWER GASTROINTESTINAL BLEEDING
BRUCE BARTON, M.D.

---

1.   **What is the overall mortality rate of a patient presenting with lower gastrointestinal bleeding?**
Approximately 10 to 15%.

2.   **Is diverticulitis the most common cause of massive lower gastrointestinal bleeding in adults?**
No. Diverticulitis or inflammation of colonic diverticulosis rarely presents with blood loss. Diverticulosis, seen in > 60% of patients over the age of 60, is the most common cause of massive hemorrhage from the lower gastrointestinal tract. Of all patients with diverticulosis only a small minority (5%) will have a major bleeding episode (see Controversies).

3.   **Can bleeding from the stomach or duodenum present with the passage of bright red blood rectally?**
Yes. The color of passed blood is a function of gastrointestinal transit time. A briskly bleeding lesion of the stomach or duodenum with subsequent quick passage of blood through the gastrointestinal tract can present with bright red

blood per rectum and often hypotension or shock. Melena (the passage of black, tarry stools) is caused by the chemical interaction of gastric acid with blood over several hours to form hematin.

4. **What are the classic nonhemorrhagic causes of dark stools?**
    Inquiries as to the ingestion of iron, licorice, or bismuth-containing compounds must be made at the initial evaluation of a patient who presents with dark stools.

5. **What two radionuclide tests are currently available for identifying bleeding in the gastrointestinal tract?**
    The 99m-Tc sulfur colloid scan and the 99m-Tc red cell scan are currently available and have different potential benefits. The sulfur colloid scan is similar to arteriography in that it must be used in the actively bleeding patient for the study to be positive. Its advocates claim that this test can detect bleeding rates as low as 0.1 ml per minute. Therefore, if the sulfur colloid scan is negative, invasive arteriography can be avoided. Because the tagged red cell scan offers persistent intravascular radioactivity (24 hours), imaging can be accomplished even in the nonactively bleeding patient. This remains the test's strongest contribution. A major pitfall lies with the test's inability to provide accurate information on the origin of bleeding detected in delayed scans.

6. **Why does the sulfur colloid scan have limited utility in the evaluation of upper gastrointestinal hemorrhage?**
    The reticuloendothelial system in the liver and spleen clears this radionuclide from the circulation, resulting in high background in the upper abdomen, which renders evaluation of the stomach and duodenum difficult.

7. **How does one work up the origin of a bleed from the lower gastrointestinal tract that requires multiple-unit transfusions?**
    See Controversies.

8. **What is the success rate in the localization of the site of colonic bleeding with such a protocol?**
    Eighty percent to 90% can be identified by angiography or colonoscopy.

9. **Is colonoscopy useful in the management of a patient actively bleeding from the lower gastrointestinal tract?**
    The benefit of colonoscopic evaluation of the patient with active bleeding will be largely dependent upon the volume of bleeding and the experience and skill of the examiner.

10. **Is carcinoma of the colon commonly associated with massive gastrointestinal hemorrhage?**
    No. Bleeding associated with colonic neoplasia is usually occult in nature and is best determined by chemical analysis, such as the guaiac test or the commercially prepared Hemoccult test.

11. **Is the barium enema of diagnostic value in the *initial* work-up of lower gastrointestinal bleeding?**
    No. Because barium is radiopaque, it may obscure angiographic attempts at localization of the bleeding source for several days.

12. **What is the most common site of bleeding colonic diverticula?**
    While colonic diverticula are most prevalent in the left side of the colon, bleeding diverticula occur more often on the right side. Whether some bleeding "right-sided diverticula" are actually bleeding arteriovenous malformations, remains controversial.

13. **In what percentage of patients will colonic bleeding of diverticular origin cease after resuscitative measures alone?**
In approximately 75% of patients so treated, the bleeding will cease and, in the majority of patients who stop bleeding, no further bleeding occurs.

14. **What rate of blood loss into the bowel is necessary for accurate localization of bleeding by arteriography?**
A rate of blood loss of at least 1.5 to 2 cc/minute is necessary for angiography to be of use.

15. **What is the therapeutic value of catheter-directed infusion of vasopressin in the management of lower gastrointestinal bleeding?**
The technique is largely successful in patients with bleeding diverticulosis. Attempts to control bleeding from other sources with this therapy are less reliable.

16. **If catheter-directed infusion of vasopressin is unsuccessful, are any other therapeutic modalities available before the catheter must be removed?**
Yes. Transcatheter embolization of a bleeding vessel is possible using Gelfoam pledgets or autologous clot. While infarction of bowel using this technique is possible, it is of definite value in the poor surgical risk or where vasopressin therapy is contraindicated.

17. **Where are arteriovenous malformations of the colon located?**
The cecum is the most common location, but they have been found in the ileum, ascending colon, and hepatic flexure. When present, there are usually several.

18. **What are the generally accepted indications for operative intervention in the management of lower gastrointestinal bleeding?**
Patients requiring greater than five units of whole blood within the first six hours despite aggressive medical or angiographic management should undergo exploratory surgery. Surgery should be performed in any patient who rebleeds after initial stabilization with conservative therapy.

19. **What techniques can be utilized intraoperatively to localize the source of lower gastrointestinal bleeding?**
The surgeon must inspect the entire gut for mass lesions. If no source is obvious, manual evacuation of bowel lumen contents is carried out followed by segmental isolation using clamps. Multiple colotomies can be made as an adjunct to this procedure. Recent studies have advocated use of the intraoperative Doppler to locate arteriovenous malformations.

20. **What is the proper surgical treatment of a patient with known diverticulosis, chronic intermittent rectal bleeding, and arteriovenous malformation?**
Both right hemicolectomy and subtotal colectomy have been advocated. There is growing evidence, however, that right hemicolectomy alone may be adequate.

21. **What is the role of "blind" subtotal colonic resection in the management of the patient with massive lower gastrointestinal bleeding?**
In the small subgroup of patients in whom aggressive work-up has failed to demonstate a bleeding source (< 10%), subtotal colonic resection may be

required. Mortality with this procedure is reported to be 10% or greater. However, in the patient who continues to bleed despite vasopressin infusion after localization, a more limited colonic resection can be performed with less surgical mortality.

22. **What is the most common cause of massive rectal bleeding in the pediatric age group?**
    Meckel's diverticulum.

23. **How much blood loss is required for a stool guaiac test to be positive?**
    Approximately 10 ml per day must be lost.

24. **What is Rendu-Osler-Weber disease?**
    Also known as hereditary hemorrhagic telangiectasia, this syndrome is transmitted as an autosomal dominant trait and is characterized by increased fragility of the small arteries and veins of the plain and mucous membranes of the nasopharynx and gastrointestinal tract, resulting in bleeding. Pulmonary arteriovenous malformations and hepatic cirrhosis are other features of this disease.

CONTROVERSIES

25. **Etiology of massive lower gastrointestinal hemorrhage.**
    While traditional teaching describes colonic diverticulosis and angiodysplasia as the commest causes of gastrointestinal hemorrhage, recent series do not uniformly agree. Chemotherapy for neoplastic disease and immunosuppression as well as hematologic abnormalities may be more prevalent causes of hemorrhage than previously accepted. Potentially exsanguinating hemorrhage, however, remains the hallmark of diverticulosis.

26. **Work-up of lower gastrointestinal bleeding.**
    No universally accepted diagnostic plan is available. Hemorrhage of the upper tract proximal to the ligament of Treitz must be ruled out by nasogastric aspiration or endoscopy. This is followed by an attempt to evaluate the rectum proctoscopically. Upon completion of these measures, angiography of the celiac and mesenteric vessels is necessary. If the origin of hemorrhage is still elusive, barium enema and/or colonoscopy may be helpful. Diverticulosis demonstrated radiographically would offer a presumptive diagnosis and would possibly limit the extent of resection at surgery.

BIBLIOGRAPHY

1. Alavi, A., et al.: Localization of gastrointestinal bleeding: Superiority of 99m Tc-sulfur colloid compared with angiography. A. J. R., 137:741, 1981.
2. Bakey, S.J., et al.: Vascular ectasias of the colon. Surg. Gynecol. Obstet., 149:353, 1979.
3. Bar, A.H., et al.: Angiography in the management of massive lower gastrointestinal tract hemorrhage. Surg. Gynecol. Obstet., 150:226, 1980.
4. Baum, S., et al.: Angiographic diagnosis and control of large bowel bleeding. Dis. Colon Rectum, 17:447, 1974.
5. Giacchino, J.L., et al.: Changing perspective in massive lower intestinal hemorrhage. Surgery, 86:368, 1979.
6. Matolo, N.M., et al.: Selective embolization for control of gastrointestinal hemorrhage. Am. J. Surg., 138:840, 1979.
7. McKusick, K.A., et al.: 99m Tc red blood cells for detection of gastrointestinal bleeding: Experience with 80 patients. A. J. R., 137:1113, 1981.

8.   Rahn, N.H., et al.: Diagnostic and interventional angiography in acute gastrointestinal hemorrhage. Radiology, 143:361, 1982.
9.   Talman, E.A., et al.: Role of arteriography in rectal hemorrhage due to arteriovenous malformations and diverticulosis. Ann. Surg., 190:203, 1979.
10.   Wright, H.K. , et al.: Controlled, semielective, segmental resection for massive colonic hemorrhage. Am. J. Surg., 139:535, 1980.

49. COLORECTAL POLYPS
G. VAN STIEGMANN and J. H. SUN

1. **What is a polyp?**
    A polyp is an elevation of the mucosal surface, usually consisting of a rounded projection into the lumen of the colon or rectum. The word "polyp" has Greek derivation and means "many feet." Polyps occur throughout the gastrointestinal tract but are most common in the colon and rectum.

2. **What is the difference between a sessile and a pedunculated polyp?**
    A pedunculated polyp is one whose head is attached by a stalk to the mucosa of the colon or rectum. The stalk is usually covered with normal mucosa. The term "sessile" refers to a polyp resting on a broad base. In either type, the muscularis mucosa is the important landmark for differentiation of invasive from noninvasive carcinoma. Lymphatics and vascular channels do not extend across the muscularis mucosa; hence, carcinoma developing on the mucosal side of this border is considered carcinoma in situ (also referred to as severe atypia or dysplasia). Such lesions do not metastasize.

3. **Which polyps have malignant potential?**
    Adenomatous polyps of the colon and rectum are recognized for their potential as precursors of cancer. Three types of adenomatous polyp are recognized histologically: tubular adenoma, villotubular adenoma, and villous adenoma. Polyps containing more than 75% tubular (glandular) elements are called *tubular*, those containing more than 75% villous elements are called *villous*. When more than 25% of the polyp consists of both tubular and villous components, it is called villotubular. Adenomatous polyps are thought to occur as a result of failure of the colonic epithelium to suppress DNA synthesis, resulting in a proliferative lesion that accumulates in the colonic mucosa, forming a clinical polyp. Polypoid cancers may represent degeneration of larger adenomatous polyps.

4. **Do carcinoid polyps have malignant potential?**
    Carcinoid tumors of the rectum may present clinically as elevations of the mucosa. These lesions grow in the submucosa as nodules and represent cancer of substantial malignant potential if larger than 2 cm in diameter.

5. **Which polyps have no malignant potential?**
    Hyperplastic (metaplastic) *polyps* are the most common polyps in the colon and rectum. These are usually small (1 to 5 mm) and constitute over 90% of the polyps in the colon and rectum that are smaller than 3 mm. Unlike adenomatous polyps, hyperplastic polyps are formed by a failure of normally matured mucosal cells to spread over the mucosal lumen. These cells accumulate at the intestinal surface of the colon, forming a polypoid lesion. *Hamartomas* are abnormal collections of normal tissue. Such hamartomas have excess proliferation of the

muscularis mucosa; others consist of excess connective tissue. *Inflammatory polyps* are commonly seen in diseases such as ulcerative colitis, granulomatous colitis (Crohn's disease), and schistosomiasis. These polyps represent islands of healing or healed mucosa, are not premalignant, and parallel the severity of the underlying inflammatory process. *Lipomas* may present as do carcinoids, with submucosal growth and a nodular lump projecting into the mucosal lumen. Occasionally lipomas may also occur in polypoid form with a head and stalk. Lipomas have no significant malignant potential.

6. **At what age do polyps occur?**
Adenomatous polyps of the colon and rectum occur infrequently under age 30. The incidence increases with age, with some autopsy series reporting a high incidence (70%) in patients over 45. This figure is based on careful postmortem examination under magnification, however, and hardly represents the true clinical incidence. A reasonable figure for polyps of clinical significance is 25% in patients over age 60.

7. **How often are colorectal polyps multiple?**
Approximately 10% of patients will harbor more than one adenomatous polyp at the time an initial polyp is discovered. Another 25% will develop additional adenomatous polyps in the following four-year period.

8. **Where do most colorectal polyps occur?**
The majority of colorectal polyps (two thirds) occur in the rectum, sigmoid colon, and descending colon. The remaining third are distributed between the right and transverse colons.

9. **What is a juvenile polyp?**
Juvenile polyps occur in the colon and rectum of infants, children, and adolescents. Histologically, they consist of large mucus-filled dilated glands with excess connective tissue. Some believe these polyps develop in response to inflammation, while others conclude they represent variations of hamartomas. The common presenting symptom of juvenile polyps is rectal bleeding. Abdominal pain resulting from intussusception may also occur. These polyps may be treated conservatively and frequently undergo autoamputation.

10. **What clinical syndromes are associated with colorectal polyps?**
Familial polyposis is a hereditary (dominant, non-sex-linked) trait characterized by multiple adenomatous polyps throughout the colon and rectum. Patients with familial polyposis often have a family history of the disease or of rectal cancer. Those lacking a family history but found to harbor multiple adenomatous polyps may represent a mutation, and subsequent generations are expected to be at risk. Bleeding, diarrhea, and abdominal pain are common presenting features. These patients have a nearly 100% incidence of cancer if left untreated.

Gardner's syndrome consists of osteomas of the skull and mandible with multiple epidermoid cysts and soft tissue tumors of the skin in addition to multiple adenomatous polyps of the colon. The risk of cancer in patients with Gardner's syndrome is, for practical purposes, equal to those with familial polyposis.

Peutz-Jeghers syndrome consists of multiple hamartomatous polyps throughout the entire gastrointestinal tract. Patients with this disease are not at high risk for malignant change.

11. **What is the proper treatment and timing of treatment for these syndromes?**

Polyps develop in patients with familial polyposis and Gardner's syndrome at or after puberty. Nearly all who will develop polyps have them by young adulthood. Because of the high risk of cancer, the current recommended treatment is panproctocolectomy with rectal mucosectomy and ileoanal anastomosis. Patients with Peutz-Jeghers syndrome do not merit a prophylactic colectomy.

12. Does the size of the polyp influence its malignant potential?
Adenomatous polyps harbor carcinoma in direct proportion to their size. An adenoma of 0.5 to 0.9 cm will be cancerous in 1 to 2% of patients; of 1 to 1.9 cm, in 3 to 5%; and of > 2 cm, in 20 to 40%. Risk is highest for patients with villous adenoma and lowest for those with pure tubular adenomas.

13. How is the diagnosis of a colorectal polyp made?
Colorectal adenomatous polyps seldom produce symptoms until they enlarge. Bleeding is the most common symptom and is usually occult. Screening for colon polyps with fecal occult blood tests has a 40% specificity (true negative) but only a 30% sensitivity (true positive).
Colonoscopy and flexible sigmoidoscopy provide the most sensitive tests for detecting colonic polyps. Colonoscopy is the gold standard; however, it is costly, often uncomfortable, and has small but significant risks. Flexible sigmoidoscopes, which are 60 cm long, will reach about two thirds of colorectal polyps. The sensitivity and specificity are operator-dependent; however, in the hands of an experienced endoscopist, the detection rate should approach 98%. Barium enema (also an operator-dependent examination) is very accurate for polyps that are 5 mm or larger if performed with the double-air contrast technique. Problems in interpretation most often arise from the inability to differentiate a polyp from a small piece of fecal material adherent to the mucosa.
We recommend colonoscopic examination of patients suspected of having polyps or at high risk for same. Patients in whom colorectal (adenomatous) polyps have been detected and removed are at higher risk (approximately two- to three-fold) and should undergo endoscopic examination of the colon at least every 2 to 3 years.

14. Which polyps should the colonoscopist remove?
Virtually all polyps discovered at colonoscopy or sigmoidoscopy that are larger than 3 mm should be removed. Removal is accomplished with a diathermy snare device so that the pedunculated polyp is transected at the base of the stalk. The polyp then is either removed en masse with the endoscope or aspirated through the suction channel and recovered from the suction device. Histologic examination of all polyps is imperative, and each polyp should be submitted and labeled separately with specific information regarding the site from which it has been removed.

15. What is the success rate of colonoscopic polypectomy?
Virtually all polyps smaller than 2.5 cm in diameter that are pedunculated can be removed endoscopically. Larger ones or those with a very short stalk and broad base may be excised using special endoscopic techniques; however, great caution must be employed to avoid undue risk of perforation. Broad-based and sessile polyps generally cannot be removed endoscopically. Biopsies from broad-based polyps such as villous adenomas must be viewed with caution. Unless total removal of the lesion is accomplished, the presence or absence of cancer cannot be ascertained.

16. What are the complications of endoscopic polypectomy?

Perforation during endoscopic polyp removal occurs with a frequency of 1% or less. Bleeding may occur more often; however, most bleeding following polypectomy is self-limited. Persistent bleeding requires reexamination and an attempt at electrocoagulation of the bleeding polyp stalk. Laparotomy for control of hemorrhage is seldom required.

17. What is the proper treatment of a villous adenoma of the rectum?
Villous adenomas of the middle and upper third of the rectum are often large and involve a substantial portion of the circumference of the bowel. These lesions are best treated with a low anterior resection. Lesions in the lower rectum may be excised locally provided that a clear margin of surrounding normal mucosa is obtained. Discovery of invasive carcinoma in the locally resected specimen or a villous lesion too large for local removal may mandate an abdominal perineal resection. Some villous lesions may lend themselves to a posterior sacral approach, in which the rectum is entered following excision of the coccyx or division of the sphincter muscles. Careful attention to detail preserves normal rectal function in these patients and allows wide local excision of certain lesions. Smaller villous lesions in high-risk patients may also be treated with electrocautery or laser ablation.

18. Is the endoscopic removal of a polyp that contains carcinoma considered adequate treatment?
Polyps with clear-cut carcinoma in situ are adequately treated by endoscopic polypectomy. In addition, most agree that a well-differentiated invasive carcinoma which has no sign of vascular or lymphatic invasion and is confined to the head of the polyp can be adequately treated by endoscopic removal.

19. What are the indications for colon resection following removal of a polyp?
Indications for colon resection following endoscopic polyp removal include (1) evidence of lymphatic or vascular invasion; (2) poorly differentiated invasive cancer; (3) incomplete removal of an adenoma or a carcinoma; and (4) sessile adenomas with or without invasive carcinoma.

BIBLIOGRAPHY

1. Cooper, H.S.: Surgical pathology of endoscopically removed malignant polyps of the colon and rectum. Am. J. Surg. Pathol., 7:613-623, 1983.
2. Ghazi, A., and Grossman, M.: Complications of colonoscopy and polypectomy. Surg. Clin. North Am., 62:889-896, 1982.
3. Hill, M.J., Morson, B.C., and Bussey, H.J.R.: Etiology of adenoma-carcinoma sequence in large bowel. Lancet, 1:245-247, 1978.
4. Leavitt, J., Klein, I., Kendricks, F., et al.: Skin tags: A cutaneous marker for colonic polyps. Ann. Intern. Med., 98:928-930, 1983.
5. Macrae, F.A., and St. John, D.J.B.: Relationship between patterns of bleeding and Hemoccult sensitivity in patients with colorectal cancers or adenomas. Gastroenterology, 82:891-898, 1982.
6. Shinya, H., Cooperman, A., and Wolff, W.I.: A rationale for the endoscopic management of colonic polyps. Surg. Clin. North Am., 62:861-867, 1982.

50. COLON CANCER

CHARLES M. ABERNATHY, M.D.

1. **What is the best *screening* test for carcinoma of the colon?**
    A test for occult blood in stool (Hemoccult). Screening proctoscopy has been evaluated in several extensive trials and has not been found to be cost-effective.

2. **If a patient has a positive stool occult blood or change in bowel habit, should a colonoscopy be done initially rather than proctoscopy and air-contrast barium enema?**
    Colonoscopy is rapidly replacing proctoscopy and barium enema as the initial diagnostic examination; however, it carries higher risk and expense. In patients in whom a carcinoma of the colon is definitely suspected, colonoscopy is indicated. In low yield settings, the combination of proctoscopy and barium enema is adequate.

3. **Describe the differences in presentation of right-sided versus left-sided cancer of the colon.**
    Right-sided lesions of the colon are bulky and bleed easily. Patients present with anemia and occasionally a palpable right abdominal mass. Left-sided colon cancers tend to be annulus constricting lesions, and patients present with diarrhea, then obstruction.

4. **How many colon cancers can be reached with the sigmoidoscope?**
    Traditionally, the teaching has been that two thirds of cancers can be reached with the rigid sigmoidoscope. (The widespread use of the flexible sigmoidoscope has certainly enhanced or solidified that number.)

5. **What is the (modified) Duke's classification and its impact on prognosis?**

		5-year survival
Dukes A	Limited to mucosa	80-90%
Dukes B.1	Involvement of muscularis	65%
Dukes B.2	Invasion of serosa	
Dukes C	Positive regional nodes	20-25%
Dukes D	Distant metastases	

6. **Can any patient with perforated cancer of the colon be cured?**
    Yes, but these patients have a much poorer prognosis than those with nonperforated lesions.

7. **If the preoperative work-up reveals metastases, should the primary tumor be removed?**
    Almost always, because of the high level of difficulty in managing complications.

8. **What is bowel preparation?**
    Bowel preparation has two components: Mechanical preparation (thought to be the most crucial component) consists of various methods of eliminating stool from the colon (i.e., cathartics, 3-day clear liquid diet plus low residue diet supplements, enemas, etc.). Antibacterial preparation is commonly used to suppress bacterial growth in the colon. A typical antibacterial preparation is neomycin, 1 gm, and erythromycin base, 1 gm orally at 1 p.m., 2 p.m., and 11 p.m. during the day prior to surgery. Parenteral antibiotics have also been recommended but their use is controversial.

9.   **What is the most common organism in the colon?**
      Bacteroides fragilis.

10.   **What is a Hartmann resection?**
      This technique is often used for an obstructive or perforated cancer of the
      descending/sigmoid colon. The tumor is removed, the rectal stump is closed
      (often with staples), and an end colostomy is fashioned. See figure below.
      (Adapted from Schrock, T.R.: Large intestine. In Way, L.W. (ed.): Current
      Surgical Diagnosis and Treatment, 6th ed. Los Altos, Lange, 1983, p. 631.)

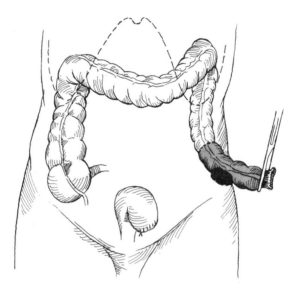

11.   **What is the role of carcinoembryonic antigen (CEA) in the
      postoperative management of cancer of the colon?**
      This test has not proved to be as specific as was hoped.   Elevated CEA
      preoperatively that returns to normal postoperatively can then be followed for a
      rise. Alkaline phosphatase level appears to be as sensitive and specific in
      detecting liver metastases. A CEA-initiated re-exploration for recurrent tumor
      (despite no other evidence of recurrence) will identify a few patients whose
      tumors can be resected for cure.

12.   **What distal margin should be obtained in resecting a carcinoma of
      the rectum?**
      The allowable, safe distal margin has been getting smaller in recent times. As little
      as 2 cm of normal bowel is now accepted by some surgeons, although most
      would be more comfortable with 5 cm.

13.   **Is there an alternative to resection in cancer of the rectum?**
      Yes. Fulguration of the tumor is an option, particularly in elderly, high-risk
      patients. Some authors have reported excellent long-term results in terms of risk,
      survival, and quality of life.

BIBLIOGRAPHY

1.   Beart, R.W., Jr., van Heerden, J.O., and Beahrs, O.H.: Evolution in the pathologic
      staging of carcinoma of the colon. Surg. Gynecol. Obstet., 146:257, 1978. Provides
      greater detail of the classification systems of carcinoma of the colon.

2. Bolt, R.J.: Evaluation of screening tests for colorectal cancer. Primary Care, 7:683, 1980. Six diagnostic tests for screening presymptomatic patients for colorectal cancer are evaluated in the light of sensitivity, expense, and patient comfort and safety. The most sensitive and specific test is that for occult blood. A good summary of screening for colorectal cancer.

3. Cohen, A.M., and Wood, W.C.: Carcinoembryonic antigen levels as an indicator for reoperation in patients with carcinoma of the colon and rectum. Surg. Gynecol. Obstet., 149:22, 1979.

4. Corman, M.L., et al.: Sphincter saving operations for rectal cancer: Contemp. Surg., 21:59, 1982. Excellent reading regarding low rectal lesions.

5. Eisenstat, T.E., et al.: Five year survival in patients with carcinoma of the rectum treated by electrocoagulation. Am. J. Surg., 143:127, 1982.

6. Goligher, J.C.: Surgery of the Anus, Rectum and Colon, 4th ed. London, Balliere Tindall, 1980. Comprehensive textbook.

7. Higgins, G.A.: Current status of adjuvant therapy in the treatment of large bowel cancer. Surg. Clin. North Am., 63:137, 1983.

8. Pihl, E., et al.: Carcinoma of the colon. Cancer specific long-term survival. A series of 615 patients treated by one surgeon. Ann. Surg., 192:114, 1978.

9. Pollett, W.G., and Nicholls, R.J.: The relationship between the extent of distal clearance and survival and local recurrence rates after curative anterior resection for carcinoma of the rectum. Ann. Surg., 198:159, 1983. Supports 2 cm margin.

10. Thorpe, C.D., Grayson, D.J., Jr., and Wingfield, P.B.: Detection of carcinoma of the colon and rectum by air contrast enema. Surg. Gynecol. Obstet., 152:307, 1981. In a retrospective review of 55 patients, the air contrast barium enema was found to be an effective method of detecting adenocarcinoma of the large intestine at all levels and at all stages.

11. Weakley, F.L.: Cancer of the rectum: A review of surgical options. Surg. Clin. North Am., 63:129, 1983. Helpful in understanding A-P resection, low anterior resection, etc.

51. ANAL DISEASE
JOSEPH C. GREER, M.D.

INTERNAL HEMORRHOIDS

1. How is diagnosis made?
History of blood on tissue or in water. Usually bright red and associated with prolapsing tissue. Pain is minimal. Itching alone is not a symptom. Confirmation of the diagnosis is made by anoscopy (cannot be made by external examination). Proctosigmoidoscopy or flexible sigmoidoscopy must be done regardless of age. Inflammatory bowel disease and tumors of the rectum may bleed without being accompained by pain.

2. What are first, second, and third degree hemorrhoids? What is the best treatment of internal hemorrhoids?
First and second degree hemorrhoids can be treated by injections or rubber bands. Isolated third degree hemorrhoids can be adequately treated by these methods. Fourth degree or multiple third degree hemorrhoids should be treated surgically. Multiple methods of surgery are acceptable, although a three-quadrant radial excision is most common. Hospital stay is 3 to 4 days. Closed or semi-closed incisions may reduce hospital stay. Complications include postoperative bleeding, strictures, and abscesses in the wound. Overtreatment of first degree plus second degree with surgery has been common.

EXTERNAL HEMORRHOIDS

3. **How is the diagnosis of external hemorrhoids made?**
    External masses are visible. Occasional bleeding may occur if necrosis of skin is present or in association with prolapsed internal tissue.

4. **How should external (?thrombosed) hemorrhoids be treated?**
    Local evacuation of isolated lesions. Conservative treatment with anti-inflammatory agents (Motrin) and heat is best for multiple lesions.

ANAL FISSURE

5. **When should anal fissure be suspected?**
    When there is a history of pain and blood in the stool on a daily basis. Pain lasts 5 minutes to all day. No history of swelling. Patient often has a history of occult blood in the stool. There may be episodes of discomfort that last only 1 or 2 days and are worse with firm stool or diarrhea. The diagnosis is often made in the office.

6. **How is the diagnosis of anal fissure confirmed?**
    Usually by external examination. Almost always in part midline. Often associated with skin tag or sentinel pyle or tag.

7. **Are anal fissures related to pregnancy?**
    They occur more commonly during the immediate postpartum period.

8. **Can anal fissures be treated nonoperatively?**
    If these fissures are of short duration, they will respond to topical steroid cream and/or suppositories.

9. **What if the anal fissure does not respond to nonoperative treatment?**
    In cases of no response or recurrence, consider operation if there are concomitant hemorrhoids or a large anal papilla.

PERIANAL ABSCESS AND FISTULA

10. **How is perianal abscess diagnosed?**
    History of anal pain with swelling of perianal tissue. Pain increases daily, and fever, chills, and myalgia occur.

11. **What are key findings on physical examination?**
    Red swollen perianal tissue or tenderness of deep perianal tissue. Posterior intermuscular abscess is not always easily determined until digital examination reveals posterior swelling of anal canal and mucosa. Anoscopy, if possible in the office, may show internal opening.

12. **What is the treatment of perianal abscess?**
    Should be drained when the diagnosis is made. There is no need to wait until it is large. Antibiotics will not cure. It is a closed-space infection and requires surgical treatment.

13. **How is the abscess drained?**
    Drainage can be done under local anesthesia; 50% will recur and 40% will develop fistula. Some prefer to do all incision and drainage of perianal abscess under general anesthesia.

CONTROVERSIES

14.   What is the best operation for anal fissure?
It must include sphincterotomy, either posterior or lateral subcutaneous.

BIBLIOGRAPHY

1.   Ferguson, J.A., et al.:   The closed technique of hemorrhoidectomy.   Surgery, 70:
     480-484, 1971.
2.   Goligher, J.C.: Surgery of Anus, Rectum and Colon, 5th ed. London, Balliere Tindall,
     1984.
3.   Salvati, E. P.:   Ligation of internal hemorrhoids. Proc. R. Soc. Med., 63:111, 1970.
4.   Turell, R., et al.: Diseases of the Colon and Anorectum, 2nd ed. Philadelphia, W. B.
     Saunders, 1969.

52. INGUINAL HERNIA
RICHARD J. SANDERS, M.D.

1.   What are the three types of inguinal hernia?
Direct, indirect, and femoral.

2.   What is the etiology of indirect?
Persistent process vaginalis.

3.   What is the etiology of direct?
Wear and tear. The fascia wore out.

4.   Which type is most common hernia in children? Adults? Women?
Indirect Indirect. Indirect (50%) femoral hernias are second at 40%.

5.   Are femoral hernias more prevalent in men or women?
Women.

6.   What is the principle of repair of a direct hernia?
Rebuild Hesselbach's triangle (the weak area medial to the epigastric vessels).
Must have a good fascia or use a prosthesis.

7.   What is the principle of repair of an indirect hernia?
Ligation of sac *and* tighten the internal ring.

8.   What is the preperitoneal approach?
Open the oblique muscles and transversalis fascia about 1 inch above the
inguinal canal to permit visualization of the inguinal area from the inside. The
spermatic cord and cremaster muscles are not seen at all, just the vas deferens
and spermatic vessels as they enter the internal ring.

9.   What are the indications for the preperitoneal approach?
It can be used for almost all hernias, but it is particularly good for incarcerated,
strangulated, sliding, recurrent, and femoral hernias. Repair of direct hernias is
difficult unless a prosthesis is used.

10.   What is the best way to visualize the internal ring?
By dividing the cremasteric fibers from the inguinal ligament for about 2 to 3 cm, below the internal ring. This permits excellent exposure of the ring and permits a tight closure.

11.   How tight should the internal ring be closed?
3 to 5 mm. The tip of a hemostat should slide in easily. If the tip of a finger can enter, it is probably too loose.

12.   In adults with the recent onset of hernia, which three body systems should be questioned carefully in the history?
Gastrointestinal, genitourinary, and respiratory. Straining to urinate (prostatism), straining to defecate (cancer of the colon), and excessive coughing (chronic pulmonary obstructive disease) can each cause increased intraabdominal pressure which, in turn, can produce a hernia. These conditions also predispose to recurrence of the hernia.

13.   What are the indications for using Dacron or Marlex mesh in hernia repairs?
A weak conjoined tendon or other tendinous and fascial layers above a direct hernia; a recurrent direct hernia; a very large direct hernia. Some surgeons will use mesh almost routinely for all direct hernias to add strength to the repair.

14.   What is the disadvantage of using mesh?
Infection. If infection develops in the wound, the mesh often must be removed to allow the infection to heal.

15.   What is the incidence of recurrence of indirect and direct hernias?
Indirect in children, 1 to 4%; indirect in adults, 5 to 10%; direct, 15 to 30%. Direct hernias recur even more often, up to 40%.

16.   What is the commonest site of hernia recurrence?
The internal ring (50%). This is caused by leaving the ring too loose or not ligating the sac high enough.

17.   What is the next commonest site of hernia recurrence?
The pubic tubercle (25%). This is a technical error from failure to place the most medial repair stitch into the periosteum over the pubic tubercle.

18.   What is the principle of treating a femoral hernia?
Remove the sac of fat and close the femoral canal with sutures.

19.   What complication occurs from closing the femoral canal too tightly?
Stenosis or occlusion of the femoral vein.

20.   What is the most likely cause and treatment of acute leg swelling immediately following a hernia repair?
Encroachment on the femoral vein by closing the femoral canal too tightly. Treat by reoperating and removing that stitch.

21.   What is an incarcerated hernia? A strangulated hernia?
A hernia that cannot be reduced is incarcerated. It is not urgent. Strangulation means compromised blood supply to bowel with possible dead bowel. This is a surgical emergency.

22. What are the borders of Hesselbach's triangle?
Laterally, the epigastric vessels; medially, the edge of the rectus sheath; and inferiorly, Poupart's ligament (the reflected inguinal ligament).

23. What is the conjoined tendon?
The combined aponeuroses of the transversus abdominus and internal oblique muscles and the transversalis fascia which lie just above the inguinal area. This tendon is usually used as the repair tissue to cover a direct inguinal hernia defect.

24. What is a Bassini repair? A McVay repair?
A Bassini repair is sewing of the conjoined tendon to the reflected inguinal ligament or the iliopubic tract. A McVay repair sews the conjoined tendon to Cooper's ligament medial to the femoral vein and to the iliopubic tract, above and lateral to the femoral vein.

25. What is the "transition" stitch?
The stitch in a Cooper ligament repair that closes the space medial to the femoral vein. It sews the conjoined tendon to tissue lying between Cooper's ligament medially and the iliopubic tract laterally.

26. What is a relaxing incision?
An incision in the deeper half of the rectus sheath, over the rectus muscle. It permits the conjoined tendon to be pulled down to the Cooper's ligament with less tension. The fascial defect created by the incision is covered above by the external oblique portion of the rectus sheath and below by the rectus muscle.

27. What nerve must be avoided in making an inguinal hernia repair incision? Where does it lie?
The ilioinguinal nerve lies just under the external oblique aponeurosis, on top of the cremasteric muscle.

28. What is a sliding hernia?
A hernia in which one wall is viscera (bowel or bladder). In such hernias, high ligation of the sac is impossible.

29. What is the significance of a hydrocele in a child as compared with an adult?
In a child, hydroceles are usually associated with indirect inguinal hernias; when repairing them, the internal ring should always be explored. In adults, this is not usually true. If you do not palpate a hernia with the hydrocele, a hernia is probably not present.

30. In children, how often is an inguinal hernia bilateral?
If a hernia presents on the left side, a right-sided hernia will also be present in 50%. If it presents on the right side, the incidence of bilaterality is much lower, about 5%.

CONTROVERSIES

31. In a child, should the contralateral side be explored when repairing a unilateral hernia?
For: Yes, especially for a left-sided hernia. Since a hernia on the right side also will be present 50% of the time, bilateral exploration will save a second anesthetic and carries almost no risk.
Against: No. Even the small risk of damaging the spermatic cord is not warranted on the asymptomatic side. It can always be repaired later if a hernia appears.

32.   **Should all people over age 35 have routine sigmoidoscopy before a hernia repair?**
For: It is good medical practice to perform sigmoidoscopy in all patients as part of a complete examination. Specifically, in patients with hernias, this could detect a colon cancer that caused the hernia from undue straining.
Against: The yield is very low. The number of adults with hernias in whom there is a significant finding on routine sigmoidoscopy is probably under 1%.

33.   **Cooper ligament repair.**
For: The ligament is strong and holds sutures well. In a femoral hernia, it must be used to close the femoral canal.
Against: In some patients, the ligament runs very deep as it moves laterally from the pubic tubercle. When the femoral vein is reached, there will be an area of laxity near the femoral vein as the transition stitch into the femoral sheath is taken.

34.   **What is the alternative to Cooper's ligament?**
The iliopubic tract. This is the thickening in the transvasalis fascia that lies below the inguinal ligament and above Cooper's ligament. It holds sutures well. It continues laterally as the femoral sheath, so no transition stitch is needed.

BIBLIOGRAPHY

1.   Griffith, C.A.: Inguinal hernia: An anatomic-surgical correlation. Surg. Clin. North Am., 39:531, 1959.
2.   Guttman, F.M., Bertrand, R., and Ducharme, J.G.: Herniography and pediatric contralateral inguinal hernia. Surg. Gynecol. Obstet., 135:551, 1972.
3.   McVay, C.G.: The hernias. In Davis, L. (ed.): Christopher's Textbook of Surgery, 9th ed. Philadelphia, W.B. Saunders, 1968.
4.   Nyhus, L.M., and Harkins, H.N.: Hernia. Philadelphia, J.B. Lippincott, 1964.

---

53. HYPERPARATHYROIDISM
R. DALE LIECHTY

---

1.   **What are the leading causes of hypercalcemia?**

Bone metastases	55%
Hyperparathyroidism	20%
Thiazide diuretics	
Hyperthyroidism	
Sarcoidosis	25%
Milk–alkali syndrome	
Cancer–endocrine syndromes	
Familial hypercalcemia, hypocalciuria	

2.   **What are the leading symptoms of hyperparathyroidism?**
Many patients with mild disease have few symptoms. For those with symptoms, a mnemonic is helpful:
   Bones: pain, fractures
   Stones: renal stones and sand
   Abdominal moans: pancreatitis, peptic ulcers, constipation
   Fatigue groans: listlessness, weakness
   Psychic overtones: depression

3. **What are the best laboratory tests to diagnose hyperpara-thyroidism?**
    Serum calcium levels (assessed 3 times) above 10.6 mg/dl
    Elevated parathormone levels
    Elevated alkaline phosphatase level
    Elevated chloride
    Decreased phosphate
    Chest x-ray (to help rule out neoplasms)

4. **Describe parathyroid embryology and anatomy.**
    Upper pair arise from branchial arch IV.
    Lower pair arise from branchial arch III.
    Normally four glands are located near four poles of the thyroid.
    Often attached to capsule.
    Supernumerary glands (5 to 11 glands) occur in up to 13% of patients.
    Less than four glands are rare, if they exist at all.
    Glands may occur ectopically:
    >   Mediastinum
    >   Intrathyroid
    >   Within paratracheal thymic tissue
    >   Within carotid sheath
    >   Above superior thyroid poles
    >   Retroesophageal
    >   Retrotracheal

5. **What is the pathology of primary hyperparathyroidism?**

Single adenoma	85%
Double adenoma	3%
Diffuse hyperplasia	11%
Cancer	<1%

6. **What localizing tests are available?**
    In the neck, thallium-technetium scans will localize parathyroid tissue (70%); ultrasound, 80%. Venous sampling for parathyroid hormone and arteriography are invasive procedures that are less accurate and carry a higher risk.

7. **What is the treatment?**
    For mild disease (calcium level < 11.0 mg/dl, no symptoms), observe every 6 to 12 months. When symptoms occur or calcium levels are over 11.0 mg/dl, neck exploration is suggested.

8. **How does the surgeon approach the parathyroid glands?**
    Explore four thyroid poles; identify all glands. If three normal glands are found but the fourth is missing, on the side of the missing gland, explore paratracheal areas (excise all suspicious tissue), look behind the trachea and esophagus, excise the thymus gland, excise suspicious thyroid nodules or perform thyroid lobectomy. If adenoma is still missing, close the wound. Obtain localizing studies (arteriogram; thallium-technetium scan; ultrasound) if hypercalcemia persists.

9. **What is the cure rate for experienced surgeons?**
    After the first operation, 95% of the patients become eucalcemic; after second operations, only 34% will become eucalcemic.

10. **What are the complications?**
    Recurrent laryngeal nerve injuries: temporary, 3%; permanent, <1%.
    Hypocalcemia: temporary, 40% ; permanent, 3%.

11. **Why do many patients with normal parathyroid tissue left in place become temporarily hypocalcemic after excision of the adenoma?**
"Hungry bone" syndrome, edema of viable parathyroid tissue. Permanent injury to remaining parathyroid glands is rare.

12. **What physical signs are important in indicating postoperative hypocalcemia?**
Chvostek's sign: Tapping the facial nerve trunk elicits spasms of the facial muscles. _Trousseau's sign:_ Occluding the brachial artery for 3 minutes with a blood pressure cuff may induce carpal spasms, indicating latent tetany.

13. **What is the treatment?**
Intravenous calcium immediately, oral calcium, (gradual discontinuation of intravenous calcium), and vitamin D therapy for permanent hypoparathyroidism.

14. **What are the consequences of permanent hypoparathyroidism?**
Cataracts (80%), mental deterioration, fatigue, paresthesias, and irritability are common.

15. **Who performed the first parathyroidectomy for hyperparathyroidism?**
Mandl in 1925.

CONTROVERSIES

16. **Operation for patients with low calcium levels (11 to 11.5 mg/dl).**
For: Difficult and expensive to follow patients for long periods; most will eventually get "soft bones" or other symptoms.
Against: Some patients have lived comfortably for years with elevated serum calcium levels.

17. **Routine preoperative localization studies (thallium–technetium scan or ultrasound)?**
For: Assurance that adenoma is there; might indicate double adenomas or hyperplasia.
Against: Expense (each test costs more than $150); only 70% will localize, excellent surgical cure rate of 95% without routine tests.

18. **Avoid mediastinal exploration at first operation.**
For: Some patients will have microadenomas that should show on frozen sections, but may be missed. Permanent sections will often disclose these. Some adenomas may be devascularized at operation.
Against: One operation and anesthetic, avoids second hospitalization.

BIBLIOGRAPHY

1. Haussler, M.R., and McCain, T.A.: Basic and clinical concepts related to vitamin D metabolism and action. N.Engl. J. Med., 297:974, 1041, 1977.
2. Johnston, I.D.A., and Thompson, N.W.: Endocrine Surgery. London, Butterworth, 1983.
3. Kaplan, E.L.: Surgery of the Thyroid and Parathyroid Glands. Edinburgh, Churchill Livingstone, 1983.
4. Liechty, R.D., and Weil, R.: The Anatomy of Parathyroid Hyperplasia. Surgery, 96:1099-1102:1984.
5. Paloyan, E., Lawrence, A.M., and Straus, F.H.: Hyperparathyroidism. New York, Grune and Stratton, 1973.

6. Purnell, D.C., Scholz, D.A., and Beahrs, O.H.: Hyperparathyroidism due to single gland enlargement. Arch. Surg., 112:369, 1977.
7. Saxe, A.W., and Brennan, M.F.: Strategy and technique of reoperative parathyroid surgery. Surgery, 89:417, 198l.
8. Wells, S.A., Gunnells, C.J., Shelburne, J.D., et al.: Transplantation of the parathyroid glands in man: Clinical indications and results. Surgery, 78:34, 1975.

54. HYPERTHYROIDISM
R. DALE LIECHTY, M.D.

1. **What are the chief symptoms and signs of hyperthyroidism?**
Goiter, increased appetite, weight loss, fatigue, exophthalmos, tachycardia, palpitations, nervousness, heat intolerance, diarrhea, lagophthalmos, increased pulse pressure, moist soft skin, hyperreflexia.

2. **What are the two main types of hyperthyroidism?**
Graves' disease (diffuse hyperplasia) and Plummer's disease (toxic nodule).

3. **What is the cause of hyperthyroidism?**
Immunoglobulin, simulating thyroid-stimulating hormone (TSH), causes thyroid cells to release excess thyroxin (Graves' disease). Hyperplastic cells release excess thyroxin (Plummer's disease).

4. **What are the best laboratory tests?**
Free thyroxin (T4) levels or total T4 and T3 resin uptake. The latter two tests give the thyroid index, which corrects for protein abnormalities. In equivocal cases, the TRH-TSH test checks integrity of the hypothalamic–pituitary–thyroid axis. Failure of TSH levels to rise following administration of TSH indicates hyperthyroidism (suppression of pituitary thyrotrophs). A normal rise in TSH levels indicates a normal feedback mechanism and euthyroidism. It will also point to the rare T3 thyrotoxicosis (1 in 1000 cases) because T3 strongly suppresses TSH. A thyroid scintiscan will differentiate diffuse from nodular thyrotoxicosis.

5. **What are the main treatment options?**
Antithyroid drugs, radioiodine, and surgery.

6. **What are the advantages and disadvantages of each?**
See Controversies.

SURGICAL TREATMENT

7. **What is the origin of the superior thyroid artery?**
First branch of the external carotid artery.

8. **What is the meaning of *recurrent* in recurrent laryngeal nerves?**
Arising from the vagus nerve, the right nerve loops (recurs) around the right subclavian artery and ascends beneath the thyroid gland to the larynx. Similarly, arising from the vagus, the left nerve loops around the aortic arch and ascends to the larynx.

9. **What defects result from injury to the superior laryngeal nerve?**
    Lack of sensation in supraglottic pharynx and paresis of the cricothyroid muscle. The voice is weak and low and lacks resonance.

10. **What defects result from injury to the recurrent laryngeal nerve?**
    Paresis of the cord (weak, whispering voice).

11. **To both recurrent laryngeal nerves?**
    Paresis of both cords. Obstruction to air flow usually demands tracheostomy.

12. **Who performed the first thyroidectomy?**
    Mikulicz in 1885.

13. **What surgeon won a Nobel prize for his work with thyroid disease?**
    Kocher in 1909.

14. **What is the incidence of nonrecurrent laryngeal nerves?**
    0.6%.

15. **Which side does it usually favor?**
    Right side (usually associated with cardiac anomalies).

CONTROVERSIES

Treatment

Antithyroid drugs
  For: Avoids surgery and irradiation.
  Against: (1) high incidence of drug reactions, blood dyscrasias, skin reactions; (2) frequent visits to physician necessary; and (3) recurrence rate high when therapy is discontinued.
Surgery
  For: (1) most rapid method of permanent control; (2) avoids irradiation and long-term drug therapy; and (3) euthyroidism in 90% at 5 years.
  Against: Complications of surgery include (1) damage to recurrent laryngeal nerves in 1%; (2) damage to parathyroid glands in 1%; (3) wound complications in 1%; and (4) permanent hypothyroidism (leaving 10-gm remnants of thyroid) in less than 5% (5-year follow-up).
Radioiodine
  For: (1) avoids operation; (2) gives permanent control; and (3) avoids drug reactions.
  Against: (1) danger of irradiation; (2) hypothyroidism rate is high, 50% or more in 10 years, probably 100% in 20 years; (3) often treatment period is lengthy (up to 2 years); and (4) contraindicated in pregnancy and in the very young.

BIBLIOGRAPHY

1. Beahrs, O.H., and Sakulsky, S.B.: Surgical thyroidectomy in the management of exophthalmic goiter. Arch. Surg., 96:512, 1968.
2. Bradley, E.L., and Liechty, R.D.: Modified subtotal thyroidectomy for Graves' disease: A two institution study. Surgery, 94:955, 1983.
3   Degroot, L.J., and Larsen, P.R.: Thyroid and Its Diseases. New York, John Wiley and Sons, 1984.
4. Farnell, M.B., van Heerden, J.A., McConahey, W.M., et al.: Hypothyroidism after thyroidectomy for Graves' disease. Am. J. Surg., 142:535, 1981.

5.   Johnston, I.D.A., and Thompson, N.W.: Endocrine Surgery. London, Butterworth, 1983.
6.   Kaplan, E.L.: Surgery of the Thyroid and Parathyroid Glands. Edinburgh, Churchill Livingstone, 1983.
7.   Lazarus, J., McGregor, A., and Hall, R.: Pathogenesis, diagnosis and management of Graves' disease. In Kaplan, E.L. (ed.): Surgery of the Thyroid and Parathyroids. Edinburgh, Churchill Livingstone, 1983.
8.   Michie, W., Hamer-Hodges, D.W., Pegg, C.A.S., et al.: Beta-blockade and partial thyroidectomy for thyrotoxicosis. Lancet, 1:1009, 1974.
9.   Michie, W., Pegg, C.A.S., and Bewsher, P.D.: Prediction of hypothyroidism after partial thyroidectomy for thyrotoxicosis. Br. Med. J., 1:13, 1972.
10. Toft, A.D., Irvine, W.J., Sinclair, I., et al.: Thyroid function after surgical treatment of thyrotoxicosis. N. Engl. J. Med., 298:643, 1978.
11. Werner, S.C., and Ingbar, S.H.: The Thyroid, 4th ed. Philadelphia, J.B. Lippincott Co., 1978.

---

55. THYROID NODULES AND CANCER
R. DALE LIECHTY, M.D.

---

1. **What is the chief clinical difference between solitary and multiple thyroid nodules?**
    Multiple thyroid nodules are considered benign unless some finding (laryngeal nerve palsy, firmness, enlarged nodes, rapid growth) suggests malignancy. Solitary thyroid nodules are considered malignant until proven benign. A previous history of irradiation or any of the above findings strongly suggests malignancy.

2. **Does a "cold" nodule on thyroid scintiscan indicate malignancy?**
    All cysts and many benign adenomas show up as "cold" nodules; conversely, a few thyroid cancers appear as "warm" nodules. Thyroid scintiscans, therefore, are unreliable in diagnosing malignancy in nodules.

3. **What are the necessary tests to determine if a solitary nodule is solid or cystic?**
    Ultrasound will differentiate between a solid and cystic nodule, but so will needle aspiration and at a much lower cost (controversial). In addition, the fluid yields material for cytologic examination. Thus, the fine needle aspiration biopsy cytology (ABC) is the single most important test for determining the malignant potential of thyroid nodules, whether solid or cystic.

4. **Should a solitary thyroid nodule be suppressed with thyroxin for 3 to 6 months to indicate whether it is benign or malignant?**
    Suppression often fails to shrink benign nodules, and in some cases it has been reported to shrink malignant ones. Soft nodules, especially those appearing during pregnancy, will often regress on suppression. Aspiration biopsy cytology is, of course, more accurate in differentiating benign from malignant nodules.

5. **How reliable is aspiration biopsy cytology in experienced hands?**
    False-negative diagnoses, 1 to 10%. False-positive diagnoses, 0 to 2%.

6. **What is the most common cancer diagnosed by aspiration biopsy cytology?**
    Papillary cancer (ground-glass nuclei and psammoma bodies).

7. **What malignancy is the least reliably diagnosed by aspiration biopsy cytology?**
    Follicular cancer (*note:* this is why all follicular nodules are excised).

8. **What are the main types of solitary thyroid nodules?**
Nodular goiter with one dominant nodule	50%
Adenoma	20%
Cancer	20%
Thyroiditis	5%
Cysts	5%

9. **How has aspiration biopsy cytology affected the number of people who undergo thyroidectomy?**
    It has decreased the number of operations by one third and increased the yield of cancer per operation.

10. **If a thyroid nodule is a cancer, what are the types and percentages of these cancers?**
Papillary	70%
Follicular	15 to 20%
Medullary	5%
Anaplastic and lymphoma	5%

11. **How should the surgeon approach the solitary nodule?**
    1. Biopsy any significant lymph nodes in the exposed neck.
    2. Perform lobectomy on the side of the nodule and obtain frozen-section diagnosis (see Controversies).
    3. If the frozen sections indicate a benign nodule (or a papillary cancer < 1.5 cm with no involved nodes), nothing more need be done.
    4. Postoperatively, patients are given thyroid replacement (Synthroid, 100 to 200 µg) to suppress TSH.

12. **What is the most common kind of thyroiditis found within nodules?**
    Lymphocytic (Hashimoto's) thyroiditis. Although it usually appears as a diffuse, rubbery goiter, lymphocytic thyroiditis can arise asymmetrically, mimicking a solitary thyroid nodule. After excision biopsy, thyroid replacement dramatically reduces the residual thyroid enlargement.

13. **What percentage of thyroid cancers are papillary or mixed?**
    About 70%.

14. **How should larger papillary cancers be treated?**
    Larger papillary tumors demand total or near-total thyroidectomy with local excision of involved lymph nodes and postoperative radioiodine if any remaining tissue takes up radioiodine. A patient with distant metastases requires the same treatment as above. Excising the normal thyroid enhances the uptake of radioiodine in metastases. All patients should take thyroxin (Synthroid, 100 to 200 µg daily) for duration of life.

15. **What is the main difference in metastatic tendencies between papillary and follicular cancers?**
    Papillary cancers metastasize to neck nodes first. Follicular cancers metastasize distantly (hematogenously).

16. **How should follicular cancers (which represent 15 to 20% of all thyroid cancers) be treated?**

Total thyroidectomy. Radioiodine is subsequently used if there is uptake in distant metastases. With no invasion through the capsule, no vascular invasion, and no distant uptake, radioiodine treatment can be held in reserve.

17. How should medullary cancers be treated?
Total thyroidectomy and mid-neck lymph node dissection (from carotid sheath to carotid sheath). Excise all palpable lymph nodes.

18. How should undifferentiated cancers be treated?
Total thyroidectomy (if possible). External irradiation.

19. What are the 10-year survival rates for the above cancers?

Papillary	85%
Follicular	
Localized	85%
With metastases	20%
Medullary	
Negative nodes	85%
Positive nodes	45%
Anaplastic	0%

CONTROVERSIES

20. Ultrasound.
For: will differentiate cystic nodules from solid ones.
Against: expense; needle aspiration will differentiate cystic from solid lesions and yield cells for cytology.

21. Fine needle biopsy.
For: Best current method for assessing nodules preoperatively; simple; relatively inexpensive.
Against: False-negative diagnoses up to 10%.

22. Lobectomy or nodulectomy?
For lobectomy: assures adequate removal of many primary cancers. Capsule limits extension of some tumors. For occult papillary cancers, this is adequate treatment.
Against lobectomy: greater risk to laryngeal nerves and parathyroid glands, especially with inexperienced surgeons.

BIBLIOGRAPHY

1. Beierwaltes, W.H., Nishiyama, R.H., Thompson, N.W., et al.: Survival time and "cure" in papillary and follicular thyroid carcinoma with distant metastases: Statistics following University of Michigan therapy. J. Nucl. Med., 23:561, 1982.
2. Block, M.S.: Management of carcinoma of the thyroid. Ann. Surg., 185:133, 1977.
3. Cady, B.: Surgery of thyroid cancer. World J. Surg., 5:3, 1981.
4. Clark, O.H.: Total thyroidectomy. The treatment of choice for patients with differentiated thyroid cancer. Ann. Surg., 196:361, 1982.
5. Degroot, L.J., and Larsen, P.R.: Thyroid and Its Diseases. New York, John Wiley and Sons, 1984.
6. Gundry, S.R., Burney, R.E., Thompson, N.W., et al.: The importance of total thyroidectomy for Hürthle cell neoplasm of the thyroid. Arch. Surg., 118:529, 1983.
7. Hubert, J.P., Kiernan, P.D., Beahrs, O.H., et al.: Occult papillary carcinoma of the thyroid. Arch. Surg., 115:394, 1980.
8. Johnston, I.D.A., and Thompson, N.W.: Endocrine Surgery. London, Butterworth, 1983.

9. Kaplan, E.L.: Surgery of the Thyroid and Parathyroid Glands. Edinburgh, Churchill Livingstone, 1983.
10. Liechty, R.D., and Zimmerman, D.: Solitary thyroid nodules. Arch. Surg., 112:59, 1977.
11. Lowhagen, T., Willem, J.S., and Lundell, G.: Aspiration biopsy cytology in diagnosis of thyroid cancer. World J. Surg., 5:61, 1981.
12. Mazzaferri, E.L., and Young, R.L.: Papillary thyroid carcinoma: A 10-year follow-up report on the impact of therapy in 576 patients. Am. J. Med., 70:511, 1981.
13. Thompson, N.W., Nishiyama, R.H., and Harness, J.K.: Thyroid carcinoma: Current controversies. Curr. Probl. Surg., 15:1, 1978.
14. Werner, S.C., and Ingbar, S.H.: The Thyroid, 4th ed. Philadelphia, J.B. Lippincott Co., 1978.

56. SURGICAL HYPERTENSION
CHARLES W. VAN WAY, M.D.

1. What are the surgically correctable causes of hypertension?
Pheochromocytoma, coarctation of the aorta, Cushing's syndrome, primary hyperaldosteronism (Conn's syndrome), renovascular hypertension, and unilateral renal parenchymal disease.

2. What findings on history and physical examination should lead to a suspicion of pheochromocytoma?
Pheochromocytoma is characterized by labile severe hypertension, paroxysmal hypertension, a feeling of nervousness, headaches, palpitations, and a generalized appearance of hypermetabolism. There may be a recent onset of abnormal glucose tolerance, misdiagnosed as diabetes.

3. What findings suggest coarctation?
Coarctation of the aorta is suggested by diminished femoral pulses and a lower blood pressure in the legs than in the arms. There may be rib notching on chest x-ray film. The adult patient with coarctation is characteristically bandy-legged.

4. What findings suggest Cushing's syndrome?
Cushing's syndrome is suggested by obesity, typically distributed to the trunk and face. There may be striae. Weakness and muscle wasting are characteristic. There may be amenorrhea in women and impotence in men. Radiographic findings of osteoporosis are common. Back pain is frequent and pathologic fractures of the vertebral bodies are seen.

5. What findings suggest primary hyperaldosteronism?
Primary hyperaldosteronism is characterized by muscle weakness. The serum potassium is low.

6. What suggests renovascular hypertension?
Renovascular hypertension is difficult to suspect unless a flank bruit is present. Patients with an abdominal or flank bruit and hypertension have one chance in three of having renovascular hypertension. Hypertensive children, teenagers, or young adults (under age 25) are frequently found to have renovascular hypertension.

7. What suggests unilateral renal parenchymal disease?

Unilateral renal parenchymal disease is suggested by otherwise unexplained hematuria or pyuria. Generally, unilateral renal parenchymal disease is diagnosed from an intravenous pyelogram obtained for other reasons. The intravenous pyelogram is diagnostic, and no other tests are necessary.

8. **How is the diagnosis of pheochromocytoma established?**
    Pheochromocytoma is diagnosed by 24-hour urine collection for vanillylmandelic acid (VMA), metanephrines, and catecholamines. Elevated plasma catecholamines (epinephrine and norepinephrine) may be found.

9. **How is Cushing's syndrome diagnosed?**
    The best screening test is the overnight dexamethasone suppression test. Dexamethasone, given at night, will suppress the normal morning elevation in plasma cortisol. A morning plasma cortisol of < 10 μg/dl after 2 mg of dexamethasone the night before is strongly suggestive of Cushing's syndrome. Further diagnostic testing is not standardized. It includes morning and evening plasma cortisol to establish whether or not diurnal variation is present, low-dose and high-dose dexamethasone suppression tests, and the metapyrone test. The object of these tests is to distinguish bilateral adrenal hyperplasia from tumor. About 20% of patients have adrenal adenoma or carcinoma.

10. **How is primary hyperaldosteronism diagnosed?**
    Primary hyperaldosteronism is characterized by a low serum potassium with a high urinary potassium, in the absence of diuretic administration. The definitive test is 24-hour urinary aldosterone excretion or aldosterone secretion study.

11. **What is the work-up for renovascular hypertension?**
    In renovascular hypertension, two questions must be answered. First, does the patient have renal artery stenosis? Second, does the patient have hypertension because of renal artery stenosis? Three tests are involved. The first is a hypertensive intravenous pyelogram. This will fail to identify one of six patients with renovascular hypertension, but it is the most reliable screening test available. Findings characterizing renovascular hypertension are delayed function of one kidney, size discrepancy exceeding 2 cm, hyperconcentration of dye on the involved side, and ureteral notching from collaterals. Next, an aortogram is done to establish whether or not renal artery stenosis is present. If technically correct, this is nearly 100% accurate. Finally, a renal vein renin assay is done, with simultaneous sampling of the renal veins and concomitant sampling of the inferior vena cava. The ratio between the two sides should be 1.5 or greater, if unilateral disease is present. If bilateral disease is present, both sides should be markedly elevated above the inferior cava sample.

12. **How common is surgical hypertension?**
    Renovascular hypertension is present in 5 to 7% of all hypertensive patients. Aldosteronism, pheochromocytoma, coarctation of the aorta, and Cushing's disease each comprise around 0.1% of all hypertensive individuals.

13. **What is the treatment for surgical hypertension?**
    Pheochromocytoma–resection of the tumor.
    Cushing's syndrome–resection of an adrenal adenoma or carcinoma.
    Bilateral adrenal hyperplasia–either pituitary irradiation, transsphenoidal hypophysectomy, or bilateral adrenalectomy may be used.
    Primary hyperaldosteronism–removal of the adrenal adenoma.
    Renovascular hypertension–aortorenal bypass graft, preferably using a segment of saphenous vein.
    Unilateral renal parenchymal disease–nephrectomy.

14.   What are the results?
Pheochromocytoma. Operative mortality is 3 to 5%. The 5-year survival if benign is 85%. Ten to twenty percent of patients have malignant disease; in these, hypertension may be temporarily alleviated by resection, but the 5-year survival is zero.
Cushing's syndrome. Operative mortality is 2 to 5%. The cure rate is 80 to 90% with bilateral adrenal hyperplasia, 95% for adenomas, and 0% for carcinomas. Perioperative complications are common.
Hyperaldosteronism. Operative mortality is 1%. Cure rate is 75%. Drug therapy can control the hypertension in 75 to 80%.
Coarctation of the aorta. Operative mortality is 1 to 2%. Cure rate is 95%.
Renovascular hypertension. Drug therapy will control approximately 65 to 70% of patients, although this is controversial. For renal revascularization, results of operation depend upon the etiology. Fibromuscular dysplasia–mortality rate is 1%, cure rate 90%, palliation in another 5%. Atherosclerotic disease–mortality 2 to 4%, cure 80%, palliation 20%.

15.   What is Chromogranin A?
Chromogranin A is a soluble protein found in catecholamine storage vesicles, which circulates in the plasma after catecholamines have been released. It has been found to be elevated by a factor of 10 in patients with pheochromocytoma. It may be of use as screening test.

16.   What is MIBG?
^{131}I-metaiodobenzylguanidine, or "hot guano," is a radionuclide that specifically labels catecholamine precursors. It concentrates in pheochromocytoma and can be used to localize tumors. It may ultimately prove to be of therapeutic value.

17.   What is the difference between Cushing's syndrome and Cushing's disease?
Cushing's syndrome is the manifestation of cortical steroid excess. It may be iatrogenic, or produced by an adrenal cortical tumor, bilateral adrenal hyperplasia, ACTH excess, or ectopic ACTH production. Cushing's disease goes back to the original description by Harvey Cushing of the symptoms of cortical steroid excess produced by an adenoma of the pituitary.

18.   What is the cause of bilateral adrenal hyperplasia?
Harvey Cushing thought that corticosteroid excess was caused by a pituitary adenoma, which stimulated the adrenal gland. More recently, it has been thought that bilateral adrenal hyperplasia is a disease of feedback regulation. The pituitary production of ACTH is normally inhibited by cortisol. In patients with bilateral adrenal hyperplasia, this inhibition takes place at a much higher level of cortisol than normal. Most recently, after transsphenoidal hypophysectomy for bilateral adrenal hyperplasia, microadenomas have been found in a majority of patients. Cushing may have been correct after all.

19.   Which is the most dangerous of these diseases?
Pheochromocytoma. Five to ten percent have been diagnosed as a result of sudden death, usually in the operating room or following minor diagnostic procedures. The usual picture is paroxysmal hypertension followed by acute heart failure and cardiovascular collapse. Sudden cardiac arrest can be seen. Pheochromocytoma is a great mimic. It can simulate many other diseases, including diabetes mellitus, hyperthyroidism, acute anxiety attack, gram-negative sepsis, and even mental illness.

Cushing's syndrome. Besides producing hypertension, it produces glucose intolerance, poor healing, susceptibility to infection, and pathologic fracture. *Coarctation of the aorta.* Life expectancy with coarctation is 35 years, if not treated. Death results from stroke, heart failure, arrhythmias, or aortic rupture.

CONTROVERSIES

20. Should renovascular hypertension be treated surgically?
Advantages:
Curative procedure, prevents loss of renal function. Renovascular hypertension is often difficult to control with drugs.
Disadvantages:
Operative mortality, loss of kidneys despite operation. Progression of disease on same or other side may necessitate reoperation.

21. How should Cushing's syndrome secondary to bilateral hyperplasia be treated?
Bilateral adrenalectomy
For: Works immediately, 90 to 95% success rate
Against: May leave pituitary adenoma
Transsphenoidal hypophysectomy
For: Resects pituitary microadenoma, thought to be the basic cause of the dieease.
Against: Very specialized neurosurgical treatment. Late effects may include panhypopituitarism, far more difficult to treat than hypoadrenocorticalism.
Pituitary radiation
For: Nonoperative treatment
Against: Low success rate (60 to 70%). Effects of treatment may not be known for 6 months, during which time patient can get pathologic fractures of vertebral bodies, which are irreversible.

22. Should all patients with hypertension be screened for surgical hypertension?
For:
Incidence of surgical hypertension is 6 to 8% of all hypertensive individuals. Palliation can be achieved only by drug therapy.
Against:
Even a minimal work-up includes an intravenous pyelogram, urinary aldosterone, and VMA, and a dexamethasone suppression test, in addition to the standard chest x-ray film and electrocardiogram. The additional cost is at least $400 to $600. There are 20 to 30 million hypertensive individuals in the United States; such a program would cost $10 to $15 billion. Most patients can be controlled with drugs. Pheochromocytoma and Cushing's syndrome, which are dangerous, generally produce enough other symptoms to allow distinguishing them on history and physical examination.

BIBLIOGRAPHY

1. Auda, S.P., Brennan, M.F., and Gill, J.R.: Evolution of the surgical management of primary aldosteronism. Ann. Surg., 191:1-7, 1980.
2. Bigos, S.T., Somma, M., Rasio, E., et al.: Cushing's disease: Management by trans-sphenoidal pituitary microsurgery. J. Clin. Endocrinol. Metab., 50:348-354, 1980.
3. Dean, R.H.: Renovascular disorders. In Rutherford, et al.: Vascular Surgery, 2nd ed. Philadelphia, W.B. Saunders, 1984.
4. Delaney, J.P., Solomkin, J.S., Jacobson, M.E., and Doe, R.P.: Surgical management of Cushing's syndrome. Surgery, 84:465-470, 1978.

5.   Edis, A.J., Ayala, L.A., and Egdahl, R.H.: Manual of Endocrine Surgery. New York, Springer-Verlag, 1975.

6.   Farndon, J.R., Davidson, H.A., Johnston, I.D.A., and Wells, S.A.: VMA excretion in patients with pheochromocytoma. Ann. Surg., 191:259-263, 1980.

7.   Freier, D.T., Eckhauser, F.E., and Harrison, T.S.: Pheochromocytoma. A persistently problematic and still potentially lethal disease. Arch. Surg., 115:388-391, 1980.

8.   Harrison, T.B., et al.: Surgical Disorders of the Adrenal Gland. New York, Grune & Stratton, 1975.

9.   Horvath, J.S., and Tiller, D.J.: Indications for renal artery surgery: A review. J. Roy. Soc. Med., 77:221-226, 1984.

10.   Johnston, I.D.A., and Thompson, N.W. (eds.): Endocrine Surgery. London, Butterworth, 1983, chs. 5, 11, and 12 (pp. 53075, 182-188, and 112-120).

11.   Manger, W.M., and Gifford, R.W., Jr.: Pheochromocytoma. New York, Springer-Verlag, 1977.

12.   Sisson, J.C., Frager, M.S., Valk, T.W., et al.: Scintigraphic localization of pheochromocytoma. N. Engl. J. Med., 305:259-263, 1980.

13.   Van Way, C.W., Scott, H.W., Page, D.L., and Rhamey, R.K.: Pheochromocytoma. Curr. Probl. Surg., 1974.

---

57. BREAST LUMPS
JOHN SIMON, M.D.

---

1.   **How is physical examination of the breast performed?**
Each examiner must develop his own technique. However, it is important to place the patient in more than one position. For instance, initially the patient may be placed in supine position with the arms up behind the head. This flattens the breast and compresses the tissue for examination. Then the patient may assume an upright position with arms behind the head. This permits examination of the contours of the dependent breast and facilitates examination of the axilla.

2.   **What particular features should be looked for in examining the breast?**
Primarily lumps, thickened areas, or changes in the shape and contour. One may also check for asymmetries, and the nipples may be checked for rashes or discharges.

3.   **Does the feel or quality of the lump in the breast help in the diagnosis?**
Yes, but only to a degree. Very discrete, smooth nodules are more likely to be benign than are contracted, ill-defined thickened areas. However, there is a large degree of variability, and the examination alone can be very misleading at times.

4.   **Is tenderness indicative of benignity?**
Yes, but again this can be misleading. It is not a completely reliable sign.

5.   **Is it reasonable to monitor a nodule during a menstrual period?**
Yes, if the nodule or areas suggest benign disease; however, the limits of observation should be set from the outset. It is a reasonable axiom not to dismiss any lump before the diagnosis is entirely clear.

6.   **Are any diagnostic modalities commonly available to help to assess lumps in the breast?**

Indeed. The mammogram is the most important. It also gives information about the rest of the breast and the opposite breast. Ultrasound can help to differentiate cystic from solid masses. Other procedures are less available and less accurate.

7. **Do mammograms always reveal a lump or thickening in the breast?**
No, particularly in premenopausal women. *Do not dismiss a palpable lump as innocuous simply on the basis of a normal mammogram.*

8. **How are the physical examination and mammogram used to evaluate lumps in the breast?**
Both are important and often complement each other. One does not negate the other! The examiner must trust the physical examination regardless of the mammographic findings, and, conversely, one must believe the mammogram regardless of physical examination.

9. **What should be the approach when the mammogram reveals an abnormality that is not palpable?**
There are basically two options. One is to localize the lesion mammographically and do a biopsy; the other is to follow the lesions with xeromammograms. The growth pattern of carcinoma of the breast if variable, and serial mammograms would need to be carried out over a long period of time (controversial). The authors favor doing a biopsy.

10. **What are the important risk factors for carcinoma of the breast?**
Age of the patient and a positive history of carcinoma of the breast in a primary relative.

11. **If a cyst is aspirated and disappears, it that sufficient evidence of benignity?**
Yes, as long as it does not chronically recur. Incidentally, cytology of this fluid has not been a particularly helpful tool.

12. **What particular findings suggest that a biopsy is necessary?**
One must have personal guidelines, but generally any patient who has any unexplained abnormality on physical examination or on mammogram should be considered a candidate for biopsy.

13. **Are there different types of biopsies?**
Yes. Open biopsy and needle biopsy. The open, or excisional, biopsy removes the entire lesion, gives the pathologist the most tissue, and is the most accurate. The needle biopsy has gained some popularity. The major objections center around the fact that the results of a needle biopsy may represent a sampling error and may also miss the lesion. Many believe that a positive needle biopsy should be confirmed by open biopsy. Thus, why not perform an open biopsy in the first place (controversial)?

14. **What is the approach to "lumpy" breasts, especially in young women?**
This is a common occurrence and there is no perfect answer. One should use all the modalities available to examine the breast, but in some instances it comes down to the judgment and experience of the physician.

15. **Is fibrocystic disease a premalignant disease?**

Generally, with a few exceptions. Very virulent adenosis or intraductal hyperplasia perhaps is associated with an increased incidence of carcinoma. For the most part, however, fibrocystic disease does not suggest a premalignant state.

16. Should a woman with severe fibrocystic disease be considered a candidate for subcutaneous mastectomy with implant?
This is a controversial issue. The answer depends partly on the reason for performing the subcutaneous mastectomy. If it is for symptomatic relief, then in very severe cases it may be justified. Performing subcutaneous mastectomies for cancer prophylaxis, however, does not offer the degree of safety one would hope. Simply reducing the volume of the breast does not necessarily reduce the likelihood of development of carcinoma.

17. What sort of anesthesia should be used in conjunction with a biopsy procedure?
Either local or general, depending on the patient's wishes and, to some extent, the nature of the nodule. Almost all biopsies can be done on an outpatient basis.

18. If the results of breast biopsy are positive, should one proceed with a more definitive procedure at the same time?
This is a controversial issue. Unless the condition of the patient dictates otherwise, or unless the patient specifically requests this course of action, the definitive procedure is perhaps best done at a later time. This does not change the prognosis whatsoever.

Today's society is so replete with literature of all types concerning breast cancer and its management that it has become increasingly more complicated to settle on a definitive procedure with the patient in whom the results of biopsy are positive. Psychologically, it can be distressing for a woman to undergo anesthesia with the prospect of losing a breast. Discussing options with the patient when the diagnosis is certain and when the patient has accepted this, has settled down, and can think clearly and logically, helps to ensure the choice of therapy suitable to all concerned.

---

58. PRIMARY THERAPY FOR BREAST CANCER
CHARLES M. ABERNATHY, M.D.

---

1. How is the diagnosis made?
Usually *excisional* biopsy of the entire mass under local anesthesia. *Cutting* needle biopsy is acceptable; needle *aspiration* (for cytology) is debatable (see Controversies).

2. What is the role of mammography after a positive biopsy?
The only value is in identifying a contralateral breast lesion or other (multicentric) lesion in the same breast. In addition, a mammogram may be abnormal as long as 2 months after biopsy as a result of hematoma, inflammation, etc.

3. Which preoperative studies should be done before mastectomy to identify metastases?
Chest x-rays and other studies such as bone scans probably will not alter the treatment plan.

4. Does a delay between biopsy and definitive treatment adversely affect cure?
Probably not if the delay is only a few days.

5. What are the preoperative stages of breast cancer?

I	II	III	IV
≤ cm; confined to breast	2-5 cm; palpable axillary lymph node	≥ 5 cm; palpable axillary nodes (and fixed to one another or to other structures)	distant metastases; extension to skin; inflammatory carcinoma; supraclavicular or infraclavicular lymph-edema

The TNM staging considers tumor size, presence and character of axillary nodes, and distant metastases. In general, stage I disease is confined to the breast; stage II is a 2 to 5 cm breast mass in which there is suspicion of positive axillary nodes; and stage III is a mass > 5 cm with certain positive axillary nodes.

6. What are the alternatives for primary treatment?
    1. Modified radical mastectomy. Most commonly performed procedure with the most solid data regarding benefit. Can be linked with either immediate or delayed (controversial) breast reconstruction.
    2. Partial mastectomy (lumpectomy or quadrantectomy) and axillary sampling with radiation to the breast. Results appear equal to those of modified radical mastectomy but series in general are much smaller and have a shortesr duration of follow-up. Remember that breast cancer can have late metastasis and therefore at leat 10 years of follow-up is needed for good data.
    3. Primary radiation to the breast (not to be confused with postoperative radiation). Acceptable cosmetic result with similar comment on results as in 2 above.

7. What exactly is done at modified radical mastectomy?
All breast tissue is removed and an axillary dissection of the lymph nodes is carried out with or without removing pectoralis *minor* muscle. Pectoralis major muscle is spared.

8. What is the overall survival after modified radical mastectomy?
Stage I, 60 to 80% 10-year survival; Stage II, 30 to 45% 10-year survival.

9. What is the role of estrogen/progesterone receptors postoperatively?
Estrogen receptors (ER) should be obtained on all primary breast cancer specimens. They are of value if a recurrence develops and in determining adjuvant settings (i.e., patient over 65 years of age, ER positive and lymph node positive may receive tamoxifen instead of Cytoxan, methotrexate and 5-fluorouracil (CMF)). Also, a patient with stage I cancer that is lymph node negative and ER negative is at risk for relapse (33% at 10 years); thus adjuvant chemotherapy can be effective.

10. Who gets adjuvant chemotherapy?
Any patient with one or more positive lymph nodes is typically treated with adjuvant therapy (see chapter on Postsurgical Breast Cancer).

11. What should be the treatment of "lobular carcinoma in situ"?
Lobular carcinoma in situ becomes invasive in 20 to 25 percent of patients over several years, occurring with equal frequency in the contralateral and ipsilateral breast. Treatment of noninvasive lobular carcinoma is local excision and mammographic evaluation of both breasts (preferred) or total mastectomy and contralateral (mirror-image) biopsy.

12. What should be the treatment of noninvasive ductal breast cancer?
Total mastectomy. Some surgeons prefer lumpectomy and irradiation. Some would add an axillary dissection with a 1 to 2% chance of positive nodes.

CONTROVERSIES

13. Needle aspiration cytology for diagnosis of breast cancer.
For: easy to do; inexpensive.
Against: 10 to 20% false positive; 5 to 10% false negative; patient left with mass.

14. Extensive preoperative work-up for metastases (bone scan, carcinoembryonic antigen, liver function tests).
For: may initiate chemotherapy or hormone therapy after definitive therapy; important for prognosis.
Against: expensive; low yield (depends on tumor size); does not alter primary therapy.

BIBLIOGRAPHY

1.   Alpert, S., et al.: Primary management of operable breast cancer by minimal srugery and radiotherapy. Cancer, 42:2054, 1978.
2.   Ashikari, R., Huvos, A.G., and Snyder, R.E.: Prospective study of noninfiltrating carcinoma of the breast. Cancer, 39:435, 1977. Total mastectomy recommended for in-situ ductal and lobular carcinoma.
3.   Baker, E.R. The indications for bone scans in the preoperative assessment of patients with operable breast cancer. Breast: Dis. Breast, 3:43, 1977.
4.   Bonadonna, G., et al.: Are surgical adjuvant trials altering the course of breast cancer? Semin. Oncol., 5:450, 1978.
5.   Cope, O., et al.: Limited surgical excision as the basis of a comprehensive therapy for cancer of the breast. Am. J. Surg., 131:400, 1976.
6.   Fisher, B., United States trials of conservative surgery. World J. Surg., 1:327, 1977.
7.   Fisher, B., and Gebhardt, M.D.: The evolution of breast cancer surgery: Past, present, and future. Semin. Oncol., 5:385, 1978.
8.   Hickey, R.C., et al.: The detection and diagnosis of early, occult and minimal breast cancer. Adv. Surg., 10:287, 1976.
9.   Kern, W.H.: The diagnosis of breast cancer by fine-needle aspiration smears. J.A.M.A., 241:1125, 1979.
10. Knapp, R.W., and Mullen, J.T.: Triage for the breast biopsy. Am. J. Surg., 131:626, 1976. Identical 5-year survival and local recurrence rates reported after both "one-step" inpatient biopsy/mastectomy and "two-step" procedure; biopsy followed by mastectomy.
11. Lee, Y.T.: Bone scanning in patients with early breast carcinoma: Should it be a routine staging procedure? Cancer, 47:486, 1981.
12. Mann, B.D., et al.: Delayed diagnosis of breast cancer as a result of normal mammograms. Arch. Surg., 118:23, 1983.
13. Moxley, J.H., III, et al.: Treatment of primary breast cancer. Summary of the National Institutes of Health Consensus Development Conference. J.A.M.A., 224:797, 1980.
14. Veronesi, U.: Value of limited surgery for breast cancer. Semin. Oncol., 5:395, 1978. Review of clinical trials of conservative surgical treatment.

59. POSTSURGICAL BREAST CANCER
SCOT M. SEDLACEK, M.D.

1. **What is the #1 risk factor for a woman developing cancer in one of her breasts?**
Cancer in the other breast.

2. **How has the annual mortality rate in women with breast cancer changed in the last 50 years?**
There has been no change in the annual death rate (approximately 27 deaths/100,000 women).

3. **How should the postmastectomy patient be followed for disease recurrence?**
Follow-up physical examination every 3 to 4 months with a yearly chest x-ray film and mammogram of the opposite breast. Two years post mastectomy, follow-up may be prolonged to every 6 months. The patient should also be taught breast self-examination. Bone scans, liver function tests, liver scans, and brain scans should be obtained when clinically indicated.

4. **Is breast cancer cured by "standard" surgical techniques?**
While it is true that patients who present with early-stage disease live longer than patients with advanced disease, even the woman with negative lymph nodes (No) and without distant metastases (Mo) has a 25% chance of disease recurrence after 10 years following radical mastectomy.

5. **Who should receive adjuvant chemotherapy?**
    1. Premenopausal women with any number of axillary lymph nodes involved with cancer.
    2. Any patient with a T3 (> 5 cm in diameter) or a nonmetastatic T4 (extension to chest wall or skin, inflammatory carcinoma, supraclavicular or infraclavicular lymph nodes, or arm edema) tumor should receive "neoadjuvant" chemotherapy and radiation therpay prior to primary surgical resection, followed by postoperative adjuvant chemotherapy for those patients with lymph node involvement.
    3. Postmenopausal women (see Controversies).

6. **What is the role of estrogen (ER)/progesterone (PgR) receptors?**
    1. Prognosis. Patients with receptor-positive cancers have a longer disease-free survival than those with receptor-negative cancers. PgR is a better predictor than is ER.
    2. Adjuvant therapy. Receptor status can identify a population of women who are at greater risk for relapse and thus may be more likely to benefit from adjuvant chemotherapy.
    3. Hormonal therapy. Patients with metastatic disease and receptor-positive cancers are good candidates for some type of hormonal therapy.

7. **Why should ER and PgR be repeated with a loco-regional recurrence or metastatic disease?**
The discordance of receptors between the primary tumor and recurrence is quite high. The greater the time interval between the two biopsies, the greater the chance of a change in receptor status. It is just as common for a tumor to change from receptor positive to negative as from negative to positive.

8. **What should be done for women with loco-regional recurrences?**
    Since approximately 50% of patients with a loco-regional recurrence also have concomitant metastatic disease, a complete metastatic work-up should be performed. This is followed by either complete surgical excision, if possible, or radiation therapy. Within 2 years, 80% of these patients will have subsequent progression of disease following an isolated single recurrence.

9. **Who should receive hormonal therapy?**
    Response to hormonal therapy depends on receptor status. More than two thirds of patients with both receptors positive will respond, whereas one third of patients with either receptor positive will respond. Therefore, receptor-positive patients are good candidates for some type of hormonal manipulation. Response to primary hormone therapy in unselected patients (unknown receptor status) is approximately 30%.

10. **What are the possible hormonal therapies in metastatic breast cancer?**
    Tamoxifen, an antiestrogen, is the most commonly used hormonal agent in the U.S. Secondary treatments include progestins (megestrol acetate) and aminoglutethimide (medical adrenalectomy). Oophorectomy is typically employed in the premenopausal patient who for some reason (compliance, side effects) cannot take oral hormonal agents.

11. **What potential side effect may be seen with almost any type of endocrine therapy?**
    Tumor flare. This is manifested by either an increase in tumor size and/or tumor bone pain. Hypercalcemia is the most life-threatening manifestation. This syndrome typically occurs 2 weeks after instituting therapy.

12. **What should be done for a woman with breast cancer and a symptomatic, malignant pleural effusion?**
    Attempts at repeated thoracentesis may be tried initially. If the fluid cannot be drained or recurs rapidly, then chest tube placement with drainage of all fluid followed by instillation of a sclerosing agent to perform pleurodesis is warranted. Agents used are tetracycline, talc, nitrogen mustard, quinacrine, and thiotepa. Talc may be the best agent listed.

13. **What percentage of women with metastatic breast cancer can be expected to respond to combination cytotoxic chemotherapy?**
    50 to 70%. The response rate depends on the dose intensity of the drugs. Adriamycin is the single most active agent.

CONTROVERSY

14. **Adjuvant chemotherapy in postmenopausal women with positive axillary lymph nodes.**
    For:
    1. Women who have received at least 85% of the predicted doses of chemotherapy have a significant decrease in disease recurrence.
    2. Prolongation of disease-free interval 1 to 4 years following adjuvant chemotherapy.

Against:
1. Significant cost and morbidity,
2. No statistically significant benefit in overall survival.
3. Hormonal therapy in ER-positive postmenopausal women may be just as good as chemotherapy but without the side effects.

BIBLIOGRAPHY

1. Allegra, J.C.: Rational approaches to the hormonal treatment of breast cancer. Semin. Oncol., 10(Suppl. 4):25-28, 1983. Concise review on the multitude of possible endocrine modalities employed in women with metastatic breast cancer.
2. Bonadonna, G., and Valagussa, P.: Adjuvant systemic therapy for resectable breast cancer. J. Clin. Oncol., 3:259-275, 1985. This is a major review article covering the last 15 years of adjuvant therapy of breast cancer patients by one of the foremost researchers in the field.
3. Clark, G.M., McGuire, W.L., Hubay, C.A., et al.: Progesterone receptors as a prognostic factor in stage II breast cancer. N. Engl. J. Med., 309:1343-1347, 1983. Disease-free survival was investigated in women post mastectomy with positive axillary lymph nodes. The progesterone receptor (PgR) was better at predicting outcome than the estrogen receptor (ER). Also when multiple prognostic factors were modeled using multivariant analysis, only the PgR level and the number of positive lymph nodes (1 to 3 versus > 3) were statistically significant, independent risk factors for relapse.
4. Fentiman, I.S., Reubens, R.D., and Hayward, J.L.: Control of pleural effusion in patients with breast cancer: A randomized trial. Cancer, 52:737-739, 1983. A controlled randomized trial in 37 evaluable patients with pleural effusions secondary to breast cancer. Nitrogen mustard achieved control in 9 of 17 (56%) patients, whereas in 18 of 20 (90%) treated with talc, control of malignant effusion was achieved.
5. Holdaway, I.M., and Bowditch, J.V.: Variation in receptor status between primary and metastatic breast cancer. Cancer, 52:479-485, 1983. When patients developed a local recurrence or a metastatic focus, repeat biopsies with ER and PgR determinations were performed. The ER changes in 54% of cases, while the PgR reversed in 35% of repeated biopsies. In over half of these cases, the change was from a receptor negative primary site, to a receptor-positive recurrent site.
6. Hryniak, W., and Bush, H.: The importance of dose intensity in chemotherapy of metastatic breast cancer. J. Clin. Oncol., 2:1281-1288, 1984.
7. Leff, A., Hopewell, P.C., and Costello, J.: Pleural effusion from malignancy. Ann. Intern. Med., 88:532-537, 1978. Review on the mechanisms of pleural fluid formation, characteristics, diagnosis and treatment of recurrent effusions.
8. Raemaekers, J.M., Beex, L.V., Koendears, A.J., et al.: Concordance and discordance of estrogen and progesterone receptor content in sequential biopsies of patients with advanced breast cancer: Relation to survival. Eur. J. Cancer Clin. Oncol., 20:1011-1018, 1984. Repeat biopsies of the primary tumor were performed ≥ 6 weeks after stopping hormone therapy. The ER changes status in 19% of patients while the PgR changes in 28%. Nearly all patients received some type of intervening therapy (i.e., chemotherapy, radiotherapy, hormonal therapy). Again, as in Holdaway's paper, a significant percentage converted from negative to positive.

---

60. MELANOMA
WILLIAM R. NELSON, M.D.

PREOPERATIVE

1. **What are the different types of moles or nevi?**
Intradermal, junctional, compound, and Spitz nevi, and nevi of the dysplastic nevus syndrome.

2. **What is a Spitz nevus?**
    This was formerly called juvenile melanoma. It has a characteristic cellular appearance and may mimic an early melanoma. It is completely benign.

3. **What characteristics typify the patient with melanoma?**
    The great majority of patients have auburn or reddish-brown hair and fair, poorly tanning skin.

4. **Does sunlight have any effect upon production of melanoma?**
    The great majority of melanomas occur in sun-exposed areas in sun-sensitive individuals. A small number of melanomas develop on the soles of the feet and near the genitalia.

5. **Do blacks ever get melanomas?**
    The numbers are small, but they can develop melanoma and, if they do, the lesions are often on unexposed and lightly pigmented areas such as the soles of the feet and the palms of the hands.

6. **In which part of the world is melanoma most common?**
    Australia and especially the northern part of the continent, where light-skinned descendants of the original settlers are exposed to the tropical sun.

7. **Which moles should be removed?**
    Growing and darkening nevi should be considered for removal, especially in sun-sensitive patients. Itching is a sign of early malignant change; ulceration is a very late sign. Melanoma may be familial in origin, and children of patients with melanomas should be carefully screened for very dark nevi.

8. **Should nevi be biopsied or should they always be totally excised?**
    It was once felt that incisional biopsy was contraindicated in all lesions suspected of being melanomas. Today it is believed that any large lesion requiring complex repair may be wedge-biopsied safely. The best method, however, is total excision of the lesion with a narrow margin of normal skin plus primary repair. Thorough pathologic study is essential.

9. **What are the types of melanoma and is the term "malignant melanoma" a redundancy?**
    The term "malignant melanoma" should be abandoned since melanoma is a malignant lesion. Types of melanoma are superficial spreading, nodular, lentigo maligna, and site-specific such as melanomas arising in giant hairy nevi, acral-lentiginous (volar plantar and subungual), mucosal, anorectal, conjunctival, ocular, and genital. We might also add unknown primary or disappearing primary lesions which may result in metastases. The outlook in this latter group is very poor, even though the primary tumor may have totally regressed.

10. **What is the importance of the Clark and Breslow classifications of melanoma invasion?**
    Clark has selected five levels of thickness in the skin and the breakdown is as follows:
    Level I: An intradermal melanoma that does not metastasize; might be better termed "atypical melanotic hyperplasia" since it is really a benign lesion.
    Level II: A melanoma that penetrates the basement membrane into the papillary dermis.
    Level III: A melanoma that fills the papillary dermis and encroaches on the reticular dermis in a "pushing" fashion.

Level IV: A melanoma that invades the reticular dermis.
Level V: A melanoma that works its way into the subcutaneous fat.
The Breslow method requires an optical micrometer fitted to the ocular position of standrard microscopes. This latter technique is an even more exact determination of tumor invasion.

11. **What are the chances of metastases to nodes in the different degrees of melanoma invasion in the skin?**
In comparing several series published, primary melanomas less than 1.5 mm thick spread to nodes in 7% of cases, whereas 23% of level II lesions over 1.5 mm have microscopic regional metastases. One author stated that 62% of level III lesions are less than 1.5 mm in thickness. In level II melanomas, 9% positive nodes were found in the combined series compared with 14% overall in level III lesions, 28% in level IV, and 39% in level V.

INTRAOPERATIVE

12. **How does the surgeon determine which node-bearing region to dissect when the primary tumor is in the mid-lateral chest?**
Spread to the axilla occurs from lesions above Sappey's line, which slopes gradually from the level of L2 to a point 2 cm above the umbilicus. If a band 5 cm wide is used for Sappey's line, then it is fairly accurate to use this as a dividing line between axillary and inguinal spread. Radioactive materials have been injected to better localize the spread from a melanoma.

13. **Should the primary melanoma be removed in continuity with the lymph nodes?**
Only if the lesion is near a lymph node area. As an example, a mid-thigh melanoma can be excised in continuity with the nodes, whereas a lesion below the knee cannot (see Controversies).

14. **After radical groin dissection, what should be done to protect the femoral vessels?**
Transposition of the sartorius muscle must be done to cover these structures.

15. **When should a node be dissected and what type of procedure should be carried out?**
See Controversies.

16. **When is chemotherapeutic isolation-perfusion used in the primary treatment of melanoma?**
See Controversies.

POSTOPERATIVE

17. **Can serious edema of the lower extremity be prevented after radical groin dissection?**
This can be kept to a minimum with the use of tailor-made support stockings, but some swelling occurs in most individuals who have this kind of surgery.

18. **How can extensive skin slough be prevented following radical groin dissection?**
The time-honored S incision resulted in many wound complications. Today it is preferable to use a double parallel technique with one incision above and one below the groin and, if properly executed, this will result in little or no skin slough (see Controversies regarding deep groin dissection).

19. **When is lymph node dissection indicated in melanoma?**
There has been quite a change in the thoughts of some surgeons regarding this matter. Certainly, in patients with resectable nodes that are enlarged, radical node dissection should be carried out. If no nodes are palpable, one should consider node dissection if the primary lesion is near a node-bearing region in lesions over 1.2 mm in thickness. The area between 0.7 and 1.2 mm is a gray zone but certainly metastases do occur in lesions of this depth. If the lesion is less than 0.7 mm or is in the the general level II area, no dissection is necessary.

20. **What type of node dissection should be done in general?**
In elective cases, the so-called functional dissection can be done, which preserves vital muscles and nerves. A modified dissection could be done in the neck with preservation of the sternocleidomastoid muscle, jugular vein, and spinal accessory nerve when nodes are not enlarged. Not all will agree with this, however.

21. **When is deep groin dissection indicated along with superficial removal of the nodes?**
Many have abandoned the deep dissection unless there are positive nodes obviously present. Generally, the deep dissection should be done if nodes in the area of the femoral canal are tested by frozen section and are found to be positive. On the other hand, Das Gupta performs deep and superficial node dissections on all patients being subjected to lymph node removal. He has found cases in which deep nodes were involved but not the superficial ones in tumors of the lower extremity.

22. **How would you treat a level IV lesion located directly between the scapulae on the posterior trunk?**
This remains controversial. Many would perform bilateral axillary dissections for deep melanomas whereas others would do merely a wide resection.

23. **When is skin graft indicated in patients having wide resections of a melanoma?**
In deep level III lesions and beyond, the wide excision generally results in a defect too large for primary repair. Most surgeons would perform a skin graft here. Others might attempt flap rotation or other means of approximation of skin edges. Superficial tumors can be excised with primary repair.

24. **Is chemotherapy or radiation indicated in the treatment of melanoma?**
Adjunctive chemotherapy has not proved effective in melanoma, and in patients with dissemination, DTIC (dacarbazine) has been helpful in about 20% (many of these were patients with pulmonary metastases who experienced at least partial regression). The drugs have been very disappointing in the management of this disease. Chemotherapeutic isolation-perfusion is effective in many patients with satellitosis of an extremity. Radiation therapy is helpful only in decreasing the size of large masses. Lentigo maligna lesions of a superficial type have been eradicated with radiotherapy, but most of these are treated by surgical excision.

25. **After surgery for curable melanoma, what follow-up procedures are indicated?**
Besides frequent physical examinations, chest x-rays, and liver function tests, gallium scans may be helpful; however, this is controversial. In patients with a poor prognosis, these scans can detect isolated metastases in soft tissue and brain before symptoms have developed. In rare instances, resection of such lesions can be carried out for palliation.

26. Is amputation ever indicated in the treatment of melanoma?
In selected cases, amputation of locally advanced lesions may be palliative. This applies to patients with huge, fungating masses or with massive satellitosis confined to the extremity where isolation-perfusion chemotherapy has failed.

27. What about the use of immunotherapy in melanoma?
In advanced melanoma, immunotherapy has been very disappointing. Interferon has helped some patients. Administration of monoclonal antibodies may be the answer for the future.

28. Is it possible to cure a patient with metastatic melanoma of unknown primary origin?
If metastases are confined to one node-bearing region, radical dissection should be done and cures have been reported to occur from 15 to 20%.

29. Which patients with positive nodes can still be considered to have a fairly good prognosis?
In the study by Day et al., a group of patients with primary lesions of 0.8 to 3.5 mm in whom less than 20% of the removed nodes were positive for melanoma metastases had an 80% 5-year disease-free survival despite these evidences of spread. This adds credence to the node dissection approach as an elective method. This is supported by the work of Balch, who showed marked benefit from elective node dissection in patients with lesions 1.5 to 4.0 mm in thickness. Day et al., in 643 patients with melanomas, found that patients with lesions less than 3.5 mm who underwent positive therapeutic node dissections when nodes were clinically palpable had a 5-year disease-free survival of 31% as compared with the same survival of 59% in patients undergoing elective (prophylactic) node dissections where positive nodes were found and the primary lesion was less than 3.5 mm. In a World Health Organization study which has turned many surgeons away from elective node dissection, the only subgroup that showed a trend of benefit was the 1.5 to 4.5 group. Thus some subgroups will benefit from elective node dissection because of metastases confined to a single node-bearing area.

BIBLIOGRAPHY

1. Balch, C.M., Soong, S., Murad, T., et al.: A multifactorial analysis of melanoma. II. Prognostic factors of clinical stage I disease. Surgery, 86:343-345, 1975.
2. Balch, C.M., Soong, S., Murad, T., et al.: A multifactorial analysis of melanoma. III. Prognostic factors in melanoma patients with lymph node metastases (stage II). Ann. Surg., 193:377-388, 1981.
3. Balch, C.M., Wilkerson, J.A., Murad, T., et al.: The prognostic significance of ulceration in cutaneous melanoma. Cancer, 45:3012-3017, 1980.
4. Breslow, A.: Thickness, cross sectional area, and depth of invasion in the prognosis of cutaneous melanoma. Ann. Surg., 172:902, 1970.
5. Breslow, A.: Tumor thickness, level of invasion and node dissection in stage I cutaneous melanoma. Ann. Surg., 182:572-575, 1975.
6. Clarke, W., et al.: The histogenesis and biological behavior of primary human malignant melanomas of the skin. Cancer Res., 29:705, 1969.
7. Cosimi, A.B., Sober, A.J., Mihm, M.C., and Fitzpatrick, T.B.: Conservative surgical management of superficially invasive cutaneous melanoma. Cancer, 53:1256-1259, 1984.
8. Das Gupta, T.K., Bowden, L., and Berg, J.: Malignant melanoma of unknown primary origin. Surg. Gynecol. Obstet., 117:341, 1963.

9.   Davis, N.C.: Cutaneous melanoma: The Queensland experience. Curr. Probl. Surg.,
      13:1, 1976.
10.   Fee, H.J., Robinson, D.S., Sample, W.F., et al.: The determination of lymph shed by
      colloidal gold scanning in patients with malignant melanoma: A preliminary study.
      Surgery, 84:626-632, 1978.
11.   Harrist, R.J., Rigel, D.S., Day, C.L., et al.: "Microscopic satellites" are more highly assoc-
      iated with regional lymph node metastases than is primary melanoma thickness.
      Cancer, 53:2183-2187, 1984.
12.   McBride, C.M.: Advanced melanoma of the extremities: Treatment of isolation-perfusion
      with a triple drug combination. Arch. Surg., 101:122-126, 1970.
13.   McNeer, G., and Das Gupta, T.: Prognosis in malignant melanoma. Surgery, 56:512-518,
      1964.
14.   Nisce, L.Z., Hilaris, B.S., and Chu, F.C.H.: A review of experience with irradiation of brain
      metastases. A.J.R., 111:329-333, 1971.
15.   Pack, G.T., Lenson, N., and Gerber, O.M.: Regional distribution of moles and melano-
      mas. Arch. Surg., 65:862-870, 1952.
16.   Reimer, R.R., Clark, W.H., Greene, M.H., et al.: Precursor lesions in familial melanoma.
      J.A.M.A., 239:744-746, 1978.
17.   Stehlin, J.S., Giovanella, B.C., Ipolyi, P.D., et al.: Results of hyperthermic perfusion for
      melanoma of the extremities. Surg. Gynecol. Obstet., 140:339-345, 1975.
18.   Sugarbaker, E.V., and McBride, C.M.: Melanoma of the trunk: The results of surgical
      excision and anatomic guidelines for predicting nodal netastasis. Surgery, 80:22-30,
      1976.
19.   Wanebo, H.J., Woodruff, J., and Fortner, J.G.: Malignant melanoma of the extremity: A
      clinicopathologic study using levels of invasion. Cancer, 35:666-667, 1975.

61. PAROTID TUMORS
WILLIAM R. NELSON, M.D.

1.   **How is a parotid tumor diagnosed?**
     A well-defined mass in the parotid gland as determined by physical examination is
     a parotid tumor until proven otherwise. Mumps, suppurative parotitis, stone in the
     parotid duct, and bilateral diffuse parotid enlargement would be excluded.

2.   **What is the most common location of a parotid tumor?**
     In the superficial lobe just beneath the lobe of the ear.

3.   **What is the most common cause of a mass high in the parotid in
     front of the tragus of the ear?**
     An enlarged parotid lymph node. In older patients, especially those with a history
     of skin cancer, such a mass must be considered a site of metastatic cancer until
     proved otherwise.

4.   **What is the ratio of malignant to benign tumors of the parotid?**
     At least 60% of tumors of the parotid are benign.

5.   **Name the types of benign tumors of the parotid.**
     Mixed tumor (the term "benign mixed tumor" has been dropped, since these
     lesions do recur locally and can be considered as local types of cancer), Warthin's
     tumors, oxyphilic adenoma, oncocytoma, and benign lymphoepithelial lesion.

6. **Name the types of malignant tumors in order of frequency.**
Mucoepidermoid carcinoma, malignant mixed tumor, acinic cell carcinoma, adenocarcinoma, adenoid cystic carcinoma, and epidermoid carcinoma.

7. **Should parotid tumors be biopsied before surgery?**
Rarely, if ever, is biopsy indicated preoperatively. In situations in which a malignant tumor seems certain, needle biopsy could be carried out in order that plans could be made for nerve removal and grafting, if necessary. Otherwise, a parotid lobectomy is the method of choice, with dissection and preservation of the facial nerve followed by frozen section.

8. **Do tumors occur in the deep lobe of the parotid, and if so, how are they treated?**
Deep lobe tumors are uncommon, since this portion is only about one fifth of the total parotid substance and this lies beneath the nerve. Superficial parotid lobectomy is first performed with dissection and preservation of the nerve followed by removal of the tumor in the deep lobe area along with any remaining deep lobe tissue.

9. **What is the significance of partial or complete nerve paralysis in the presence of a parotid tumor?**
If the paralysis has come on gradually (and is not Bell's palsy) in a patient with a parotid tumor, the diagnosis is cancer.

10. **Is it possible to cure patients who come in with nerve paralysis from a parotid cancer?**
Many patients have been cured if the tumor can be totally eradicated even though nerve paralysis was present on admission.

11. **Do tumors of the parotid occur in children?**
There are uncommon instances of this, but the types of tumors seen in children are exactly similar to those seen in adults.

12. **Are there any known etiologic factors in the production of parotid tumors?**
The only known factor is radiation. Tumors of the major and minor glands have developed in patients in past years who were treated for benign skin conditions of the face and neck. There is no proof that inflammatory disease of the parotid or stones in the parotid duct have produced tumors.

13. **Should all apparently benign tumors of the parotid be removed?**
The only exceptions to removal would be in instances of very aged of infirm patients with longstanding parotid lesions of apparently benign type. In rare instances, aspiration biopsies have been performed to confirm the diagnosis of a mixed tumor in situations in which surgery would be life-threatening.

INTRAOPERATIVE

14. **If cancer is found in a parotid lobectomy specimen, what is the next step in treatment?**
Except in the unusual very low-grade and very well-localized cancers, a total parotidectomy is indicated with dissection and preservation of the facial nerve. If nerve branches are involved, they may have to be sacrificed, but the entire nerve is not removed unless there is obvious involvement of this nerve.

15. **Is radical neck dissection necessary in these cases?**
In high-grade cancers, certainly the nodes of the upper neck should be removed along with the total parotid gland but a formal neck dissection is not done, unless there is clinical evidence of metastatic disease in the nodes.

16. **When is nerve graft used in the treatment of parotid cancer?**
If a branch or the entire nerve is involved, resection would have to be performed and frozen sections obtained from the nerve ends. A nerve graft using the greater auricular nerve from the opposite side of the neck is indicated and, of course, this should be sutured in place, if possible, by microsurgery.

17. **Is it possible to remove a parotid tumor without dissecting the facial nerve?**
This should never be done. A parotid lobectomy should be performed in any case of a parotid tumor and the nerve should be carefully identified and dissected out.

18. **What is the most common type of nerve injury seen in parotidectomy?**
Injury to the ramus marginalis mandibularis, the lowest branch of the nerve in the face that innervates the depressor muscles of the lower lip. This nerve must be carefully preserved during the operation and, if it is not injured, weakness of the lower lip, a common complication even of careful surgery, will clear within 4 to 6 weeks.

19. **Is bone resection ever indicated in the treatment of malignant parotid tumors?**
This is rarely necessary and will be carried out only in the presence of a deep recurrence of cancer or in an instance in which cancer has actually invaded the mandible.

20. **Is it possible to reduce the incidence of temporary post-parotidectomy facial nerve palsy when the nerve has been preserved?**
If great care is taken with nerve dissection, postoperative palsy should be minimal. Coagulation of bleeders near the nerve, careless suctioning around the nerve itself, and unnecessary pulling and stretching of the nerve can result in several weeks of distressing palsy.

POSTOPERATIVE

21. **When is radiation therapy indicated after treatment of a parotid cancer?**
In all except the very low-grade cancers, radiation therapy should be used following total parotidectomy and removal of the upper neck nodes.

22. **What is the cure rate in cancer of the parotid?**
In the low-grade cancers, the cure rate can approach 80 to 90%, but in one overall series, the 5-, 10-, and 15-year determinate cure rates were approximately 62, 54, and 47%, respectively.

23. **What is Frey's syndrome?**
Also called "gustatory sweating," this phenomenon occurs with eating in some 30 or more percent of patients who have had parotidectomy. This is thought to arise from regeneration of parasympathetic fibers within the auriculotemporal

nerve, resulting in stimulation of the sweat glands when the parotid gland has been removed.

24. Does salivary fistula ever occur following superficial parotid lobectomy?

If all except a few fragments of the superficial lobe are removed cleanly, fistulas should not occur. The deep lobe itself is rarely, if ever, the source of salivary leak following removal of the superficial lobe.

CONTROVERSIES

25. Is chemotherapy of advantage in patients who have had radical removal of cancers of the parotid followed by radiation therapy?

At this time, additional chemotherapy has not made any great impact upon cure rate in these malignant lesions. Not all agree that adjuvant chemotherapy is essentially without effect. The study of Rentschler and his group at the M.D. Anderson Hospital in Houston demonstrates some definite effects of chemotherapy but these were of short duration. Pulmonary lesions did regress with Adriamycin but the responses were only partial. Combination chemotherapy with three and four drugs was also used in some advanced cases, but the instances of tumor regression of significant degree were few and far between.

26. Do mixed tumors turn into true cancers?

Most believe that truly malignant mixed tumors can develop from the benign type after many years, but this is certainly not a common phenomenon. Many advanced mixed tumors are benign even though they may have achieved incredible growth. On the other hand, the incidence of malignant mixed tumors is quite a bit higher in older patients than in those under 60. This along with studies in the pathology laboratory has given credence to the theory that carcinomatous transformation does occur in unusual settings. O.H. Beahrs and a group at the Mayo Clinic have well documented this phenomenon.

27. Can spontaneous return of facial function occur following removal of the facial nerve?

This is a rare happening but it has been well recorded in isolated cases. The exact mechanism has not been determined, but a takeover by fifth nerve fibers and regrowth of facial nerve fibers are possibilities. The exact mechanism of facial function return following total removal of the seventh nerve is still not well worked out. Martin and Helsper discuss this in great detail in their paper on spontaneous return. Fifth nerve takeover was considered by these authors to be the most likely mechanism. One patient with spontaneous return underwent injection of the fifth nerve for neuralgia and temporary rapid loss of facial function occurred with the local anesthetic.

BIBLIOGRAPHY

1. Beahrs, O.H., Woolner, L.B., Kirklin, J.W., and Devine, K.D.: Surgical management of parotid lesions: A review of 760 cases. Arch. Surg., 75:605, 1957.
2. Beahrs, O.H., Woolner, L.B., Kirklin, J.W., and Devine, K.D.: Carcinomatous transformation of mixed tumors of the parotid gland. Arch. Surg., 75:605, 1957.
3. Conley, J.J.: Facial nerve grafting and treatment of parotid gland tumors. Arch. Surg., 70:359-366, 1955.
4. Guillamondegui, O.M., Byers, R.M., Luna, M.A., et al.: Aggressive surgery in treatment for parotid cancer: The role of adjunctive postoperative radiotherapy. A.J.R., 123:49-54, 1975.

5. Hanna, D.C., Gaisford, J.C., Richardson, G.S., and Bindra, R.N.: Tumors of the deep lobe of the parotid gland. Am. J. Surg., 116:524-527, 1968.
6. Kolson, H., and Aslam, P.: Accuracy and value of needle biopsy of the parotid gland. Arch. Otolaryngol., 87:75-79, 1968.
7. Martin, H.: Surgical removal of parotid tumors. CIBA Clin. Symp., 13:121-131, 1961.
8. Martin, H., and Helsper, J.T.: Spontaneous return of function following surgical section or excision of the seventh cranial nerve in the surgery of parotid tumors. Ann. Surg., 151:538, 1960.
9. Patey, D.H., and Thackray, A.C.: The pathological anatomy and treatment of parotid tumour with retropharyngeal extension (dumb-bell tumours). Br. J. Surg.,44:352-358, 1957.
10. Perzik, S.L., and Fisher, B.: The place of neck dissection in the management of parotid tumors. Am. J. Surg., 120:355-358, 1970.
11. Rentschler, R., Burgess, M.A., and Byers, R.: Chemotherapy of malignant major salivary gland neoplasms: A 25-year review of M.D. Anderson Hospital experience. Cancer, 40:619-624, 1977.
12. Spiro, R.H., and Martin, H.: Gustatory sweating following parotid surgery and radical neck dissection. Ann. Surg., 165:118-127, 1967.

---

62. DEBULKING (CYTOREDUCTIVE) SURGERY
SCOT M. SEDLACEK, M.D., and PAUL A. BUNN, JR., M.D.

---

1. **What is cytoreductive surgery?**
A procedure whereby a surgically incurable malignant neoplasm is partially removed without curative intent in order to make subsequent treatment with chemotherapy or radiotherapy more effective, and therefore possibly increase the number of complete responses and ultimately survival.

2. **Why is it needed when chemotherapy is known to have efficacy in certain tumors?**
Cytotoxic chemotherapeutic agents kill cancer cells by first-order kinetics, meaning a given dose will kill a constant fraction of cells regardless of tumor size. Current effective chemotherapy can accomplish a 2 log cell kill (90% cell kill = 1 log cell kill, 99% cell kill = 2 log cell kill). Tumors typically do not become detectable until there are 10^9 cells.

```
          30 doublings              10 doublings
1 cell--------------------> 10^9 cells --------------------> 10^12 cells----------------> host dies
undetectable               palpable                          bulky disease
                           1 cm^3 1 gm                       1 L, 1 kg
```

Thus, despite a 99% eradication of all cancer cells with a course of chemotherapy, the tumor would decrease only from 10^{12} to 10^{10} cells. Thus the chance of eradicating certain cancers is greater when the cell population size is small.

3. **How does tumor size relate to cytotoxic chemotherapeutic drug resistance?**
Temporary drug resistance may develop in very large tumors due to areas of relative hypoxia, thus not exposing the cells to the same therapeutic concentrations of the drugs administered as other cells with adequate vascular supply. Also, the Goldie-Coldman hypothesis states that drug resistance via cellular mutations is more likely with large cell numbers.

4. **What is required for maximum effectiveness of cytoreductive surgery postoperatively?**
    Having effective chemotherapy and/or radiotherapy for that particular cancer.

5. **In what types of malignant diseases has cytoreductive surgery been of benefit?**
    Ovarian and testicular carcinomas along with Burkitt's lymphoma.

6. **In ovarian carcinoma, what is the single most important prognostic factor following cytoreductive surgery?**
    The presence of a residual tumor mass with a largest diameter $\leq$ 1.0 to 1.5 cm. Stage and abdominal spread is less important than the size of the largest residual tumor nodule. Survival is the same for patients with residual tumor reduced to < 1.5 cm as for patients whose largest metastases were < 1.5 cm prior to surgery. There is a 20% survival at 80 months if the residual tumor is $\leq$1.5 cm, and a 0% survival at 38 months if the residual tumor is > 1.5 cm.

7. **How does residual tumor size relate to outcome at the time of second-look operations in ovarian cancer?**
    In patients with residual tumors $\leq$ 2 cm following cytoreductive surgery, who are given postoperative chemotherapy, 30% have no residual cancer at the time of second-look laparotomy. In patients with residual tumors > 2 cm, only 16.7% have negative second-look laparotomies.

8. **What sequence of therapies should be used in nonseminomatous testicular carcinoma and bulky disease (stage II or stages B3 and C)?**
    Cytoreductive chemotherapy followed by surgical resection and cytoreduction in patients with bulky retroperitoneal lymph node involvement. Surgical resection prior to chemotherapy in these patients is a very difficult procedure because the tumor surrounds vital structures (blood vessels and the ureters), thus leading to excess bleeding, disruption of tissue planes, and possible tumor dissemination. This may ultimately lead to a poorer prognosis in patients treated in such a manner (see Controversies).

9. **What is the major factor predisposing to treatment failure in patients with seminoma following radiotherapy?**
    Tumor volume. Eight of twenty-one (38%) patients with retroperitoneal metastases > 5 cm in diameter relapsed following radiotherapy. Recommend cytoreductive surgery before radiotherapy in patients with bulky abdominal disease (stages B3 and C).

10. **How is American Burkitt's lymphoma different from African Burkitt's lymphoma?**
    The overwhelming majority of children with the American variety present with massive abdominal disease, not the typical cervical node involvement seen in African Burkitt's lymphoma. It is the patient with bulky abdominal disease in whom surgical cytoreduction should be attempted.

11. **What special considerations must be taken into account in patients with bulky abdominal disease from Burkitt's lymphoma prior to attempted surgical cytoreduction?**
    Burkitt's lymphoma is one of the most rapidly growing malignant tumors in humans. It has a 90 to 100% growth fraction (actively dividing cells) and an acutal mean doubling time of 66 hours. Therefore, if 90% of the tumor is surgically removed (1 log reduction) and the chemotherapy is not administered for 11 days

postoperatively, by the time the drugs are given the tumor will have had time to grow to 160% of its original volume (see Controversies).

12. **What life-threatening complication may occur in patients with massive abdominal Burkitt's lymphoma given cytotoxic chemotherapy without prior surgical cytoreduction?**
Acute tumor lysis syndrome. Because of the high growth fraction and cell doubling time, these tumor cells are exquisitely sensitive to chemotherapeutic agents. Thus a massive cell kill generates potentially life-threatening situations:

> Hyperkalemia-----------------> arrhythmias
> Hyperphosphatemia ------> hypocalcemia and tetany
> Hyperuricemia ---------------> acute renal failure

13. **What unusual operative risk should the anesthesiologist be reminded of prior to surgery in patients with Burkitt's lymphoma?**
The potential for malignant hyperthermia.

CONTROVERSIES

14. **Sequence of therapies in nonseminomatous testicular cancer with bulky retroperitoneal disease.**

Chemotherapy Before Surgery:
  For:
  1. Convert surgically unresectable disease into resectable lesions.
  2. Determine effectiveness of preoperative chemotherapy and thus necessity for a change in chemotherapy if viable carcinoma is persistent (one third of patients will have persistent carcinoma after initial chemotherapy).
  3. Determine necessity for any further therapy. (None if only fibrosis and/or mature teratoma are found at time of surgery.)
  Against:
  1. Potential tumor seeding.
  2. Compromised blood supply postoperatively to area, making subsequent radiation or chemotherapy more difficult (and possibly less effective).
  3. Potentially two thirds of patients will have benign disease and thus surgery is unnecessary (one third with fibrosis only, one third with mature teratoma only).

15. **Role of cytoreductive surgery in patients with Burkitt's lymphoma.**
  For:
  1. Less acute tumor lysis syndrome following surgical cytoreduction.
  2. Improved response to chemotherapy and less chance of relapse for patients who are able to undergo surgical cytoreduction prior to chemotherapy.
  Against:
  1. Risk of tumor regrowth during recovery thus requiring immediate administration of chemotherapy in the postoperative period.
  2. Risk of poor wound healing and secondary infection if chemotherapy is given soon after surgery.
  3. Artifactual benefit seen with cytoreductive surgery because of patient selection (only patients with "operable" disease considered). All studies are retrospective and uncontrolled.

BIBLIOGRAPHY

1. Brunner, N., Rorth, M., Schultz, H., et al.: Secondary surgery in advanced testicular germ cell tumors. Scand. J. Urol. Nephrol., 17:283-285, 1983. Secondary surgery in 24 patients with residual tumor following intensive chemotherapy. Residual mass completely resected in 20, with 18 of 20 alive with no evidence of disease. Four patients had incomplete resection, of whom 2 have died from disease recurrence.

2. Griffiths, C.T.: Surgical resection of tumor bulk in the primary treatment of ovarian carcinoma. Natl. Cancer Inst. Monogr., 42:101-104, 1975. Survival studies in 102 patients with stages II and III ovarian carcinoma. The most important factors as determined by multivariant analysis were histologic grade and size of largest residual tumor mass after operation. Survival time was inversely proportional to residual mass size under 1.6 cm.

3. Hacker, N.F., Berek, J.S., Lagasse, L.D., et al.: Primary cytoreductive surgery for epithelial ovarian cancer. Obstet Gynecol., 61:413-420, 1983. UCLA experience in 47 patients with stage III or IV ovarian carcinoma. Able to obtain optimal cytoreduction ($\leq$ 1.5 cm) in 31 of 47 (66%) patients. Survival for patients with residual tumors > 1.5 cm, 0.5-1.5 cm, and < 0.5 cm was 6,18, and 40 months, respectively.

4. Janus, C., Edward, B.K., Sariban, E., and Magrath, I.T.: Surgical resection and limited chemotherapy for abdominal undifferentiated lymphomas. Cancer Treat. Rep., 68:599-605, 1984. Decription of the National Cancer Institute protocol using intensive chemotherapy following cytoreductive surgery. Chemotherapy was given the same day as surgery. Of 14 patients described, 12 were diagnosed as having Burkitt's lymphoma. Only two patients have relapsed, one of whom dies, while the second is alive and free of disease. Thus, 13 of 14 are alive without evidence of disease 25 to 63 months after presentation.

5. Magrath, I.T., Lwanga, S., Carswell, W., and Harrison, N.: Surgical reduction of tumor bulk in management of abdominal Burkitt's lymphoma. Br. Med. J., 1:308-310, 1974. Report from Uganda concerning 25 patients in whom surgical cytoreduction was attempted prior to chemotherapy. Nine patients had near complete removal of tumor and 16 had little over half of the tumor removed. Only the group with $\geq$ 90% of abdominal disease removed showed a statistically significant prolongation in survival. There was no advantage to partial resection.

6. Merrin, C., Takita, H., Beckley, S., and Kassis, J.: Treatment of recurrent and widespread testicular tumor by radical reductive surgery and multiple sequential chemotherapy. J. Urol., 117:291-295, 1977. Roswell Park experience with 37 patients with stage II and III disease treated with prechemotherapy cytoreductive surgery. Discusses therapeutic rationale behind combined approach.

7. Silberman, A.W., Surgical debulking of tumors. Surg. Gynecol. Obstet., 155:577-585, 1982. This is the only comprehensive review on cytoreductive surgery discussing cancers of the testis, ovary, kidney, brain, lymphomas, sarcomas, endocrine-related tumors, and chordomas.

8. Smith, J.P., and Day, T.G., Jr.: Review of ovarian cancer at the University of Texas Systems Cancer Center, M.D. Anderson Hospital and Tumor Institute. Am. J. Obstet. Gynecol., 7:984-992, 1979. The records of 2115 patients with ovarian carcinoma were reviewed. The most important prognostic factor was the size of the largest tumor mass that remained after initial surgery.

9. Ziegler, J.L.: Burkitt's lymphoma. N. Engl. J. Med., 305:735-745, 1981. The classic review article on history, etiology, clinical features, staging, treatment, and immunology of Burkitt's lymphoma. Surgical cytoreduction and the acute tumor lysis syndrome are discussed.

63. HODGKIN'S DISEASE
L. MICHAEL GLODE, M.D.

1. **Contrast the incidence curves for Hodgkin's disease and the non-Hodgkin's lymphomas.**
For Hodgkin's disease, there is a bimodal incidence with one peak in the 20's and a second in the 60's. Non-Hodgkin lymphomas rise steadily in incidence from childhood through 80 years of age.

2. **Are there any clues when a patient presents that may tip you off to suspect one or the other type of lymphoma?**
Hodgkin's is a "centripetal" disease which tends to start in the axial nodes and spread to adjacent groups. Non-Hodgkin's lymphomas are often multicentric and involve nodes which are frequently spared in Hodgkin's such as the epitrochlear nodes, Waldeyer's ring, and gastrointestinal tract.

3. **What do you suspect in a young woman who presents with mediastinal widening on a routine chest film?**
This is a classic presentation for nodular sclerosing Hodgkin's. In advanced cases, there may be local problems associated with the mass such as the superior vena cava syndrome, dysphagia, or hoarseness.

4. **What are the staging tests used for Hodgkin's disease?**
Any non-nodal involvement other than the spleen indicates stage IV disease. Therefore, one of the first tests used is bilateral bone marrow biopsies. If positive, one need only pursue work-up of other potential problem areas such as renal obstruction. A chest x-ray is mandatory. Lymphangiography in good hands is about 85% accurate in diagnosing periaortic nodes below the renal arteries; however, CT scanning is more sensitive for upper abdominal nodes.

5. **When should a work-up be done for an enlarged lymph node?**
Most patients will have a few lymph nodes palpable in the axillary and inguinal regions on careful examination. About half of individuals will have soft, flat nodes 0.5 to 1.0 cm in size, in the head and neck region. A careful history in a young patient will frequently reveal the presence of an antecedent upper respiratory infection, and physical examination, particularly of the scalp, can be useful in identifying the etiology of enlarged preauricular and posterior triangle nodes. In these cases, it is reasonable to follow the node for 4 to 6 weeks and watch for resolution. On the other hand, a spherical, hard, discrete node almost always requires biopsy. This is particularly true in older patients, and if the node is fixed or matted with other nodes. In heavy smokers and drinkers, firm nodes in the anterior triangle or submental region are a clue to cancers of the oropharynx. Diffuse lymphadenopathy in a young male should trigger questions about homosexuality and/or intravenous drug abuse.

6. **What is the staging system for Hodgkin's disease?**
The Ann Arbor Classification is:
 Stage I: Involvement of a single lymph node region (I) or as single extralymphatic organ site (IE)
 Stage II: Involvement of two or more lymph node regions on the same side of the diaphragm.

Stage III: Involvement of lymph node regions on both sides of the diaphragm. Spleen involvement is called IIIs.

Stage IV: Diffuse or disseminated involvement of 1 or more extranodal organs with or without nodes involved.

A = asymptomatic   B = fever, sweats, > 10% weight loss

7.   What are the pathologic subtypes of Hodgkin's disease?
They are (in rough order of frequency) nodular sclerosis (35%), mixed cellularity (33%), lymphocyte-predominant (16%), and lymphocyte-depleted (16%). Of interest, nodular sclerosis does very well in stage I or II when treated by radiation therapy alone, but has the second highest relapse rate when stage III or IV is treated with chemotherapy.

8.   Does every patient need a staging laparotomy?
Probably not. See Controversies.

9.   Other than biopsy information, what is there to gain by doing a staging laparotomy?
If there is a questionable call on the lymphangiogram, the removal of the node in question should be accompanied by leaving a visible surgical clip. In women of childbearing age, oophoropexy allows radiation therapy to be given to the "inverted Y" field, which covers the iliac and inguinal nodes without radiation damage to the ovaries.

10.   Do staging laprotomies provide any additional risks for patients other than that of the operation itself?
In patients less than 15 years of age, removal of the spleen can result in an increased risk of overwhelming bacterial sepsis.

CONTROVERSIES

11.   Staging laparotomies should be done in everyone:
For:
1.   It is the only way to be sure of the splenic and liver involvement.
2.   It can detect disease in the porta hepatis that can be missed by other techniques.
3.   In large centers, about one third of patients will have their treatment plans altered as a result of staging findings.
4.   It has low morbidity in experienced hands.
Against:
1.   Significant morbidity does occur even in experienced hands in about 10% of patients.
2.   It adds significantly to the cost of caring for a patient with Hodgkin's disease.
3.   Overwhelming infections may be seen in children who have undergone splenectomy.
4.   If you are planning to use chemotherapy anyway, the results of the laparotomy will not be of use.

BIBLIOGRAPHY

1.   Aisenberg, A.C.: Current concepts in cancer. The staging and treatment of Hodgkin's disease. N. Engl. J. Med., 299:1228-1231, 1978.
2.   Chilcote, R.R., et al.: Septicemia and meningitis in children splenectomized for Hodgkin's disease. N. Engl. J. Med., 295:798-800, 1976. A retrospective study of the problem in 200 patients, 18 of whom developed septic complications.

3.   DeVito, et al: Curability of advanced Hodgkin's disease with chemotherapy. Ann. Intern.
        Med., 92:587-595, 1980. A classic article documenting the 63% relapse free survival
        at 10 years of complete remission (80% of total group) patients. Thus, 55% of all
        patients treated with chemotherapy are cured.
4.   Pearth, et al.: Partial splenectomy for staging Hodgkin's disease: Risk of false negative
        results. N. Engl. J. Med., 299:345-346, 1978. Reviews 112 cases of splenic
        involvement at Mayo Clinic and indicates that 13 (11.6%) would have been under-
        staged by partial splenectomy. Agrees that splenctomy might be avoided in 96
        (86%) of cases with other abdominal involvement.
5.   Symposium on contemporary issues in Hodgkin's disease: Biology, staging and treat-
        ment. Cancer Treat. Rep. , 66:501-1071, 1982.

64. NECK MASSES
NATHAN PEARLMAN, M.D.

1.   **A 21-year-old women presents with a 3 to 4 cm mass below the
        angle of the mandible, and slightly anterior and adjacent to the
        anterior border of the sternomastoid muscle. What is a reasonable
        differential diagnosis?**
        Reactive lymphadenopathy, lymphoma, metastatic carcinoma, infectious
        mononucleosis, tumors (benign and malignant) of the submaxillary or parotid
        gland, carotid body tumors, and branchial cleft cyst.

2.   **Metastatic cancer? In a 21-year-old woman?**
        Yes. Both thyroid cancer and nasopharyngeal cancer are relatively common in
        this age group and are becoming more common with time.

3.   **Is there any way to narrow this list?**
        Yes. Inflammatory nodes are generally soft, bilateral, and less than 3 cm in
        diameter, as are those involved with mononucleosis. In contrast, nodes or
        masses larger than 3 to 4 cm (use a measuring device if needed) are virtually
        always tumors or metastases. Nodes involved with lymphoma are soft and are the
        consistency of the submaxillary gland, whereas those harboring carcinoma are
        relatively hard and have a consistency more like that of the thyroid. Parotid
        tumors tend to have an indistinct upper border that merges imperceptibly with
        the body of the gland itself. Tumors of the submaxillary gland tend to occupy the
        same position as those of the contralateral gland and are generally rubbery in
        consistency. Carotid body tumors are also rubbery but are often tender and
        difficult, if not impossible, to separate from the carotid pulse. These lesions also
        have a very indistinct, to absent, upper border. Branchial cleft cysts *rarely*
        present in patients over 21 years of age, often have been present for long
        periods of time, and are usually fluctuant (they also may transilluminate).

4.   **What is the *first* and most *important* test or examination to perform
        in a patient with a neck mass?**
        A complete head and neck examination. This consists of a comprehensive
        palpable and visual examination (using head lamp and mirror, or flexible
        endoscope) of the ipsilateral and contralateral neck, thyroid gland, parotid glands,
        oral cavity, tonsillar region, nasopharynx (between and cephalad to eustachian
        tube orifices), hypopharynx, piriform sinuses, and larynx. In 90% of instances,
        this will narrow the list of possibilities to one, or perhaps two, diseases and obviate
        the need for expensive, wasteful radiographic studies.

5. Most surgeons acknowledge the *eventual* need for such an examination; however, many feel awkward carrying out a mirror examination and do not have a flexible endoscope available. Instead, they immediately carry out open biopsy. What is wrong with this approach?

Open biopsy of neck nodes, without knowledge of a possible primary site, unduly complicates management of the patient when metastatic carcinoma is found and may compromise his or her chance for cure. Such a biopsy is followed by scarring of subcutaneous tissues and destruction of tissue planes used for a neck dissection. If the latter becomes necessary, the scar tissue cannot be distinguished from tumor and must be removed en bloc with the cancer. The result is a bigger operation, and complications that otherwise would have been avoided.

Notwithstanding perioperative problems, open biopsy often destroys nodal or fascial barriers holding the cancer in check and seeds the surrounding soft tissues or lymphatics with tumor cells. This, in turn, increases the chances for neck recurrence, which is almost uniformly fatal, even with irradiation. Since recurrence above the clavicles, and not distant metastases, remains the major cause of death in squamous head and neck cancer, one can understand why surgeons who deal with this problem have, for years, looked with abhorrence on preliminary open biopsies of the neck.

6. All right. I am suitably impressed with the need for a complete head and neck examination before neck biopsy. The examination reveals nothing. What now?

An examination under anesthesia. This consists of a more detailed visual and digital examination of the neck, mouth, pharynx, and larynx as well as cervicothoracic esophagoscopy and tracheobronchoscopy. If nothing is found during this examination, then blind biopsies of the nasopharynx, tonsils and tonsillar beds, base of tongue, and piriform sinuses are performed.

7. Why esophagoscopy and bronchoscopy?

If the patient is found to have a squamous head and neck cancer, there is a 10 to 20% chance that a second squamous primary tumor will be found in the aerodigestive tract.

8. Why blind biopsies of the sites listed above?

In about 10 to 15% of cases in which nothing is seen grossly, and metastatic neck nodes exist, the primary tumor will be found by blind biopsies.

9. If we are going to carry out examination under anesthesia anyway, why not proceed to that at the outset, and skip the mirror flexible endoscopic examination?

Because each of these examinations provides information not available on the other. The mirror and endoscopic examination provides more information about tongue and laryngeal function than does direct examination under anesthesia, and treatment plans depend on knowledge of such function. In addition, the mirror examination provides a good hint as to where to look for abnormalities on the direct examination; the latter often becomes a blind search without such hints owing to collapse of the tongue and pharyngeal walls once the patient is asleep. Thus, these two methods of evaluating the patient are complementary, not overlapping.

10. The patient undergoes a good mirror examination, direct examination under anesthesia, and blind biopsies, and nothing is

found. There is still no explanation for the neck node or mass. **What now?**
One might consider a needle, or aspiration, biopsy. This will often provide a diagnosis without incurring some of the problems inherent in an open biopsy.

11. **A needle biopsy is done and reveals only lymphocytes. What should the patient be told?**
The presence of lymphocytes suggests that the biopsy specimen is from a lymph node or salivary gland tumor (Warthin's). The patient will still require an operation, either lymph node excision to rule out lymphoma or removal of the tumor, but it seems unlikely that a neck dissection will also be required.

12. **What if the needle biopsy returns only fat and muscle?**
The needle probably missed the suspect node or mass. Now, an open biopsy is indicated and should be followed by an immediate neck dissection if metastatic cancer is found on frozen section.

13. **A radical neck dissection?**
Yes. The best time for this, and the patient's best chance for cure, is when normal tissue planes are intact, and this time exists only once—when the neck is entered for the biopsy. The reasons against carrying out a delayed dissection have already been enumerated. Thus, there is a time to carry out an open biopsy, but that time is not until you are ready to carry out a radical neck dissection, should carcinoma be found.

14. **Suppose this neck mass is not in the submandibular region but in the posterior neck. Do we need to go through all this preliminary work-up as for the former location?**
Yes. Although most oral or phyaryngeal tumors metastasize first to the submandibular or submaxillary region; some—notably thyroid, nasopharyngeal, and posterior hypopharyngeal or cervicoesophageal—tend to go first to posterior triangle nodes.

15. **What if the needle and/or open biopsy shows adenocarcinoma?**
Although most metastatic nodes high in the ipsilateral neck show squamous or thyroid cancer, or lymphoepithelioma, some may reveal adenocarcinoma. There is, at this point, about an equal likelihood that the patient has an otherwise occult lung cancer, or a prostatic, renal, gastrointestinal primary, or salivary gland tumor. This is the one time that further work-up makes sense to try to locate such a primary tumor before proceeding with a neck dissection.

16. **What if the needle or open biopsy shows undifferentiated carcinoma?**
Proceed with a neck dissection. The patient has either a melanoma, which has undergone spontaneous regression or will never be found, or an undifferentiated variant of a squamous head and neck cancer.

17. **Is there anything else to offer the patient with metastatic squamous or undifferentiated carcinoma after a neck dissection?**
Yes. Postoperative irradiation. Experience suggests recurrence rates in the neck can be reduced from 25 to 35% with surgery alone, to 5 to 10% using surgery and preoperative and postoperative irradiation.

18. **What if the primary tumor is never found?   Does this influence prognosis?**

Assuming that an obvious oral, pharyngeal, or laryngeal primary tumor was not missed (unfortunately, this occurs more often than is optimal), the answer is "No." The primary tumor, if truly small or occult, will probably be included in the port used for postoperative irradiation and cured by such treatment. The patient's prognosis in such cases is determined primarily by whether or not the tumor recurs in the neck or distant sites (lung, bone, or liver).

19. **This is all well and good for seemingly solid tumors or nodes in the anterior or posterior triangles of the neck.   What about those in the midline or those that are "obviously" nothing more than branchial cleft cysts?**

True midline lesions, if located cephalad to the isthmus of the thyroid gland, are unlikely to be anything other than thyroglossal duct remnants. In such cases, much of the work-up and treatment outlined earlier can be omitted and the patient taken directly to surgery. On the other hand, the noncompulsive physician will be "surprised" by unsuspected cancer 3 to 4 times more often than he or she will encounter true branchial cleft cysts in the adult. The message is, or should be, crystal clear: branchial cleft cysts are uncommon in adults, cancer is not. Much more damage has been done in the past by blithely assuming that the former was present, than by worrying about the latter. Until this changes, one should err on the side of completeness rather than on the side of expediency.

20. **What is the role of adjuvant chemotherapy?**

The use of adjuvant chemotherapy for head and neck cancer remains to be determined. Some studies suggest that preoperative/preradiation chemotherapy in advanced (stage III/IV) disease improves survival; however, no prospective study to confirm this has yet been published. In contrast, there is evidence to show that postoperative/postradiation chemotherapy does *not* contribute to improved survival.

BIBLIOGRAPHY

1. Barrie, J.R., Knapper, W.H., and Strong, E.W.: Cervical nodal metastases of unknown origin.   Am. J. Surg., 120:466-470, 1970.
2. Batsakis, J. G.:   The pathology of head and neck tumors: The occult primary and metastases to the head and neck, Part 10. Head Neck Surg., 3:409-423, 1981.
3. Cady, B., Sedgwick, C. E., Meissner, W.A., et al.:   Changing clinical, pathologic, therapeutic, and survival patterns in differentiated thyroid carcinoma. Ann. Surg., 184:541-553, 1976.
4. Clark, R.M., Rosen, I.B., and Laperriere, N.J.: Malignant tumors of the head and neck in a young population. Am. J. Surg., 144:459-462, 1982.
5. Coker, D.S., Casterline, P.F., Chambers, R.G., et al.: Metastases to lymph nodes of the head and neck from an unknown primary site. Am. J. Surg., 134:517-522, 1977.
6. McGuirt, W.F., and McCabe, B.F.: Significance of node biopsy before definitive treatment of cervical metastatic carcinoma. Laryngoscope, 88:594-597, 1978.
7. Strong, E.W., Henschke, U.K., Nickson, J.J., et al.: Preoperative x-ray therapy as an adjunct to radical neck dissection. Cancer, 19:1509-1515, 1966.
8. Vikram, B., Strong, E.W., Shah, J.P., et al.: Failure in the neck following multimodality treatment for advanced head and neck cancer. Head Neck Surg., 6:724-729, 1984.

65. ARTERIAL INSUFFICIENCY
ROBERT RUTHERFORD, M.D.

1. **Arteriosclerotic occulusive disease (AOD) involving the lower extremities, also known as arteriosclerosis obliterans, progresses in severity through three distinct clinical stages. What are they?**

   I — claudication; II —ischemic rest pain; and III — ischemic tissue necrosis.

   Comment: The Frenchman Fontaine originally described these clinical stages to which a 0 or asymptomatic stage has been added to allow categorization of the not uncommon situation of occlusive disease evidenced by pulse deficits in elderly, sedentary patients who do not exercise enough to claudicate. The final stage of ischemic tissue loss is commonly subdivided into two subtypes, nonhealing ulcers and gangrene. The ulcers may result from focal ischemic infarcts or may be *initially* due to other factors (pressure, neuropathy, venous insufficiency, trauma), but *do not heal* because of diffuse pedal ischemia caused by arteriosclerosis obliterans. Similarly, one may have *focal* gangrene without diffuse pedal ischemia, as in atheromicroembolism or ("the blue toe syndrome") or digital artery thrombosis. It is important to distinguish these patients who are capable of local healing and those with ulcers or gangrene *and* diffuse pedal ischemia, who will not heal unless their circulation is improved by some therapeutic intervention.

2. **Describe claudication and the clinical features that distinguish it from other forms of extremity.**

   Claudication is extremity pain or discomfort *regularly* produced by *the same degree* of exercise and relieved *promptly* by rest.

   Comment: Claudication may occur in the calf, the buttock, the hip or thigh, or the foot, in that order of frequency. Calf claudication is typically a cramping pain, but buttock, hip or thigh claudication may not be very painful; most often it is an aching discomfort associated with a feeling of weakness. The rare foot claudication is typically a severe metatarsalgia associated with a "wooden" numbness. The more proximal the location of the claudication, the more proximal the distribution of the responsible ischemic lesions. Sporadic calf cramps occur at rest, after exercise and, particularly at age extremes, nocturnally as one stretches during periods of arousal from sleep. Buttock, hip or thigh discomfort, aggravated by exercise, may occur with arthritis of the hip, but the presence of pain at rest and for prolonged periods after exercise and the lack of precise relationship with duration and degree of exercise distinguish it from the claudication. Narrowing of the neurospinal canal by osteoarthritic hypertrophic changes of the lumbar spine cause cauda equina compression and an aching numbness of the hips and thighs when the lordosis of erect posture further narrows the canal. Thus, patients may regularly experience weakness and discomfort when they get up and walk. But stopping does not relieve their distress *unless they sit,* and standing *without* walking (exercise) for the same duration also brings on these symptoms. Other forms of metatarsalgia do not have the clear-cut relationship to duration of exercise and prompt relief by rest that is observed in those with foot claudication due to severe infrapopliteal occlusive disease as seen in diabetics or those with Buerger's disease.

3. **What are the clinical features of *ischemic rest pain*, especially those which distinguish it from other forms of foot pain?**

   Severe forefoot pain which is usually relieved by dependency and associated with the "trophic" changes of chronic ischemia.

Comment: In the claudicator, limb flow at rest is *normal* and there are no trophic changes except for some muscle atrophy in those who stop walking. In the more severe degree of ischemia that produces pain at rest, the pain is in the most distal part (forefoot) and cannot be relieved by analgesics. However, in the chronic situation when there has been no tissue loss as yet, pain is relieved by dependency. Thus, when the patient is up, sitting, or standing, he may experience no pain, but when he lies down to rest or sleep, the gravitational "boost" in arterial pressure perfusing the foot is lost and, as time passes, ischemic pain awakens the patient. Eventually such patients may learn to sleep with the foot down on a chair beside the bed, in a chaise lounge or, on a physician's advice, with the head of the bed elevated. The perfusion of tissues is no longer normal at rest and as a result trophic changes develop, i.e., slow-growing, thickened nails, thin atrophic skin, lack of skin appendages—hair growth, sweat, and oil gland production—and loss of subcutaneous fat. These changes associated with pallor and collapsed veins when the patient is supine produce a cadaveric, skeletonized appearance to the foot. However, when the foot is down, dependent rubor may develop, as the chronically vasodilated peripheral bed is filled and, once tissue oxygen needs have again been met, red blood pools in postcapillary venules. This combination of dependent rubor and cadaveric pallor on elevation is called "Buerger's sign."

4. **What is the natural history of claudication in terms of eventual limb loss?**

The 5-year limb loss rate with expectant therapy is in the 5 to 10% range.

Comment: Several major studies show that about 75% of claudicators, over a 5-year follow-up period, will be relatively stable or improve or worsen only slightly. Of the 25% requiring therapeutic intervention, 5 to 8% will lose their limbs because of acute progression before limb salvage surgery can be applied. The remaining 17 to 20% will have been operated upon during the interim period for increasing symptoms. Importantly, during that same 5-year period, close to 40% will have suffered a significant new complication of arteriosclerosis (myocardial infarction, stroke, mesenteric ischemia, ruptured aneurysm) with an overall mortality of almost 25%. Cessation of tobacco abuse can significantly affect this outcome, reducing the amputation rate to a negligible level compared with 12% in those who continue to smoke. Other than this, regular exercise to the point of claudication to maximize collateral development and the efficiency of rate-limiting enzymes involved in oxydative metabolism, and antiplatelet drugs to retard progression by thromboembolic events, there is little to offer these patients. The benefit of pentoxifylline and vasodilators is limited at best.

5. **What are the classic signs and symptoms of acute arterial insufficiency?**

The five P's: pain, pulselessness, pallor, paralysis, and paresthesias.

Comment: Admittedly a bit contrived and by no means all universally present, this pentad provides a useful reminder in evaluating patients presenting with acute extremity symptoms. Sudden shooting *pain* down the extremity is common at the moment of embolism and is often associated with numbness and weakness which may diminish quickly. Thrombosis tends to be silent at the outset. However, if severe ischemia persists, typical ischemic rest *pain*, as described above, soon develops. *Pulses* will be absent beyond the level of occulusion. *Pallor* is common at the outset, but after a few hours may give over to a mottled cyanosis. Temperature changes may be more marked than the color change, but alas, coolness does not begin with "P." *Paralysis* will develop in time if severe ischemia persists, beginning in the distribution of the peroneal nerve, but early on the signs may be subtle, such as weakness of dorsiflexion of the toe or foot. Weakness of intrinsic muscle comes first, but is hard to test for. It should be remembered that considerable motion of the toes and ankle may persist because the origins of the responsible muscles are far proximal and may not suffer from as severe a degree of ischemia. *Paresthesias* and a sensation of increasing numbness warn of serious consequences should the ischemia not be promptly relieved. Sensory loss may be subtle at first. Loss of appreciation of light touch, vibration and sense of position should be tested for rather than perception of pain, pressure or two point discrimination. Depending on the presence and degree of sensory and motor changes, acutely ischemic limbs may be categorized as (a) *viable*, (b) *threatened* but salvageable, or (c) with major *irreversible* ischemic changes. Marbling of the skin and muscle rigor are obviously very late signs.

6.   **In what way are the indications for surgical intervention for acute or chronic ischemia related to clinical staging?**

Operative intervention may be indicated in acute ischemia even if the extremity is *viable*, if simple embolectomy will suffice. Otherwise, as for chronic ischemia, only if truly *disabling* claudication persists beyond 2 to 3 months and the patient is a reasonable anesthetic risk would reconstruction be undertaken. Operative intervention is *mandatory* for the acutely or chronically *threatened* limbs (the latter including Fontaine's stages II and III, which are combined under the term "limb salvage"). Major amputation is the only option when *irreversible* ischemic change preclude salvage of a functional foot.

Comment: Like any other surgery, the indications for arterial reconstruction must be justified on the basis of a risk-to-benefit analysis. The risk of loss of life or limb weighs heavily in such deliberation. When the benefit is only increased walking distance, the risk of surgery must be small and the durability of the procedure and the longevity of the patient must both be prolonged, i.e., extended benefit must be anticipated.

7.   **How does the coexistence of diabetes affect the distribution of arterial occlusive disease, its natural history, and surgical indications?**

The distribution of arterial lesions is greater in arteries of *supply* than in arteries of *conduction*. The outlook for life and limb is poor, and surgery is indicated *only* in limb salvage situations.

Comment: Arteriosclerosis in diabetics more commonly affects arteries of supply, e.g., the infrapopliteal branches, the profunda femoris, and hypogastric arteries. Diabetics have about 5 times the risk of limb loss as that of diabetics (34% versus 8% in five years), although much of this is also due to neuropathy and local sepsis. Once arterial occlusive diseases become apparent, life expectancy is greatly shortened (38% mortality in 10 years versus 10% for nondiabetics), primarily owing to the greater visceral artery involvement with arteriosclerosis (e.g., coronary, carotid, renal, mesenteric disease). Diabetics also have a lower operability rate (because of infrapopliteal disease) and patency rate (because of poor runoff) than nondiabetics. In one report the 5-year survival after amputation in diabetics was 39% (versus 75% for nondiabetics) and the risk of losing the other leg approached 50%. For all these reasons, arterial reconstruction should be limited to limb salvage indications in diabetics; it cannot be justified for claudication.

8.   **When dealing with proximal (aortoiliac) occlusive disease, one has three therapeutic options which offer decreasing risk but also decreasing (degree and duration of) benefit. What are they?**

Aortobifemoral bypass (ABF), axillobifemoral bypass, and percutaneous transluminal angioplasty (TLA).

Comment: Aortobifemoral bypass has almost completely replaced aortoiliac bypass or endarterectomy as the direct reconstructive approach to A-I occlusive disease. It carries about a 3% mortality, 2% risk of amputation, and a 5-year patency approaching 90%. Axillobifemoral bypass (which is subcutaneous bypass from axillary to femoral artery plus a suprapubic crossover graft from femoral to femoral artery) carries a lower risk, but because it is reserved for very high-risk patients, its operative mortality is paradoxically higher than for ABF bypass. With the aid of thrombectomy, 75% 5-year patency rates can be achieved but the actual primary patency rate is between 33 and 50%. This operation should be reserved for categorically high-risk patients and those with "hostile" intraabdominal pathology (multiple adhesions, ostomies, radiation damage, malignancy, inflammatory bowel disease, etc.). The single femorofemoral graft has a better success rate (75 to 85% 5-year patency) and is the operation of choice in unilateral iliac artery occlusive disease, which is not suitable for transluminal angioplasty. TLA give 2-year patencies that are equivalent to the 5-year patency for femorofemoral bypass (75 to 85%) if applied to favorable lesions—ideally, discreet (< 5 cm) *common* iliac stenoses. Its major advantage is a negligible mortality and minimal morbidity. Complete occlusions, extensive disease, or multiple lesions, especially involving the external iliac artery, do much less well (50 to 60% success) and should be treated by bypass grafting.

9. **Infrainguinal bypasses fare less well than proximal bypasses, with a direct correlation with length of graft, i.e., the more distal the distal anastomosis, the worse the patency rate. There is also a correlation with type of graft used in such bypasses. Can you identify and rank the graft options for infrainguinal bypass?**

In situ saphenous vein > reverse saphenous vein > other (e.g., lesser saphenous, cephalic) vein > umbilical vein = PTFE (expanded polytetrafluoroethylene) > Dacron.

Comment: Saphenous vein carefully harvested from the same leg and reversed to avoid valve obstruction of flow has been the "gold standard" in femoropopliteal bypass (5-year patency close to 75%). Unfortunately, it is also the ideal graft for coronary disease, which many of these patients have or will develop. Furthermore, the vein may be unsuitable or unavailable in 20 to 25% of cases (too narrow or short, bifid, already used, stripped out for varicose veins, damaged by phlebitis, etc.). In situ bypass, in which the vein is left in place, the valves are rendered incompetent with valvulotomies, and the major branches are ligated to avoid arteriovenous fistulas, offers significantly better patency rates (+10%), and better vein utilization (because smaller and bifid veins can be used). Its major advantages show up in distal bypass to the peroneal or tibial arteries. Human umbilical vein (HUV)–stripped, digested with ficin, tanned with glutaraldehyde, and reinforced with Dacron mesh–and PTFE grafts give roughly equivalent results and are clearly inferior to saphenous vein (-10% at AK popliteal level, -20% at BK popliteal level, and -30% at peroneal tibial level), where they achieve at best a 25% 5-year patency. The externally supported, small caliber Dacron velour graft with an uncrimped end (EXS graft) may achieve similar results, but all other Dacron grafts are at least 10% worse than PTFE or HUV.

10. **Why do grafts fail (occlude) and in what way is the cause of failure related to time of implantation?**
Grafts can fail because of poor inflow, poor outflow (runoff), or structural changes in the graft itself or at its two anastomoses. In temporal sequences the commonest causes of graft failure are technical, surface thrombogenicity combined with low flow (0 to 30 days), neointimal fibroplasia (1 to 18 months), structural changes in vein grafts, valve site stenosis, segmental fibrosis (1 to 18 months), or

aneurysm or new atheromatous change (> 18 months), dilation or aneurysmal change in Dacron, PTFE or HUV graft (> 36 months). The risk of late graft thrombosis correlates with poor runoff, continued tobacco abuse, and coexistence of a hypercoagulable state (AT III or protein C or S deficiency).

11. **What are the relative roles of noninvasive vascular testing and arteriography in the evaluation of patients with arteriosclerosis obliterans with and without therapeutic intervention?**

Noninvasive testing will detect, localize, and gauge the functional severity of arteriosclerotic occlusive lesions and is ideal for screening and follow-up monitoring. Arteriography yields two-dimensional, anatomic detail (i.e., morphologic not physiologic information), which is needed only in patients already determined to be probable candidates for therapeutic intervention (i.e., arterial reconstruction or transluminal angioplasty).

Comment: Segmental limb pressures and plethysmography can detect and localize ASO lesions with 97% accuracy. Arteriography is like an up-to-date road map—you only need it if you are going to make the trip (operate).

12. **Why are vascular surgeons so conservative with claudicators and so aggressive in limb salvage situations?**

The 5-year loss of limb with expectant treatment of claudication is just over 5%; the immediate postoperative limb loss after some reconstructive procedures is almost half of this, leaving little margin for safe benefit (see also question 4). In limb salvage, major amputation is inevitable, and in the elderly, rehabilitation with prosthesis and maintaining an enjoyable, independent existence is unlikely. Arterial reconstruction actually carries a *lower* mortality than major amputation for arteriosclerotic gangrene and keeps most patients independent and active.

13. **What are the main reasons for the significantly lower operative mortalities, lower rates of limb loss and better patency rates enjoyed in the 80's as compared with one or two decades ago?**

Surgical technique is responsible for lower amputation rates but not the lower operative mortality. Better postoperative care with invasive monitoring and hemodynamic manipulation must be credited for most of this, although the selective use of low-risk alternatives has also contributed. Better patency rates relate to better grafts, but also to more aggressive postoperative surveillance, with periodic monitoring using noninvasive tests and intervening by local revision or PTA *before* graft occlusion occurs.

14. **What is the most common arteriosclerotic occlusive lesion in the lower extremity? Why is it *now* being bypassed less frequently than other sites?**

The superficial femoral artery (at the adductor canal) is the single most common occlusive lesion in the lower extremity arterial tree (over 50%), but as an isolated, well-collateralized lesion, it will cause at worst only 2-block claudication and so is not very disabling. More disabled patients (e.g., half-block claudicators or those with rest pain or ischemic lesions) invariably have multilevel disease. If the additional block is *proximal*, e.g., iliac stenosis, it may be bypassed or dilated alone, with enough improvement that the SFA occlusion may be left alone. Similarly, if the additional block is *parallel*, i.e., in the profunda femoris, a profundaplasty or dilation may suffice. Usually only when the additional occlusive lesions are in the distal vessels is femoropopliteal or tibial bypass indicated. Because of the additional incidence of isolated aortoiliac disease and its common association with superficial femoral occlusion, proximal bypass (direct or extra-anatomic) or dilation is twice as common as infrainguinal bypass.

66. CAROTID DISEASE

WILLIAM PEARCE, M.D., and MARY MOCKUS, PH.D.

PREOPERATIVE

1. **What diseases may affect the carotid arteries?**
   Atherosclerosis, fibromuscular dysplasia, radiation damage, and Takayasu's arteritis.

2. **What does a carotid bruit signify?**
   It is a marker for generalized atherosclerosis; not a risk factor for ipsilateral stroke. A bruit may originate from carotid stenosis.

3. **Describe a bruit produced by an internal carotid artery stenosis.**
   Cervical bruit, which begins in systole and extends into diastole, is unaffected by superficial temporal artery occlusion.

4. **Will a severe internal carotid artery stenosis produce a bruit?**
   No. Very high-grade stenoses may have such low flow that no bruit is produced.

5. **What test should be ordered to evaluate a cervical bruit?**
   Oculoplethysmography (OPG).

6. **What is an OPG and how does it work? What are its flaws?**
   Although several varieties of OPG exist, all are based on the deep orbital circulation provided by the ophthalmic artery, the first major branch of the internal carotid artery. Only a hemodynamic lesion will produce a positive test–that is, a lesion that has narrowed the diameter of the artery >50% or a cross-section decrease of 90%.
   False positives may occur with isolated ophthalmic artery stenosis, but this is unusual. False negatives occur in the following situations: (1) Equal bilateral stenosis, although OSP/BSP should be low. (2) Well-compensated lesion via circle of Willis or external carotid artery stenosis. It is important to realize that in the symptomatic patient, the OPG will miss nonhemodynamic ulcers; angiography is then indicated.

7. **Should a patient with an asymptomatic bruit undergo surgery?**
   A bruit may be produced by stenosis of the internal or external carotid arteries, or it may be transmitted to the neck from a proximal common carotid artery stenosis or cardiac murmur. Thus, an asymptomatic bruit alone is not an indication for surgery.
   A bruit should be followed up by noninvasive vascular laboratory studies. Patients with a bruit and negative OPGs have a stroke incidence of about 1 to 2%,whereas patients with positive OPGs have a stroke incidence of about 6 to 15%. Surgery is only recommended in patients with high-grade stenosis.
   Any patient with a bruit who is facing major elective surgery should undergo noninvasive testing so that serious carotid artery stenosis can be ruled out. Other considerations in deciding whether to perform arteriography include (1) a pre-existing contraindication to carotid endarterectomy and (2) the nature of the bruit. A soft, unilateral bruit, particularly when accompanied by negative OPGs, is not an indication for an invasive study. However, a harsh, bilateral bruit, especially when associated with positive OPGs, should be followed by arteriography.

Endarterectomy is indicated if the arteriogram shows significant bilateral stenoses, unilateral stenosis with contralateral occlusion, stenosis of the artery to the dominant hemisphere, or a severely ulcerated plaque.

8. **What mechanisms produce neurologic deficits?**
(1) Artery-to-artery embolus. (2) Low-perfusion, multivessel disease. Low-perfusion states may produce both focal and nonfocal symptoms.

9. **What are the definitions of transient ischemic attack, reversible ischemic neurologic deficit, and acute stroke?**
These are clinical terms that describe a spectrum of cerebral ischemic syndromes. *Transient ischemic attack* (TIA) is a reversible neurologic deficit that lasts no longer than 24 hours. *Reversible ischemic neurologic deficit* (RIND) is a neurologic event that lasts longer than 24 hours and completely resolves within days. These definitions are clinical and may not represent actual pathology. Also, in many asymptomatic patients or in those with TIAs, there may be CT evidence of ischemic stroke.

10. **What is a crescendo TIA ? Stroke in evolution?**
Crescendo TIA: repeated neurologic events without interval neurologic deterioration. Stroke in evolution: repeated neurologic events in which neurologic function does not return to baseline between attacks.

11. **What is the natural history of a TIA?**
The annual stroke rate is 6%, with the highest risk occurring within 12 months of the initial TIA.

12. **What is the effect of aspirin on TIAs?**
Acetylsalicylic acid is a cyclooxygenase inhibitor that will decrease the incidence of both TIAs and stroke. However, the decrease in stroke is not below what can be achieved surgically, particularly in women.

13. **When posterior cerebral circulation is impaired, what symptoms occur and what extracranial arteries may be diseased?**
Ischemia to the brainstem will produce near syncope, visual disturbances, and motor paralysis. Extracranial arterial lesions that may produce vertebrobasilar insufficiency include subclavian artery stenosis, vertebral artery stenosis, carotid artery stenosis in combination with vertebral artery stenosis, basilar artery disease, and small vessel disease.

14. **What is amaurosis fugax?**
An episode of transient (minutes to hours) monocular blindness, often likened to a window shade being pulled across the eye, due to temporary ischemia.

15. **What are Hollenhorst plaques?**
Bright yellow plaques of cholesterol in the retinal vessels that have embolized from the carotid bifurcation. Clinically, this finding indicates that the atheromatous plaque in the carotid is quite friable, and other microemboli may occur spontaneously with manipulation at surgery.

16. **Why is a preoperative cardiac evaluation essential in patients with carotid disease?**
Myocardial infarction is the leading cause of death following surgery, as a result of atherosclerotic disease of the coronary arteries as well as of the carotids.

OPERATIVE

17. How many branches of the internal carotid artery are located in the neck?
None.

18. What is the landmark of the carotid artery bifurcation?
Facial vein.

19. What is the carotid sinus and what is its function?
A dilation at the origin of the internal carotid artery. The walls of the sinus are innervated by the glossopharyngeal and vagus nerves, which also innervate the carotid body. The function of the carotid sinuses is regulation of the blood pressure. Hypertension stimulates efferent impulses to vasomotor center in the medulla, inhibiting sympathetic tone and increasing vagal tone.

20. When the internal carotid artery is occluded, what branches of the external carotid artery form collaterals and reestablish circulation in the circle of Willis?
Periorbital branches of the external carotid artery form communications with the ophthalmic artery, a branch of the internal carotid.

21. What surgical procedure should be performed on a totally occluded carotid artery?
None, or an extracranial-intracranial (ECIC) bypass operation. In patients with chronic total occlusion, surgery is rarely helpful. When the occlusion is acute, the associated severe neurologic deficits and risk of creating a hemorrhagic infarct are contraindications to surgery. ECIC is indicated when there is complete occlusion of the internal carotid artery and a patent superficial temporal artery large enough to serve as a receptor artery.

22. What is a stump pressure?
The internal carotid artery back pressure obtained after clamping, indicative of the adequacy of cerebral perfusion. The safe presure for cross-clamping varies according to author, with the mean being 25 to 50 mm Hg.

23. What is a shunt and when should it be used?
A plastic conduit that diverts blood flow around the surgically opened carotid artery while endarterectomy is being performed (see Figure 1 on page 204). Several varieties are available. The use of shunts remains controversial.

24. When do neurologic events occur during carotid endarterectomies?
(1) Dissection: dislodgement of arterial wall disease. (2) Carotid artery clamping: ischemic infarct. (3) Postoperatively: intimal flap, reperfusion, and external carotid artery clot.

25. What are the complications of carotid endarterectomy?
Intraoperative complications include neurologic deficits and cerebral ischemia. New deficits or exacerbations of old ones may occur by embolization of debris during vessel manipulation or by poor flushing technique after arteriotomy closure. Cerebral ischemia may occur because of hypotension, cerebral artery thrombosis, or poor protection during cross-clamping. There may be no clinical symptoms (asymptomatic), or the ischemia may be manifested as TIA or acute stroke. The overall incidence of neurologic deficits occurring during endarterectomy is about 2 to 3%.

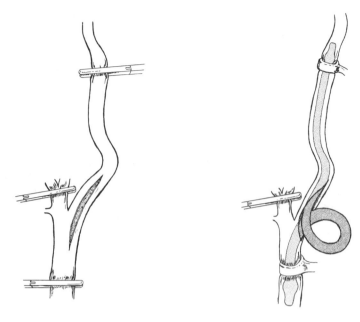

Figure 1. Intraluminal shunt for carotid artery surgery.

POSTOPERATIVE

26. **Which cranial nerves may be injured during carotid endarterectomy, and what are the clinical signs of nerve injury?**
Hypoglossal (XII): deviation of the tongue to the operated side, difficulty with speech and mastication. Vagus (X): minor swallowing difficulty, recurrent laryngeal cord paralysis, and hoarseness. Glossopharyngeal (IX): difficulty swallowing with an ipsilateral Horner's syndrome. Facial (VII): droop of the ipsilateral corner of the lip and decreased ability to smile. Superior laryngeal: easy fatigability of the voice.

27. **What is the danger of wound hematoma after carotid surgery?**
Airway compromise. The risk of wound hematoma can be reduced by careful attention to hemostasis.

28. **What are the possible causes of postoperative hypertension?**
Denervation of the carotid sinus, cerebral renin production, preexisting hypertension, and a central neurologic deficit.

29. **What is the mortality rate for stroke, and what is the cumulative recurrence rate over 5 years?**
Initial mortality is 15%, with 5-year recurrence rate of 42% for men and 24% for women.

HONORS

30. **When was the association between carotid artery disease and neurologic deficit first reported?**
In 1857 by Savory.

31. When was the first carotid endarterectomy performed and by whom?
In 1954 by Eastcott.

32. In what layer of the artery is the endarterectomy performed?
Tunica media.

CONTROVERSIES

33. Cerebral protection.
Adequate cerebral protection is essential to avoid intraoperative ischemia. Some surgeons believe that temporary clamping under local anesthesia is an adequate test of the effectiveness of the collateral circulation. Others use the stump pressure to assess the collateral circulation. Alternatives also include the use of an intraoperative electroencephalogram or a determination of regional cerebral blood flow (rCBF) by the 133-Xe method (usually not available). Because none of these methods is 100% accurate, many surgeons will routinely use an intraoperative shunt, while others will use it selectively or rarely, if at all.

34. Intraoperative shunts.
For: Ensures adequate cerebral protection in all patients.
Against: Prolongs time of operation, results in increased manipulation of friable vessel, not usually necessary.

BIBLIOGRAPHY

1. Baker, W.H., Dorner, D.B., and Barnes, R.W.: Carotid endarterectomy: Is an indwelling shunt necessary? Surgery, 82:321, 1977.
2. Bove, E.L., et al.: Hypotension and hypertension as consequences of baroreceptor dysfunction following carotid endarterectomy. Surgery , 85:633, 1979.
3. Brodac, G.B., et al.: Spontaneous dissecting aneurysm of cervical cerebral arteries: Report of six cases and review of the literature. Neuroradiology, 21:149, 1981.
4. Brandyh, D.E., and Thiele, B.C.: Safe intraluminal shunting during carotid endarterectomy. Surgery, 93:260, 1983.
5. Hajner, C.D.: Minimizing the risks of carotid endarterectomy. J. Vasc. Surg., 1:392, 1984.
6. Kartchner, M.M., and McRae, L.P.: Carotid occlusive disease as a risk factor in major cardiovascular surgery. Arch. Surg., XX:117, 1982.
7. Sacco, R.L., Wolf, P.A., Konnel, W.B., et al.: Survival and recurrence following stroke: The Framingham Study. Stroke, 13:290, 1982.
8. Thompson, J.E., Potman, R.D., and Talkington, C.M.: Asymptomatic carotid bruit: Long-term outcome of patients having endarterectomy compared with unoperated controls. Annu. Surg., 188:308, 1978.
9. Wolf, P.A., Kannel, W.B., et al.: Asymptomatic carotid bruit and the risk of stroke: The Framingham Study. J.A.M.A., 245:1442, 1985.

---

67. ACUTE ARTERIAL OCCLUSION
GLENN L. KELLY, M.D.

---

1. What are the causes of acute arterial occlusion?
Usually an embolus (of cardiac origin [30%], from a proximal aneurysm [2%] or of undetermined origin [30%]) or thrombosis (of an arteriosclerotic stenosis [30%] or aneurysm [2%]). Other infrequent causes are venous thrombosis, vasospasm,

extrinsic compression or paradoxical embolism through a cardiac defect. Emboli of cardiac origin are usually associated with atrial fibrillation or recent myocardial infarction.

2.   **What are the symptoms and findings?**
There is usually sudden coolness followed by ischemic pain. When tissue hypoxia is extreme, there is numbness and paralysis. In the case of emboli, there may be a history of antecedent cardiac symptoms. Arterial thrombosis often is preceded by symptoms of claudication or rest pain.
On examination the proximal pulse is absent, there is pallor, and reduced capillary and venous refill. Diagnosis may be confirmed when Doppler flow is absent or Doppler pressure is markedly reduced.

3.   **Is diagnostic arteriography necessary?**
See Controversies.

4.   **Is it important to distinguish between embolism and thrombosis?**
It may be. Emboli can be expeditiously removed by surgery with a high expectation of circulatory recovery. Because emboli contain old, organized fibin, they are less successfully dissolved by lytic enzymes. Conversely, thrombi usually are associated with underlying occlusive or aneurysmal disease, which will require repair or bypass during or after thrombectomy. However, thrombi are usually less well organized, making them more responsive to enzymatic lysis.

5.   **What is the treatment?**
After prompt evaluation and stabilization, full-dose intravenous heparin will help prevent clot propagation prior to surgery. With the patient under local anesthesia, thromboembolectomy should be performed, using a Fogarty balloon catheter. Emboli to the upper extremity should be treated in the same manner as those occurring in the leg. Completion arteriography is important so that unrecognized residual clots can be avoided. Postoperative heparin therapy can help prevent recurrent embolism or thrombosis. In cases in which underlying stenosis or aneurysm exists, concomitant or staged reconstructive procedures will be necessary to prevent recurrence. Occasionally patients with mild to moderate ischemia present late after an arterial occlusion. Although chances of successful thrombectomy or lysis are diminished, it is usually worthwhile to attempt these even at 2 weeks (thrombectomy) to 3 months (lysis) if the history and arteriograms suggest that occlusion is due to clot.

6.   **What are the associated complications?**
Owing to coexisting serious diseases, the mortality is 10 to 30% in this group of patients. Revascularization, especially when ischemia is severe and surgery is delayed, may lead to three other problems: (1) *Reperfusion shock* is due to systemic acidosis and hyperkalemia. This may be prevented by slow release of the vascular clamps and systemic administration of bicarbonate solution, glucose, and insulin. (2) *Compartment syndrome* from muscle edema and subsequent neurovascular compression is treated by prompt fasciotomy of the involved muscle compartment. (3) *Acute tubular necrosis* is due to release of myoglobin from damaged muscle tissue. Alkalinization of the urine and diuretics are the recommended therapy. Finally, local tissue necrosis or neuropathy due to prolonged preoperative ischemia may ensue.

7.   **What is a Fogarty catheter?**
A flexible plastic catheter with a syringe at the proximal end and a soft, inflatable latex balloon at the distal end. It is passed through the clot, then gently inflated

and withdrawn to remove the clot. It was invented in 1963 by Dr. Thomas Fogarty, a cardiovascular surgeon who also invented the friction clutch for the motor scooter.

CONTROVERSIES

8. Is preoperative arteriography always necessary?
Not usually, especially when acute onset associated with atrial fibrillation or recent myocardial infarction suggests embolism. This is best treated by rapid embolectomy without the risk, delay, and expense of arteriography. When a history of chronic ischemic symptoms or physical findings suggests thrombosis of an intrinsic arterial lesion, then arteriography can be useful in planning a concomitant or subsequent reconstructive procedure.

9. Are lytic enzymes helpful?
Streptokinase, or preferably urokinase, has had varying success (30 to 70%) in dissolving peripheral arterial clots. In certain high-risk patients in whom thrombosis is suspected and ischemic symptoms are mild, intraclot lytic therapy is necessary.

10. Heparin therapy alone?
A few authors have advocated this method over surgery, using 2000 to 4000 U of heparin per hour. Although the mortality can be reduced slightly, the amputation rate is increased; thus, this modality is not used extensively in most centers.

BIBLIOGRAPHY

1. Abbott, W.M., Maloney, R.D., McCabe, C.C., et al.: Arterial embolism: A 44-year perspective. Am. J. Surg., 143:460, 1982.
2. Blaisdell, F.W., Steele, M., and Allen, R.D.: Management of acute lower extremity arterial ischemia due to embolism and thrombosis. Surgery, 84:822, 1978.
3. Elliot, J.P., Hageman, J.H., Szilagyi, D.E., et al.: Arterial embolization: Problems of source, multiplicity, recurrence and delayed treatment. Surgery, 88:833, 1980.
4. Fisher, B.D., Fogarty, T.J., and Morrow, A.G.: Clinical and biochemical observations of the effect of transient femoral artery occlusion in man. Surgery, 68:323, 1970.
5. Fogarty, T.J., Cranley, J.J., Krause, R.J., et al.: A method for extraction of arterial emboli and thrombi. Surg. Gynecol. Obstet., 116:241, 1963.
6. Haimovici, H.: Arterial embolism, myoglobinuria and renal tubular necrosis. Arch. Surg.,100:639, 1970.
7. Hargrove, W.C., Berkowitz, H.D., Freiman, D.B., et al.: Recanalization of totally occluded femoral popliteal vein grafts with low-dose streptokinase infusion. Surgery, 92:890, 1982.
8. Patman, R.D.: Fasciotomy: Indications and techniques. In Rutherford, R.B.: Vascular Surgery, 2nd ed. Philadelphia, W. B. Saunders Co., 1984.
9. Porter, J.M., and Taylor, L.M.: Current status of thrombolytic therapy. Vasc. Surg., 2:239, 1985.
10. Savelyer, V.S., Zatevakhin, I.I., and Stepanov, N.V.: Artery embolism of the upper limbs. Surgery, 81:367, 1977.
11. Sicard, G.A., Schier, J.J., Totty, W.G., et al.: Thrombolytic therapy for acute arterial occlusion. Vasc. Surg., 1:65, 1985.
12. Spencer, F.C., and Eiseman, B.: Delayed arterial embolectomy: A new concept. Surgery, 55:64, 1972.
13. Tawes, R.L., Beare, J.P., Scribner, R.G., et al.: Value of postoperative heparin therapy in peripheral arterial thromboembolism. Am. J. Surg., 146:213, 1983.
14. Tawes, R.L., Harris, E.J., Brown, W.H., et al.: Arterial thromboembolism, a 20-year perspective. Arch. Surg., 120:595, 1985.

68. VASCULAR INJURIES
WILLIAM PEARCE, M.D., and MARY MOCKUS, PH.D.

PREOPERATIVE

1. **By what mechanisms can arterial trauma occur?**
    Blunt, penetrating, orthopedic dislocations, and iatrogenic.

2. **In civilian practice, what is the most common arterial injury?**
    Penetrating extremity injury.

3. **What is the kinetic energy of a bullet and why is it important?**

    $\dfrac{1/2\,MV^2}{g}$ The tissue energy is related to the square of the velocity.
    A high-velocity bullet will cause more damage and require more extensive debridement and repair than a bullet of smaller mass and lower velocity.

4. **What are the five "P's" of arterial insufficiency?**
    Pulse (absence of), pallor, pain, paresthesia, and paralysis. The latter two are the most important, as nerves are highly sensitive to anoxia.

5. **How often does an arterial injury present with palpable distal pulses?**
    Depending upon the location and nature of the injury, 15 to 20% of significant arterial injuries will present with distal palpable distal pulses.

6. **When should angiography be performed?**
    Multilevel injuries (i.e., a shotgun wound); wounds in proximity; wounds with decreased pulses, suspicious bruits, large hematomas, recurrent hemorrhage; and orthopedic injuries with absent or decreased pulses.

7. **What is the Allen test?**
    It is a maneuver performed to assess the circulation to the hand. The patient is instructed to make a tight fist and hold his forearm up with the elbow flexed. The examiner uses finger and thumb pressure to occlude the ulnar and radial arteries. When the hand is blanched, the patient is instructed to relax his fist, while the examiner releases one of the arteries and watches the return of color (blood flow) to the hand. The test is then repeated with release of the other artery.

8. **Occlusion of end arteries often causes death to tissues because they are the sole source of the blood supply. Where are end arteries found?**
    Kidney, spleen, spinal medulla, and brain.

OPERATIVE

9. **What are the three layers of a large artery?**
    Tunica intima, tunica media, tunica adventitia.

10. **Which layer is the thickest in a large artery?**
Tunica media. This is important because it allows the large muscular arteries to withstand the pressure of the blood as it is pumped from the heart. In addition, vessel wall recoil due to the action of the tunica media helps to propagate blood flow.

11. **What are the two types of aneurysms?**
True aneurysm: localized dilation of an artery covered by all three layers of the vessel. *False aneurysm:* usually caused by trauma. A disruption of the vessel layers that results in a pulsating hematoma covered by intima, clot, and fibrous tissue.

12. **What is an arteriovenous fistula?**
It is a direct communication between an artery and vein that bypasses the capillary bed. A fistula may develop whenever there is simultaneous injury to an artery and adjacent vein. The complications of arteriovenous fistulas, particularly of the large vessels, are tachycardia, left venticular enlargement with eventual left-sided cardiac failure, subacute bacterial endocarditis, and aneurysm of both the artery and the vein.

13. **If the nerve, artery, vein and bone are injured, what is the order of repair?**
With a short period of ischemia: bone, vein, artery, nerve. With longer period of ischemia: vein, artery, bone, nerve. In these cases, fasciotomy should be performed.

14. **List the indications for fasciotomy.**
A delay of over 6 hours between injury and repair; arterial injury with venous injury, especially to the popliteal vessels; prolonged hypotension with severe shock; massive soft tissue trauma; and massive preoperative and/or postoperative edema.

15. **What are the four compartments of the leg, and why are they important in arterial injuries to the leg?**
Anterior, laterial, superficial posterior, and deep posterior. With a significant vascular injury to the leg, edema may develop secondary to ischemia or massive soft tissue trauma. This may raise the intracompartmental pressure to such a degree that the vascular supply to the leg will be occluded. Thus, it is important to understand the anatomy of the leg in order to know what compartments may need to be opened at fasciotomy.

16. **Should a retroduodenal hematoma be explored?**
Yes, to assess damage to the duodenum.

17. **What intraabdominal vessel is most often injured?**
The inferior vena cava, in 10 to 20% of intraabdominal vessel injuries and 30 to 50% of abdominal venous injuries.

18. **Why do injuries to the iliac vessels require rapid diagnosis and surgery?**
Because they carry a high risk of rapid exsanguination, with an associated mortality rate of 30 to 90%.

19. **Why is a partially transected vessel potentially more dangerous than a completely transected one?**

A completely transected vessel is more likely to retract with spasm and clot than a partially transected one. In addition, partially transected vessels are more likely to lead to the development of fistulas, false aneuryms, and hemorrhage.

20.   What orthopedic injuries are likely to be associated with vascular injuries?

Fracture of the clavicle; fracture or dislocation of the humerus or femur; dislocation of the posterior hip, elbow, or knee.

21.   What are the steps involved in arterial repair?

Debridement, removal of distal thrombi, arterial reconstruction, and soft tissue coverage.

22.   If an arterial replacement is required, what material should be used?

Autogenous vein or hypogastric artery is preferred. Whenever possible, a synthetic graft is avoided because of the increased risk of infection associated with a contaminated traumatic wound. The use of PTFE in such wounds remains controversial.

23.   Why are venous repairs important?

Because there is a higher incidence of pulmonary embolism with ligation. Although patency may last for only 24 to 72 hours, this may be sufficient to allow the development of additional collateral venous return. Also, venous outflow obstruction may impede arterial inflow.

24.   The surgical alternatives in renal vessel injury are nephrectomy versus reconstruction. On what factors is a decision based?

Hemodynamic status and extent of associated injuries; extent of injury to vessels, ureters, and renal parenchyma; known functional level of the contralateral kidney; and duration of renal ischemia (< 3 hours).

POSTOPERATIVE

25.   In an extremity with a neurovascular injury, what injury results in the major disability?

Injury to the nerve. Injury to the vascular system may be repaired, and with time the establishment of collaterals may increase flow to the extremity. Injuries to the nerves of an extremity, however, may be impossible to repair, leading to significant disability.

26.   If an arterial injury is not repaired and is ligated, what is the chance of amputation?

Femoral	81%
Popliteal	72%
Tibial	69%
Subclavian	29%
Axillary	43%
Brachial	56%

27.   What are the complications of arterial trauma when it is not repaired?

Thrombosis, false aneurysm, and stenosis. Thrombosis is caused by activation of the clotting cascade after full or partial transection of a vessel. This can lead to stenosis of the vessel, total occlusion, infection, or the propagation of emboli. All of the problems further compromise tissue that has already been traumatized.

28.   What is the bullet embolus?
Arterial embolus consisting of a bullet fragment. The fragments of a shotgun blast or a bullet that enters a major artery may travel through the arterial system and become lodged in a vessel, creating stenosis or total occlusion. The bullet may serve as a site for false aneurysm thrombus, and infection may develop also. The location of the embolus is determined by arteriogram, and management included prompt removal and repair of the artery.

29.   In patients with major intraabdominal injuries who require massive blood transfusions, what coagulation abnormalities may develop?
Dilutional thrombocytopenia; factor V or VII deficiency; hypothermia; hypocalcemia unless transfusion rate exceeds 100 ml/minute; and occasionally disseminated intravascular coagulation.

30.   What is causalgia and how may it be treated?
Pain that often occurs soon after a traumatic, crushing injury to an extremity, characterized by burning, cutaneous dysesthesias, and varying degrees of vasomotor dysfunction and atrophy. It is treated by sympathectomy.

Honors

31.   Who performed the first venous interposition for arterial injury?
Goyanes in 1906.

32.   Who performed the first end-to-end repair?
John Murphy.

BIBLIOGRAPHY

1.   Gaspar, M.R.: Arterial Trauma. In Gaspar, M.R., and Barker, W.F. (eds.): Peripheral Arterial Disease, 3rd ed. Philadelphia, W. B. Saunders Co., 1981.
2.   Millikan, J.S., et al.: Vascular trauma in the groin: Contrast between iliac and femoral injuries. Am. J. Surg., 142:695, 1981.
3.   Moore, E. E., Eiseman, B., and Van Way, C.W.: Critical Decisions in Trauma. St. Louis, C. V. Mosby Co., 1984.
4.   Rich, N.M., and Spencer, F.C.: Vascular Trauma. Philadelphia, W.B. Saunders Co., 1978.
5.   Sagalowsky, A.I., McConnell, J.D., and Peters, P.C.: Renal trauma requiring surgery: An analysis of 185 cases. J. Trauma, 23(2):128, 1983.

---

69. ABDOMINAL AORTIC ANEURYSM
CHARLES M. ABERNATHY, M.D.

---

1.   How is the diagnosis of abdominal aortic aneurysm made?
Physical examination. Abdominal pulsation is present in 70% of patients; aorta is *upper* abdominal organ with bifurcation at umbilicus; some are diagnosed on radiography (intravenous pyelogram or upper gastrointestinal series obtained for other reasons) because calcium in wall of aneurysm can be seen (70%). Occasionally the patient will feel the aneurysm or will complain, "My heart is beating in my abdomen."

2.   How is diagnosis confirmed? Is aortogram required?

Ultrasound. *Size* of aneurysm is the *key* item for further therapeutic decisions. Abdominal plain film (i.e., cross-table lateral) will outline the aneurysm when it is calcified (70%). The use of aortography is controversial (see Controversies).

3. **What is a "meandering artery"?**
Appears on the aortogram when the inferior mesenteric artery is the primary source of intestinal blood supply.

4. **Should antibiotics be given prophylactically?**
Yes, in which case the infection rate is 0.9% as opposed to 7% without the use of antibiotics.

5. **Why is size important?**
The key measurement is 6 cm. The incidence of rupture is much higher when the aneurysm is 6 cm. Below 6 cm can be "watched" with follow-up visits scheduled every 6 months. Ultrasound should be used for sizing aneurysms. In patients who are good surgical risks, aneurysms as small as 4.5 cm should be repaired; the chance of rupture is 20% 3 years after surgery. Even aneurysms 4 cm have a small but definite incidence of rupture.

6. **What does surgery involve?**
Abdominal aortic aneurysms are 90% *infra*renal. The aneurysm is opened and replaced with a *tube* or *bifurcation* graft, usually to the common iliacc vessels (see Controversies).

7. **What is the risk of operation?**
In good-risk patients (i.e., no history of myocardial infarction, under 70 years of age, no diabetes), mortality is 5%. In poor-risk patients, mortality rises to 20%.

8. **What is the risk of rupture if not operated?**
For aneurysms >6 cm, there is a 43% risk of eventual rupture.

9. **What are the technical details of the operation?**
(1) "Declamping hypotension" is possible after the graft is in and the aortic clamp is released; the patient needs an extra fluid load before the clamp is removed. This also prevents acidosis; (2) Big "bites" of suture should be used for anastomoses; (3) Leave in the aneurysm sac to avoid dissection posterior to the aneurysm and to use in covering the graft.

10. **What complications are specific to the operation?**
    1. Renal failure (4 to 7%).
    2. Rare paraplegia from spinal ischemia while the aorta is cross-clamped.
    3. Infected graft (1 to 2%). The graft must be removed; usually the aorta is ligated below the renal vessels and flow to legs is established using an axillary-bifemoral graft.
    4. Aortoduodenal (or small bowel) fistula. The patient with upper gastrointestinal bleeding who underwent prior aneurysm resection usually will have premonitory bleeding. Minimal help is afforded by diagnosis by upper gastrointestinal series, arteriography, and endoscopy; emergency surgery is similar to that described for an infected graft (above).
    5. Acute colonic ischemia. This should be suspected when postoperative stool Hemoccult is positive and diarrhea is present. Sigmoidoscopy or colonoscopy will facilitate diagnosis.

11. **Are there any alternatives to graft replacement of aneurysm?**

1. Follow with ultrasound.
2. Axillary-bifemoral graft and thrombosis of aneurysm using either ligation of outflow or ligation of neck (proximal of aneurysm) and outflow.

CONTROVERSIES

12. Preoperative aortography.
For:
1. Indicates whether aneurysm extends above renal arteries so that surgeon is prepared for a more difficult operation, and outlines anatomy of renal arteries and visceral branches.
2. Demonstrates aortic outflow and presence of arterial occlusive disease (might influence whether or not graft extends to common femoral artery), as well as any vascular anomalies.
Against: Some morbidity (1%); occasional rise in BUN secondary to administration of contrast medium; added cost and time.

13. Type of graft.
Woven Dacron graft
For: Doesn't leak *through graft* at time of operation (ideal for ruptured aneurysms where blood loss must be kept at a minimum).
Against: Harder to sew (stiff); may not grasp "pseudointima" (desired for increased patency, though not usually a problem at aortic level) because of smaller "holes" in fabric.
Knitted Dacron graft
For: Larger interstitial holes, easier for body to incorporate than woven, easier to sew.
Against: Must be pre-clotted (not always successful, increased intraoperative blood loss).
Other: Gortex, antibiotic-impregnated grafts on the horizon.

BIBLIOGRAPHY

1. Bernhard, V.M.: Management of graft infections following abdominal aortic aneurysm replacement. World J. Surg., 4:679, l980.
2. Bush, H.L., Jr.: Renal failure following abdominal aortic reconstruction. Surgery, 93:107, 1983.
3. Crawford, E.S., et al.: Infrarenal abdominal aortic aneurysm. Factors influencing survival after operation performed over a 25-year period. Ann. Surg., 193:699, 1981.
4. Darling, R.D., and Brewster, D.C.: Elective treatment of abdominal aortic aneruysms. World J. Surg., 4:661, 1980.
5. Dielh, J.T., et al.: Complications of abdominal aortic reconstruction: An analysis of perioperative risk factors in 557 patients. Ann. Surg., 197:49, 1983.
6. Fielding, J.W.L., et al.: Diagnosis and management of 528 abdominal aortic aneurysms. Br. Med. J., 283:355, 1981.
7. Hertzer, N.R.: Diagnosis and management of abdominal aortic aneruysms. Compr. Ther., 6:55, 1980.
8. Leather, R.P., et al.: Nonresective therapy of abdominal aneurysm. Use of acute thrombosis axillofemoral bypass. Arch. Surg., 114:1401, 1979.
9. Nuno, I.N., et al.: Should aortography be used routinely in the elective surgery of abdominal aortic aneurysm? Am. J. Surg., 144:53, 1982.
10. O'Donnell, R.F., Jr., Darling, R.C., and Linton, R.R.: Is 80 years too old for aneurysmectomy? Arch. Surg., 111:1250, 1976.
11. Thompson, J.E., et al.: Surgical treatment of abdominal aortic aneurysm: Factors influencing mortality and morbidity–A 20-year experience. Ann. Surg., 181:654, 1975.

70. RUPTURED ABDOMINAL AORTIC ANEURYSM
RICHARD J. SANDERS, M.D.

1. **Differentiate between the terms "dissecting aneurysm," "leaking aneurysm," and "ruptured aneurysm."**
   "Leaking" and "ruptured" are terms usually used to describe abdominal aortic aneurysms. "Dissecting" is usually reserved for thoracic aortic aneurysms that dissect a false lumen and whose hallmark is occlusion of branch vessels (i.e., coronary, carotid, renal) as the dissection occurs.

2. **What is the classic, and often the only, symptom of a ruptured abdominal aneurysm?**
   Pain, often in the back, but it can be abdominal or in the left flank.

3. **What physical findings are seen with a ruptured abdominal aortic aneurysm?**
   Sometimes none, but often a widened aortic pulsation can be felt in the abdomen. Tenderness above and to the left of the umbilicus is common. Hypotension, with or without tachycardia, may be seen.

4. **When the diagnosis is suspected, how soon should the patient be operated on?**
   30 to 60 minutes. If the patient is hypotensive, he should be taken to the operating room immediately, a pressure suit applied to the lower body, and resuscitation begun while awaiting the blood. If the patient is normotensive, a period of 15 to 30 minutes can be safely taken so that the diagnosis can be verified.

5. **What diagnostic tests should be ordered to confirm the diagnosis?**
   If the patient is hypotensive and an abdominal examination reveals an aneurysm, no further studies are necessary. If the patient is normotensive, a cross-table lateral x-ray film, ultrasonogram, or CT scan of the abdomen can be obtained, whichever will be faster.

6. **What diagnostic tests are indicated?**
   Complete blood count, BUN, creatinine, blood sugar, electrolytes, electrocardiogram, and chest x-ray film. Ten units of whole blood should be typed and cross-matched. Packed red blood cells should not be used, as they are too hard to pump in. If the patient is in shock, cross-matching the blood is the only necessary emergency procedure; the other tests can be run later. The chest x-ray film and electrocardiogram can be done en route to the operating room but can be omitted if the patient is in shock.

7. **Once in the operating room, when can the patient be anesthetized?**
   General anesthesia often results in hypotension, or even cardiac arrest. Therefore, the following should be done before the patient is anesthetized:
   1. 6 units of blood should be in the room, 2 units being administered intravenously.
   2. Prepare the abdomen, and apply the drapes with the patient awake.
   3. If the patient has been hypotensive, use a pressure suit over the lower half of the body until ready to wash the skin.

4. Foley catheter in bladder.

5. Large-bore needle (16-gauge; minimum, 18-gauge) in two different veins.

6. Systemic heparinization (to avoid distal thrombosis when aorta is occluded). This is given before the skin is incised.

8. In most hospitals, what is the reason for the delay in beginning the operation?
Cross-matching the blood. However, other causes of delay are taking unnecessary diagnostic x-rays, locating operating room personnel, and finding an anesthesiologist.

9. After the abdomen is opened, what is the next step and how is it done?
Obtaining proximal control of the aorta. The quickest way is to use an aortic compressor, placed against the aorta, just below the diaphragm. The aorta and the esophagus are compressed against the spine by pressure. A sponge stick can substitute for an aortic compressor.

10. What is the second step?
Open the posterior peritoneum, dissect the mesentery, and isolate the aorta below the renal arteries by finger dissection. The aorta is clamped at this spot and the aortic occluder, above the renals, can be removed. If the patient's blood pressure is stable, the iliac arteries can be dissected before the aorta.

11. What is the major complication to occur when the common iliac arteries are dissected?
Injury and bleeding from the common iliac veins. In some series, this is the #1 cause of death.

12. What graft material is used to replace a ruptured aortic aneurysm?
Woven Dacron or PTFE to avoid bleeding through the graft. A knitted graft will be difficult to preclot as the patient was heparinized when the incision was made. In addition, because the operation usually proceeds so quickly, there is little time for preclotting.

13. What is the mortality in ruptured aortic aneurysms? What are the causes of death?
20 to 80%. Early deaths are from hypotension, shock, and myocardial failure. Later deaths are due to myocardial infarction, renal failure, and bleeding stress ulcers.

14. Can paraplegia occur following rupture of an aortic aneurysm? What is the mechanism?
Yes. The blood supply to the spinal cord, the artery of Adamkiewicz, usually arises at the level of C6, T2, or T10, from branches of the intercostal arteries. In a few patients, this artery arises at L2 and the blood supply to the spinal cord is occluded during clamping of the abdominal aorta.

BIBLIOGRAPHY

1. Hiatt, J.C.G., Barker, W.F., Machleda, H.L., et al.: Determinants of failure in the treatment of ruptured abdominal aortic aneurysm. Arch. Surg., 119:1264-1268, 1984.

71. VENOUS DISEASE
ROBERT RUTHERFORD, M.D.

1. **Why do people get varicose veins?**

    Most commonly because of congenital absence of valves proximal to the saphenofemoral junction.

    Comment: There are no valves in the vena cava or common iliac vein, and only one or two valves in the external iliac and common femoral veins. The most constant of those is the sentinel valve just above the saphenofemoral junction. Anatomic studies show this is absent on one side or the other in approximately one third of patients. Doppler studies show saphenofemoral reflux in 16% of asymptomatic children of parents with varicose veins. This inherent weakness becomes manifest by the development of varicose veins in a much lower percentage of patients and most of them are female. The common denominator here is pregnancy, which causes increased back pressure, increased blood volume, and relaxation of vascular smooth muscle. Once the saphenous begins to dilate and its upper valves become incompetent, downward progression, with dilation of the next lower segment and its valve continues until the high ambulatory back pressure is transmitted out into thinner wall tributaries, which become dilated and tortuous (i.e., varicose). Varicose veins may also be *secondary* to high pressure of other causes, e.g., deep venous and perforator incompetence (the postphlebitic syndrome) or arteriovenous (AV) fistulas. Their differentiation is relatively easy.

2. **How can one distinguish primary varicose veins due to uncomplicated saphenofemoral incompetence from those secondary to deep venous and perforator incompetence (i.e., the postphlebitic syndrome)?**

    The former has a saphenous distribution, a positive tourniquet test, *no* morning ankle edema, and *no* stasis sequelae (dermatitis or ulceration).

    Comment: If one empties the leg by elevation and then applies a high thigh tourniquet, patients will not fill their varicosities on standing again for 20 to 30 seconds but will rapidly fill in a retrograde fashion with the tourniquet off or released. Rapid reflux after pumping the calf with the leg dependent can be demonstrated plethysmographically and can be controlled by repeating the study with a thigh tourniquet. Venous Doppler examination will confirm saphenofemoral reflux and competent deep veins.

3. **How, when, and in whom should varicose veins be treated?**

    Varicose veins causing discomfort or serious cosmetic embarrassment deserve treatment. The earlier treated, the better the result. The varicose tributaries may be obliterated by either surgical stripping or sclerotherapy, with equally good *initial* results, but recurrence will be infrequent only if the back pressure is interrupted by *high ligation.*

    Comment: Many doctors advise their female patients with varicose veins to postpone treatment until they have finished having children. This approach is wrong, as it allows for more extensive varicose degeneration so that it is harder to achieve a good cosmetic result with few incisions. Furthermore, the patient suffers unnecessarily for several more years; and since when standing, retrograde flow is down the saphenous and into perforators, it runs the risk of causing perforator incompetence, which in turn jeopardizes control by the standard surgical technique of high ligation and stripping. Performed early, the latter can be carried out through a groin and an ankle incision. Varicose tributaries require either multiple additional incisions or adjunctive sclerotherapy. Incompetent perforators will be missed if only the main greater saphenous is stripped.

4.   **What are the characteristics of venous edema that distinguish it from other causes of leg swelling?**
     Venous edema is brawny and nonpitting, and is usually associated with the typical *discoloration* of venous stasis. It is associated with a *tight, heavy* aching discomfort that is relieved by elevation.
     Comment: Very early on, the legs of patients with different forms of edema may be difficult to distinguish from each other, but by the time of presentation, most can be identified on the basis of the presence or absence of pain, pittting, discoloration, and its distribution and response to elevation. Venous edema is associated with the described discomfort, which is produced by venous distention. Because protein-rich fluid and red cells are extravasated during periods of venous hypertension, the subcutaneous tissues are thickened by fibrin and discolored by hemoglobin pigment and the inflammatory reaction they incite. The swelling is greatest at the ankle and the foot is *relatively* spared. It responds to elevation. In contrast, lymphedema is painless, almost pale without discoloration, and though it yields on pressure, it does not "pit." It has been described as "spongy." It is *not* relieved by elevation and is maximally distributed distally, right down to the toes. Edema of central or systemic origin, occurring in the absence of venous or lymphatic obstruction, commonly stems from two basic causes, cardiac failure or hypoalbuminemia, both of which are easily confirmed. When rapidly progressive, the skin becomes tense, shiny, and even pigmented, but the hallmark of this type of edema is its pitting with pressure.

5.   **What is the etiology of a venous stasis ulcer, and how can it be distinguished from other leg ulcers?**
     Venous hypertension rather than stasis causes the ulcers of venous insufficiency. They are usually located around the malleoli and surrounded by typical "stasis dermatitis."
     Comment: Ambulatory venous hypertension, secondary to valvular incompetence and/or persistent obstruction following deep venous thrombosis, causes extravasation of fluid rich in red cells, fibrinogen, and other proteins into subcutaneous tissue. Inflammation and scarring result and interfere with capillary flow to the skin, which becomes atrophic and breaks down easily. Venous hypertension retards capillary inflow and may even open arteriovenous shunts that bypass the skin. With minor trauma, the skin breaks down and, as long as the venous hypertension goes unrelieved (i.e., until patient elevates legs and uses elastic compression bandages or stockings), it cannot heal and further enlarges. Ischemic ulcers have poor granulations, do not bleed when manipulated, are usually more distally placed, and are associated with absent pulses and ischemic rest pain, which is made worse by–not relieved by–elevation. Neurotrophic ulcers are painless. located over pressure points, and associated with neuropathy, usually diabetic in origin.

6.   **Which contributes most to the "postphlebitic syndrome": venous obstruction or valvular incompetence?**
     Valvular incompetence.
     Comment: After deep venous thrombosis, collateralization occurs and, with bed rest, the initial edema subsides. Eventually most thrombosed veins recanalize, but even though the resulting lumen is large enough to relieve obstruction in most cases, the valves are scarred or plastered down against the

side wall of the vein. Whenever the patient is up out of bed, *venous hypertension* quickly develops because incompetent valves disable the ability of the "venomotor pump"of the calves to force blood upward against the relentless force of gravity. Brawny edema, stasis dermatitis, and ulceration eventually develop. In a smaller percentage of patients, usually those with iliofemoral thrombophlebitis, recanalization is incomplete and obstructive symptoms predominate.

7. **What is "venous claudication"?**
Pain with ambulation caused by venous outflow obstruction.
Comment: When recanalization fails to occur after iliofemoral venous thrombosis (close to 30%, but more commonly on the left), sufficient collaterals usually develop so that, at rest, there is no obstruction to venous outflow. However, with exercise (even walking at a normal pace), arterial inflow increases and may exceed the capacity of venous outlflow channels. Pressure builds up in the venous system until a "heavy," "tight," or "bursting" pain is experienced and forces the patient to rest. Because pain is associated with exercise and is relieved by rest, it has been termed "venous claudication." Patients with this problem have prominent venous collaterals and even swollen thighs, but may have little of the distal "stasis" changes seen in those with valvular incompetence. Patients with both obstruction and valvular reflux are particularly difficult to manage.

8. **What is the natural history of deep venous thrombosis, i.e., how many untreated (or noncompliant) patients develop significant "stasis sequelae"? How successfully can one prevent this by nonoperative measures?**
Half the patients will have "stasis" dermatitis with 5 years, half will have "stasis" ulcers by 10 years. A postphlebitic regimen consisting of external elastic support and intermittent leg elevation will prevent these sequelae or control them once they develop in close to 100% of *compliant* patients, *if* they do not have obstruction in addition to valvular incompetence.
Comment: The key here is proper patient education *and* compliance. Many patients are allowed to discontinue treatment at the final office visit when anticoagulants are discontinued, and they ask about the need to continue with elevation and elastic support at a time when their legs are not swollen or discolored. This is not surprising, as stasis sequelae take time to develop (median time for first stasis ulcer is 2-1/2 years) and patient has been elevating legs and wearing elastic support. In addition, the advice to elevate and wear elastic support is rarely explained in sufficient detail to insure compliance. Unfortunately, few patients are told to elevate above heart level at regular intervals (e.g., 10 minutes out of *every* 2 hours) or that elastic stockings retard rather than prevent swelling and, without elevation, will soon become too tight and cause, rather than relieve, discomfort.

9. **Won't a complete stripping of varicose veins also take care of incompetent perforators?**
No, most such perforators communicate with the posterior arch and are not affected by stripping of the main saphenous vein.

10. **What is the accuracy of clinical diagnosis of deep vein thrombosis? What are the relative roles of noninvasive studies and venography?**
Less than 50%, in three major series with venographic confirmation. Venography, while still the gold standard, is expensive, difficult to interpret, often

does not visualize well the iliac veins, profunda system, or soleal plexus, cannot be performed at the bedside in seriously ill patients, and carries a significant morbidity (extravasation, phlebitis). Two vascular laboratory tests, venous Doppler examination, and venous plethysmography, are close to 90% accurate for *proximal* deep vein thrombosis, i.e., venous thrombosis at or above the popliteal level. They combine for an accuracy of over 95% and are fast, inexpensive, noninvasive, and can be performed at bedside or in the clinic. The decision to admit and treat with heparin or follow as an outpatient can thus be made without venography, which is performed only if these tests disagree with each other or there is a strong clinical impression to the contrary. The fact that these tests do not detect calf vein thrombi with adequate accuracy (25 to 30%) has little practical significance. Clots in this location do not produce fatal emboli and outpatient management is appropriate.

11. What are phlegmasia alba dolens and phlegmasia cerulea dolens, and what is the practical significance of distinguishing between them?

Iliofemoral venous thrombosis, if mild, produces a bland, pale, swollen limb (literally, painful white swelling). More extensive thrombosis, involving tributaries that might otherwise serve as collaterals, produces massive swelling and cyanosis (literally, pain purple swelling). The latter condition can produce a compartmental syndrome and/or venous gangrene because venous outflow obstruction is severe, even reducing arterial inflow by 25 to 40%. Thrombectomy and fasciotomy may be required to stem this threat. Thrombectomy is indicated only in phlegmasia alba dolens in active young patients presenting within 24 to 48 hours, where it offers the best chance of preventing postphlebitic sequelae.

12. What measures are effective in preventing DVT, and to which patients should they be applied?

Low-dose heparin with or without dihydroergotamine, external pneumatic compression, Coumadin, dextran, and antiplatelet drugs have been shown to be effective in certain groups of patients at risk and, therefore, must be used selectively.

Comment: Low-dose subcutaneous heparin (500 U every 8 to 12 hours) is the most widely used but has been disappointing in hip surgery and prostatectomy. The addition of dihydroergotamine, which improves venous tone and flow, appears to improve efficacy. Coumadin is of proven effectiveness, but it takes time to achieve stable therapeutic levels. Because of the greater risk of hemorrhage in surgical patients, its use is restricted to very high-risk patients. Intravenous dextran is equally effective but more difficult to administer and requires close monitoring. Compression boots are quite effective and can be used if there are no leg incisions and in conjunction with antithrombotic drugs. Patients who require neurosurgery, prostatectomy, or hip surgery are good candidates for this approach. Antiplatelet drugs appear to be effective only in males undergoing orthopedic or general surgery procedures. In addition to the type of surgery, risk factors for postoperative venous thromboembolism include age, obesity, varicose veins or history of deep vein thrombosis, cardiac decompensation, anticipated long period of bed rest, malignancy, oral contraceptives, family history, and trauma. Unfortunately, none of the prophylactic measures is effective in the trauma setting and antithrombotic drugs are specifically contraindicated.

13. Why do almost three fourths of cases of iliofemoral venous thrombosis occur on the left side?

Because of compression of the left iliac vein by the right iliac artery.

Comment: This also explains the higher rethrombosis rate after thrombectomy on the left side. Occasionally this condition gives preocclusive symptoms, usually intermittent left leg edema, and surgical correction is advised *if* resting pressure gradients exist across the indented segment.

14. **Does the efficacy of nonoperative therapy of the postphlebitic syndrome preclude surgical intervention?? When is operative intervention indicated, and what surgical options deserve consideration?**
Operative intervention for the postphlebitic syndrome is *limited* to selected refractory patients and/or those in whom compliance is not compatible with their occupational pursuits. While still controversial and incompletely evaluated, the following may be indicated in carefully selected patients: relief of obstruction by venous bypass, interruption of incompetent perforator veins, and/or restoring valvular competence to a key segment of the deep venous system (i.e., the femoral or popliteal vein) by valvuloplasty, venous interpostion graft, or transpostion of competent segments.

---

72. CORONARY ARTERY DISEASE
ALDEN H. HARKEN, M.D.

---

1. **What causes angina?**
Although 25% of patients sustaining a myocardial infarction do so asymptomatically, angina typically results when myocardial oxygen demand exceeds supply.

2. **What are the determinants of myocardial oxygen demand (MVO2)?**
Braunwald has identified 9 independent determinants of MVO2 in the laboratory. Clinically, increasing heart rate, contractility, and wall tension are the major stimulants of oxygen demand.

3. **How do you treat angina?**
Most patients with atherosclerotic coronary artery disease live with a relatively fixed myocardial blood flow and resultant oxygen supply. The treatment of angina must therefore be directed toward reducing cardiac oxygen demand. Nitroglycerin may dilate coronary arteries a bit, but primarily reduces afterload and therefore decreases ventricular wall tension, contractility, and resultant oxygen demand. Beta-blockers, such a propranolol, decrease heart rate, contractility, and resultant oxygen demand. Calcium channel blockers may reduce afterload and prevent superimposed coronary vasoconstriction.

4. **What are the indications for coronary artery bypass grafting?**
Failure of medical therapy: When a patient with chronic stable angina and documented coronary artery disease is limited in his daily activities, he may reasonably request coronary artery bypass grafting. Following surgery, the patient can anticipate a 60% chance of no angina on no medication, while 90% of patients following surgery are improved.

Prevention of subsequent myocardial infarctions: The annual risk of lethal myocardial infarction is 11% for left main coronary artery disease and 3% incrementally for each of the three major coronary arteries. Thus, the annual mortality for single-vessel coronary artery disease is 3%; for double-vessel coronary artery disease, 6%; and for triple-vessel coronary artery disease, 9%. Following "complete" surgical revascularization, the annual myocardial infarction mortality decreases to 2%. Thus, coronary artery bypass grafting probably decreases myocardial infarction and resultant mortality in patients with coronary artery diseases of at least two vessels.

5. **Does coronary artery bypass grafting improve myocardial function? Is coronary artery bypass grafting useful in patients with congestive heart failure?**
Unfortunately, coronary artery bypass grafting does not seem to improve left ventricular function. Reversible ischemic left ventricular dysfunction seems to be unusual.

6. **Is coronary artery bypass grafting valuable in preventing ventricular arrhythmias?**
No.

7. **Does everyone with an acute myocardial infarction need a coronary artery bypass grafting procedure?**
An acute myocardial infarction almost invariably indicates atherosclerotic coronary artery disease. If a patient has had one myocardial infarction, there is certainly a high risk of a second. It is probably not necessary to catheterize everyone who has had a myocardial infarction. There are testing procedures, however, that can uncover imminent myocardial ischemia. A "submaximal" exercise stress test prior to hospital discharge can examine both electrophysiologically and symptomatically whether a patient still has jeopardized myocardium. If indeed this stress test is positive, most cardiologists would proceed with subsequent catheterization in a nonurgent fashion. If a patient has postinfarction angina or ominous coronary anatomy, then he may become a candidate for coronary artery bypass grafting.

8. **What group (anatomic) of patients with coronary artery occlusive disease are at highest risk of having further problems postoperatively?**
Astonishingly enough, the number of occluded coronary arteries is probably not a risk factor so long as all vessels are revascularized at the time of surgery. As with all vascular disease, the patients with diffuse disease and poor run-off will be the group at high risk of further problems.

9. **What is done at coronary artery bypass grafting?**
This is an arterial bypass grafting procedure. A saphenous vein (internal mammary artery, brachial artery, or Gortex graft) is anastomosed from the ascending aorta to the coronary artery distal to the atherosclerotic obstruction. Internal mammary arteries can be used only on the anterior surface of the heart. Both saphenous veins and mammary arteries have very good patency (90% at one year). Free radial artery grafts and Gortex grafts are substantially less effective, with a 1-year patency of approximately 50 to 60%.

10. **What are the technical pitfalls of coronary artery bypass grafting?**
As with all vascular surgery, the technical pitfalls revolve around compromised proximal or distal anastomoses. In almost all instances, a continuous layer of

monofilament sutures are used for both anastomoses. If either the coronary artery or the aorta is heavily atherosclerosed, the anastomosis may well be compromised and nonpatent. At the coronary artery level, an attempt is made to find a portion of coronary artery that is free of atherosclerosis. If this can be accomplished, the anastomosis is characteristically good. If it cannot, the atherosclerosis may well crumble or dissect and compromise the anastomosis.

11.   What is the risk of coronary artery bypass grafting?

The risk of coronary artery bypass grafting relates almost exclusively to ventricular function. In an elective patient with good ventricular function, the 30-day operative mortality is consistently less than 1%. As left ventricular function deteriorates, the operative mortality increases substantially.

12.   What can you do if a patient cannot be weaned from cardio-pulmonary bypass?

If a patient cannot maintain his own circulation without an external mechanical assist device (cardiopulmonary bypass machine), then the surgeon is really treating shock. As with any kind of shock, the steps are (1) replete volume until left- and right-sided filling pressures are adequate; (2) when intravascular volume is adequate, initiate pharmacologic support with epinephrine or dopamine; and (3) when volume and drugs are insufficient, resort to an intraaortic balloon, a mechanical heart, a transplanted heart. . .or prayer.

BIBLIOGRAPHY

1.   Buccino, R.A., and McIntosh, H.D.: Aortocoronary bypass grafting in the management of patients with coronary artery disease. Am. J. Med., 66:651, 1979.

2.   CASS Principal Investigators, et al.: Coronary artery surgery study (CASS): A randomized trial of coronary artery bypass surgery: Survival data. Circulation, 68:939-950, 1983.

3.   de Feyter, P.J., Serruys, P.W., van den Brand, M., et al.: Emergency coronary angioplasty in refractory unstable angina. N. Engl. J. Med., 313:342, 1985.

4.   Dobrin, P., Canfield, T., Moran, J., et al.: Coronary artery bypass. The physiological basis for differences in flow with internal mammary artery and saphenous vein grafts. J. Thorac. Cardiovasc. Surg., 74:445, 1977.

5.   European Coronary Surgery Study Group: Coronary artery bypass surgery in stable angina pectoris: Survival at two years. Lancet, 1:889-893, 1979.

6.   European Coronary Surgery Study Group: Long-term results of prospective randomised study of coronary artery bypass surgery in stable angina pectoris. Lancet, 2:1173-1180, 1982.

7.   Gersh, B.J., Kronmal, R.A., Schaff, H.V., et al., and the Participants in the Coronary Artery Surgery Study: Comparison of coronary artery bypass surgery and medical therapy in patients 65 years of age or older. N. Engl. J. Med., 313:217, 1985.

8.   Klocke, F.J., and Wittenberg, S.M.: Heterogeneity of coronary blood flow in human coronary artery disease and experimental myocardial infarction. Am J. Cardiol., 24:782, 1969.

9.   Kloster, F.E., Kremkau, E.L., Ritzmann, L.W., et al.: Coronary bypass for stable angina. A prospective randomized study. N. Engl. J. Med., 300:149, 1979.

10. Murphy, M.L., Hultgren, H.N., Detre, K., et al.: Treatment of chronic stable angina. N. Engl. J. Med., 297:621, 1977.

11. Pelletier, L.C., Pardini, A., Renkin, J., et al.: Myocardial revascularization after failure of percutaneous transluminal coronary angioplasty. J. Thorac. Cardiovasc. Surg., 90:265, 1985.

12. Principal Investigators of CASS, et al.: The National Heart, Lung and Blood Institute Coronary Artery Surgery Study (CASS). Circulation, 63 (Suppl. 1):1-81, 1981.

13. Takaro, T., Hultgren, H.N., Lipton, M.J., et al.: The VA cooperative randomized study of surgery for coronary arterial occlusive disease. II. Subgroup with significant left main lesions. Circulation 54 (Suppl. 3):107-117, 1976.

73. MITRAL STENOSIS

DAVID CAMPBELL, M.D., and ALDEN H. HARKEN, M.D.

1. **What is the cross-sectional area of the normal mitral valve?**
   4 to 6 sq cm.

2. **When do symptoms occur?**
   Mild, <2.5 sq cm.
   Moderate, 1 to 2 sq cm
   Severe, <1 sq cm

3. **What is the most common symptom and why?**
   Dyspnea on exertion because the ability to increase cardiac output with exercise is limited when the valve is narrowed.

4. **How is the diagnosis made?**
   Ausculatory findings of a loud, first heart sound, an opening snap, and a systolic rumble.

5. **How is the diagnosis confirmed?**
   Cardiac catheterization. In a patient with the characteristic diastolic rumble and echocardiographic findings of mitral stenosis, a diastolic gradient must be measured across the mitral valve. It is difficult to place a catheter across a stenotic mitral valve; therefore, pulmonary capillary wedge pressure and left ventricular end-diastolic pressures are measured simultaneously.

6. **How do you document mitral insufficiency at cardiac catheterization?**
   A pulmonary artery catheter may reflect a large V wave, but this is not specific for mitral insufficiency. The gold standard is dye injected into the left ventricle. If this dye is seen to regurgitate into the left atrium during ventricular systole, then mitral regurgitation is confirmed. At this point, science and subjectivism are rampantly exchanged. "Trace" and "wide open" (4+) mitral regurgitation are obvious, while 2+ and 3+ mitral regurgitation are somewhere in between. Remember, the patient's symptoms, not the catheterization, determine indications for surgery.

7. **What is the major indication for operation?**
   Development of symptoms. Mitral stenosis causes pulmonary venous hypertension and shortness of breath *early* in its natural history and fatigue *late*. Mitral insufficiency causes a decrease in cardiac output and fatigue *early* and shortness of breath *late*. The pulmonary hypertension associated with mitral valvular disease is reversible following valve surgery. It is, therefore, permissible to wait until the patient requests surgery. Alternatively, mitral valvular disease does *not* typically result in irreversible pulmonary vascular obstruction.

8. **What is the operation of choice for mitral stenosis?**
   Open versus closed commissurotomy (see Controversies).

9. **When should valve replacement be considered?**
   When the valve leaks significantly and/or the valve is heavily calcified.

10. **If valve replacement is necessary, which type of valve should be used, tissue or mechanical?**
    See Controversies.

11. During open operation, why is it a good idea to tie off the atrial appendage?
The atrial appendage can harbor clot, which can be ejected and lead to cerebral embolization after operation.

12. During open commissurotomy, how can the surgeon check to be sure that the valve is competent?
There are two major ways:
1. A special catheter can be placed across the aortic valve. The catheter has many holes in it, and some remain on either side of the valve. This rapidly fills the left ventricle when the cross-clamp is removed, causing the leaflets to balloon. Areas of leakage can then be identified.
2. Using a finger, the aortic valve can be rendered incompetent by pushing the aortic wall inward at the noncoronary cusp base of the aortic annulus. This allows the left ventricle to fill and the mitral leaflets to balloon. Any leaks will be quite visible.

13. What is the risk of mitral commissurotomy?
In good- risk patients, less than 5%; in poor-risk patients, up to 20%.

14. What are the major complications of mitral commissurotomy?
Death (1 to 3%), usually due to poor myocardial protection; significant mitral insufficiency (5%); significant residual stenosis (5 to 10%); air embolus and/or stroke (1%); bleeding (3 to 5%); and arrhythmias, particularly atrial fibrillation (20 to 40%).

15. What are the long-term results of mitral commissurotomy?
The majority of patients will have satisfactory results for 10 years or more, and 30% of patients will do well for 15 years.

CONTROVERSIES

16. Closed commissurotomy.
For: Mitral valvuloplasty (commissurotomy)–the commissures may be cut back to the annulus and the chordae freed in patients with pure mitral stenosis (minimal insufficiency). The track record for this procedure is superb. One third of patients enjoy an excellent hemodynamic result for 15 years! In addition, it is fast and less expensive, and blood usually is not required.
Against:
1. Blind procedure with a higher incidence of regurgitation.
2. Higher recurrence rate (probably this really represents incompletely relieved stenosis at operation), 20 to 50% at 5 years.
3. Emboli can be dislodged and cause cerebral infarcts.

17. Open commissurotomy
For:
1. Low mortality (1 to 2%).
2. Incidence of residual stenosis and production of insufficiency is low because the valve can be visualized during the procedure.
3. Incidence of dislodgement of emboli from the left atrium is almost nonexistent.
Against:
1. More costly.
2. Blood is usually necessary.

18. **Tissue valve.**

For: The aortic valve of a pig is sterilely sewn to a metal and cloth circular stent. This valve is treated with a glutaraldehyde preservative and stored in multiple different sizes for placement in either the mitral, aortic or tricuspid position. The advantage of these tissue valves is that they do not require long-term anticoagulation in the aortic position and mitral heterograft valves need not be anticoagulated if the patient is in sinus rhythm, has a small left atrium, and has no atrial clot at the time of surgery.

Against: They tend to calcify in children and deteriorate in adults. The anxiety over tissue valve degeneration may be exaggerated, however. Structural tissue valve failure is not common, with 80% of these valves lasting for 7 to 10 years (which compares favorably with any mechanical prosthesis).

19. **Mechanical valve.**

For: Valve technology is improving such that mechanical valves are now available with almost no transvalvular gradient.

Against:

1. Higher incidence of bleeding complications such as cerebral hemorrhage.
2. Contraindicated in patients with alcohol abuse or duodenal ulcers.
3. Thromboembolism rate higher than tissue valves.
4. Valve can acutely malfunction, placing the patient in extreme danger.

Although these valves are hemodynamically superb, they can be noisy and many are not radiopaque. The big problem is that all mechanical valves in any position require chronic anticoagulation. Anticoagulation is not without risk, and the annual mortality associated with anticoagulation approximates 1%. In addition, it calls for great discipline on the part of the patient to take medication that doesn't make him feel better. However, some patients with mitral stenosis have chronic atrial fibrillation and large left atria that often require permanent anticoagulation anyway. Use of a mechanical valve should be strongly considered in this setting.

BIBLIOGRAPHY

1. Carpentier, A., Branchini, B., Cour, J.C., et al.: Congenital malformations of the mitral valve in children: Pathology and surgical treatment. J. Thorac. Cardiovasc. Surg., 72:845, 1976.
2. Carpentier, A., Chauvaud, S., Fabiani, J.N., et al.: Reconstructive surgery of mitral valve incompetence: Ten-year appraisal. J. Thorac. Cardiovasc. Surg., 79:338, 1980.
3. Chaux, A., Gray, R.J., Matloff, J.M., et al.: An appreciation of the new St. Jude valvular prosthesis. J. Thorac. Cardiovasc. Surg., 81:202, 1981.
4. Cheung, D., Flemma, R.J., Mullen, D.L., et al.: Ten-year follow-up in aortic valve replacement using the Bjork-Shiley prosthesis. Ann. Thorac. Surg., 32:138, 1981.
5. Cobb, L.A., Werner, J.A., and Trobaugh, G.B.: Sudden cardiac death. 1. A decade's experience with out-of-hospital resuscitation. Mod. Concepts Cardiovasc. Dis., 49:31, 1980.
6. Cobbs, B.W., Jr., Hatcher, C.R., Jr., Craver, J.M., et al.: Transverse midventricular disruption after mitral valve replacement. Am. Heart J., 99:33, 1980.
7. Culliford, A.T., Boyd, A.D., and Spencer, F.C.: A special rongeur for removal of extensively calcified mitral valves. Ann. Thorac. Surg., 28:605, 1979.
8. Cutler, E.C., and Levine, S.A.: Cardiotomy and valvulotomy for mitral stenosis. Boston Med. Surg J., 188:1023, 1923.
9. Geha, A.S., Laks, H., Stansel, H.C., Jr., et al.: Late failure of porcine valve heterografts in children. J. Thorac. Cardiovasc. Surg., 78:351, 1979.
10. Gross, R.I., Cunningham, J.N., Jr., Snively, S.S., et al.: Long-term results of open radical mitral commissurotomy: Ten-year follow-up study of 202 patients. Am J. Cardiol., 47:821, 1981.

11. Halseth, W.L., Elliott, D.P., Walker, E.S., and Smith E.A.: Open mitral commissurotomy: A modern re-evaluation J. Thorac. Cardiovasc. Surg., 80:842, 1980.

12. Housman, L.B., Bonchek, L., Lambert, L., et al.: Prognosis of patients after mitral commissurotomy: Actuarial analysis of late results in 100 patients. J. Thorac. Cardiovasc. Surg., 73:742, 1977.

13. Isom, O.W., Spencer, F.C., Glassman, E., et al.: Long-term results in 1375 patients undergoing valve replacement with the Starr-Edwards cloth-covered steel ball prosthesis. Ann. Surg., 186:310, 1977.

14. Isom, O.W., Culliford, A.T., Colvin, S.B., et al.: Porcine valves: Is there a difference? Presented at the American Heart Association, Miami, November 1980.

15. Jamieson, W.R.E., Janusz, M.T., Miyagishima, R.T., et al: Embolic complication of porcine heterograft cardiac valves. J. Thorac. Cardiovasc. Surg., 81:626, 1981.

16. Karp, R.B., Cyrus, R. J., Blackstone, E.H., et al.: The Bjork-Shiley valve. Intermediate-term follow-up. J. Thorac. Cardiovasc. Surg., 82:602, 1981.

17. Kay, J.H., and Egerton, W.S.: The repair of mitral insufficiency associated with ruptured chordae tendineae. Ann. Surg., 157:351, 1963.

18. Magilligan, D.J., Jr., Lewis, J.W., Jr., Jara, F.M., et al.: Spontaneous degeneration of porcine bioprosthetic valves. Ann. Thorac. Surg., 30:259, 1980.

19. Miller, D.W., Jr., Johnson, D.D., and Ivey, T.D.: Does preservation of the posterior chordae tendineae enhance survival during mitral valve replacement? Ann. Thorac. Surg., 28:22, 1979.

20. Mullin, M. J., Engelman, R. M., Isom, O. W., et al.: Experience with open mitral commissurotomy in 100 consecutive patients. Surgery, 76:974, 1974.

21. Oyer, P.E., Miller, D.C., Stinson, E.B., et al.: Clinical durability of the Hancock porcine bioprosthetic valve. J. Thorac. Cardiovasc. Surg., 80:824, 1980.

22. Pluth, J.R.: The case for the Starr-Edwards valve. Presented at the American College of Cardiology, San Francisco, March 1981.

23. Reed, G.E., Pooley, R.W., and Moggio, R.A.: Durability of measured mitral annuloplasty. Seventeen-year study. J. Thorac. Cardiovasc. Surg., 79:321, 1980.

24. Roe, B.B., Edmunds, H., Jr., Fishman, N.H., and Hutchinson, J.C.: Open mitral commissurotomy. Ann. Thorac. Surg., 12:483, 1971.

25. Selzer, A., and Cohen, K.E.: Natural history of mitral stenosis: A review. Circulation, 45:878, 1972.

26. Spencer, F.C.: A plea for early, open mitral stenosis: A review. Circulation, 45:878, 1972.

27. Starr, A., and Edwards, M.L.: Mitral replacement: Clinical experience with a ball valve prosthesis. Ann. Surg., 154:726, 1961.

28. Tandon, A.P., Sengupta, S.M., Luckacs, L., and Ionescu, M.I.: Long-term clinical and hemodynamic evaluation of the Ionescu-Shiley pericardial xenograft and the Braunwald-Cutter and Bjork-Shiley prosthesis in the mitral position. J. Thorac. Cardiovasc. Surg., 76:763, 1978.

29. Teply, J.F., Grunkemeier, G.L., Sutherland, H.D., et al.: The ultimate prognosis after valve replacement: An assessment in twenty years. Ann. Thorac. Surg., 32:111, 1981.

30. Williams, J.B., Karp, R.B., Kirklin, J.W., et al.: Considerations in selection and management of patients undergoing valve replacement with glutaraldehyde-fixed porcine bioprostheses. Ann. Thorac. Surg., 30:247, 1980.

31. Williams, W.G., Pollock, J.C., Geiss, D.M., et al.: Experience with aortic and mitral valve replacement in children. J. Thorac. Cardiovasc. Surg., 81:326, 1981.

74. AORTIC STENOSIS

DAVID CAMPBELL, M.D.

1. **What are the two most common causes of aortic stenosis?**
   Congenital anomaly and rheumatic fever.

2. **What is the most common anatomic anomaly in congenital aortic stenosis?**
   Bicuspid aortic valve.

3. **What is the most common presentation in infancy?**
   Congestive heart failure.

4. **What are the most common symptoms in the adult with aortic stenosis?**
   Syncope, dyspnea on exertion, and angina.

5. **What are the physical findings that suggest aortic stenosis?**
   In the infant systolic crescendo-decrescendo murmur, poor peripheral pulses. In the adult, systolic crescendo-decrescendo murmur, delayed pulse upstroke (pulsus parvus et tardus).

6. **What is the most feared complication of aortic stenosis?**
   Sudden death.

7. **How is the diagnosis confirmed?**
   Cardiac catheterization. In children, associated lesions such as patent ductus arteriosus and coarctation of thoracic aorta can be identified. In adults, the status of the coronary arteries is important to assess since atherosclerotic heart disease is a common finding in older patients.

8. **When is an operation indicated?**
   Development of symptoms, progression of left ventricular hypertrophy, or measured gradient of 50 to 60 mm Hg.

9. **What is the best method to use for aortic valvotomy in infants under 3 months of age?**
   See Controversies.

10. **Is aortic valvotomy for congenital aortic stenosis curative?**
    Usually not; most of these children will ultimately need aortic valve replacement later in life.

11. **Can aortic valvotomy be used for calcific aortic stenosis?**
    No! Aortic valve replacement is the procedure of choice in the adult.

12. **What are the technical details of aortic valve replacement?**
    It is done on cardiopulmonary bypass. The left ventricle is quite thickened, so special care must be taken to avoid injury to the myocardium. The left ventricle should be vented to decrease wall tension, and the heart should be quieted with cold potassium cardioplegia. Care must be taken during debridement of the calcified valve and annulus to prevent dislodgement of calcium particles into the ventricle, which can later be ejected as calcium emboli. Finally, when suturing the valve, care must be taken to avoid interference with the left coronary orifice.

13. **If a valve replacement is necessary in a child, what type of valve should be used?**
A mechanical valve should be used in children under 15 years of age, as the incidence of rapid calcification is very high in tissue valves, which leads to early failure. Calcification of a tissue valve can occur more rapidly than normal in young adults between the ages of 15 and 30 and, therefore, use of a tissue valve in this group is controversial.

14. **What are the techniques to manage a small aortic annulus?**
    1. Kono aortoventriculoplasty: With this technique the ventricular septum is split along the aortic annulus. A patch is then sewn in to enlarge the aortic annulus usually by two valve sizes or more.
    2. Patch plasty through the aortic annulus toward the mitral valve: An incision is carried through the center of the noncoronary annulus toward the annulus, of the mitral valve but not onto the valve. A V patch is then sewn into position. This enlarges the annulus about one valve size.
    3. Manouguian patch plasty into the anterior leaflet of the mitral valve: This technique extends an incision described above onto the mitral valve. This allows the annulus to be enlarged about two valve sizes.

15. **What is the operative morality?**
In good-risk patients, less than 3%. In patients with poor ventricular function, 15 to 20%.

16. **What are the complications of aortic valve replacement?**
Low cardiac output (3 to 5%), higher for patients with preoperative congestive heart failure; bleeding requiring reexploration (5%); heart block (1 to 2%); and stroke (1%) due to air or calcium left in the heart following closure of the aortotomy.

17. **What are the long-term results of aortic valve replacement?**
Excellent, unless the patient has had preoperative congestive heart failure or severe coronary artery disease. Ten-year survival ranges from 60 to 75%.

CONTROVERSIES

18. **Knife valvotomy using inflow occlusion for infants under three months of age.**
    For:
    1. Low mortality (10%).
    2. Low incidence of low cardiac output.
    Against:
    1. Time-limited. Procedure must be performed very rapidly.
    2. 20% incidence of significant aortic regurgitation.

19. **Knife valvotomy using cardiopulmonary bypass for infants under three months of age.**
    For: Allows plenty of time to accomplish operation.
    Against: Higher incidence of low cardiac output postoperatively.

20. **Use of a tissue valve in young adults between ages 15 to 30.**
    For: Anticoagulation is not necessary, thus the risk of significant bleeding complications in this group of very active patients is avoided. Also, for females in the childbearing years the advantages are obvious.
    Against: There is a somewhat higher incidence of early valve dysfunction owing to calcification so that valve replacement might be necessary before 10 years.

BIBLIOGRAPHY

1. Barratt-Boyes, B.G., Roche, A.H.G., Brandt, P.W.T., et al.: Aortic valve replacement–a long-term follow-up in an initial series of 101 patients. Circulation, 40:763, 1969.

2. Bjork, V.O., and Henze, Z.: Ten years' experience with the Bjork-Shiley tilting disc valve. J. Thorac. Cardiovasc. Surg., 78:331, 1979.

3. Blank, R.H., Pupello, D.F., Bessone, L.N., et al.: Method of managing the small aortic annulus during valve replacement. Ann. Thorac. Surg., 22:356, 1976.

4. Bonow, R.O., Kent, K.M., Rosing, D.R., et al.: Aortic valve replacement without myocardial revascularization in patients with combined aortic valvular and coronary artery disease. Circulation, 63:243, 1981.

5. Braun, L.O., Kincaid, O.W., and McGoon, D.C.: Prognosis of aortic valve replacement in relation to preoperative heart size. J. Thorac. Cardiovasc. Surg., 65:381, 1973.

6. Callard, G.M., Flege, J.B., Jr. and Todd, J.C.: Combined valvular and coronary artery surgery. Ann. Thorac. Surg., 22:338, 1976.

7. Chaux, A., Gray, R.J., Matloff, J.M., et al.: An appreciation of the new St. Jude valvular prosthesis. J. Thorac. Cardiovasc. Surg., 81:202, 1981.

8. Cohn, L.H., Mudge, G.H., Pratter, F., and Collins, J.J., Jr.: Five- to eight-year follow-up of patients undergoing porcine heart-valve replacement. N. Engl. J. Med., 304:258, 1981.

9. Copeland, J.G., Griepp, R.B., Stinson, E.B., and Shumway, N. E.: Long-term follow-up after isolated aortic valve replacement. J. Thorac. Cardiovasc. Surg., 74:875, 1977.

10. Copeland, J.G., Griepp, R. B., Stinson, E. B., et al.: Isolated aortic valve replacement in patients older than 65 years. J.A.M.A., 237:1578, 1977.

11. Crosby, I. K. Ashcraft, W.C., and Reed, W.A.: Surgery of the proximal aorta in Marfan's syndrome. J. Thorac. Cardiovasc. Surg., 66:75, 1973.

12. Curcio, C.A., Commerford, P.J., Rose, A.G., et al.: Calcification of glutaraldehyde-preserved porcine xenografts in young patients. J. Thorac. Cardiovasc. Surg., 81:621, 1981.

13. Deboer, A., and Midell, A.I.: Isolated aortic valve replacement: Analysis of factors influencing survival after replacement with the Starr-Edwards prosthesis. Ann. Thorac. Surg., 17:360, 1974.

14. Hancock Laboratories, Inc. (Vascor Labs) Anaheim, California: Durability assessment of the Hancock porcine bioprosthesis: A multicenter retrospective analysis of patients operated on prior to 1975. April 1980.

15. Hatcher, C.R., Jr.: Aortic valve replacement: The problem of the small aortic annulus. Editorial from the Division of Thoracic and Cardiovascular Surgery, Emory University School of Medicine, Atlanta, Georgia, 1981.

16. Hehrlein, F.W., Gottwik, M., Fraedrich, G., and Mulch, J.: First clinical experience with a new all-pyrolytic carbon bileaflet heart valve prosthesis. J. Thorac. Cardiovasc. Surg., 79:632, 1980.

17. Henrlein, F.W., Gottwik, M., Mulch, J., et al.: Heart valve replacement with the new all-pyrolytic bileaflet St. Jude Medical prosthesis. J. Cardiovasc. Surg., 21:395, 1980.

18. Herr, R.H., Starr, A., Pierie, W.R., et al.: Aortic valve replacement: A review of six years' experience with the ball valve prosthesis. Ann. Thorac. Surg., 6:199, 1968.

19. Jamieson, W.R.E., Janusz, M.T., Miyagishima, R.T., et al.: Embolic complications of porcine heterograft cardiac valves. J. Thorac. Cardiovasc. Surg., 81:626, 1981.

20. Jamieson, W.R.E., Janusz, M., Munro, A.I., Early clinical experience with the Carpentier Edwards porcine heterograft cardiac valves. J. Thorac. Cardiovasc. Surg., 81:626, 1981.

21. Karp, R. B., Cyrus, R.J., Blackstone, E.H., et al.: The Bjork-Shiley valve: Intermediate term follow-up. J. Thorac. Cardiovasc. Surg., 81:602, 1981.

22. Kirklin, J.W.: The replacement of cardiac valves (Editorial). N. Engl. J. Med., 304:291, 1981.

23. Kirklin, J.W., and Kouchoukos, N.T.: Aortic valve replacement without myocardial revascularization (Editorial). Circulation, 63:252, 1981.

24. Konno, S., Imai, Y., Iida, Y., et al.: A new method for prosthetic valve replacement in congenital aortic stenosis associated with hypoplasia of the aortic valve ring. J. Thorac. Cardiovasc. Surg., 70:909, 1975.

25. Lawrence, R.S., Mena, I., Jengo, J.A., et al.: Noninvasive evaluation of late left ventricular function after aortic valve replacement. J. Thorac. Cardiovasc. Surg., 79:504, 1980.

26. Lee, G., Grehl, T.M., Joye, J.A., et al.: Hemodynamic assessment of the new aortic Carpentier-Edwards bioprosthesis. Cathet. Cardiovasc. Diagn., 4:373, 1978.

27. Macmanus, Q., Grunkemeier, G.L., Lambert, L.E., et al.: Year of operation as a risk factor in the late results of valve replacement. J. Thorac. Cardiovasc. Surg., 80:834, 1980.

28. Magilligan, D.J., Jr., Lewis, J.W., Jr., Jara, F.M., et al: Spontaneous degeneration of porcine bioprosthetic valves. Ann. Thorac. Surg., 30:259, 1980.

29. Manouguian, S., and Seybold-Epting, W.: Patch enlargement of the aortic valve ring by extending the aortic incision into the anterior mitral leaflet. J. Thorac. Cardiovasc. Surg., 78j:402, 1979.

30. Manouguian, S., Abu-Aishah, N., and Neitzel, J.: Patch enlargement of the aortic and mitral valve rings with aortic and mitral double valve replacement. J. Thorac. Cardiovasc. Surg., 78:394, 1979.

31. Mori, T., Kaashima, Y., Kitamura, S., et al.: Results of aortic valve replacment in patients with a narrow aortic annulus: Effects of enlargement of the aortic annulus. Ann. Thorac. Surg., 31:111, 1981.

32. Najafi, H., Ostermiller, W.E., Jr., Javid, H. et al.: Narrow aortic root complicating aortic valve replacement. Arch. Surg., 99:690, 1969.

33. Nicks, R., Cartmill, T., and Bernstein, L.: Hypoplasia of the aortic root: The problem of aortic root replacement. Thorax, 25:339, 1970.

34. Nicoloff, D.M., and Emery, R.W.: Current status of the St. Jude cardiac valve prosthesis. Contemp. Surg., 15, 1979.

35. Norman, J.C., Cooley, D.A., Hallman, G.L., and Nihill, M.R.: Left ventricular apical-abdominal aortic conduits for the left ventricular outflow tract obstructions: Clinical results in nine patients with a special composite prosthesis. Circulation, 54 (Suppl.):100, 1976.

36. Ott, D.A., Coelho, A.T., Cooley, D.A., and Reul, G.J., Jr.: Ionescu-Shiley pericardial xenograft valve: Hemodynamic evaluation and early clinical follow-up of 326 patients. Cardiovasc. Dis., 7:137, 1980.

37. Oyer, P.E., Miller, D.C., Stinson, E.B., et al.: Clinical durability of the Hancock porcine bioprosthetic valve. J. Thorac. Cardiovasc. Surg., 80:824, 1980.

38. Oyer, P.E., Stinson, E.B., Reitz, B.A., et al.: Long-term evaluation of the porcine xenograft bioprosthesis. J. Thorac. Cardiovasc. Surg., 78:343, 1979.

39. Pentely, G., Morton, M., and Rahimtoola, S.H.: Effects of successful, uncomplicated valve replacement on ventricular hypertrophy, volume, and performance in aortic stenosis and in aortic incompetence. J. Thorac. Cardiovasc. Surg., 75:383, 1978.

40. Pipkin, R.D., Buch, W.S., and Fogarty, T.J.: Evaluation of aortic valve replacement with a porcine xenograft without long-term anticoagulation. J. Thorac. Cardiovasc. Surg., 71:179, 1976.

41. Pupello, D.F., Blank, R.H., Bessone, L.N., et al.: Surgical management of the small aortic annulus: Hemodynamic evaluation. Chest, 74:163, 1978.

42. Riddle, J.M., Magilligan, D.J., and Stein, P.D.: Surface morphology of degenerated porcine bioprosthetic valves four to seven years following implantation. J. Thorac. Cardiovasc. Surg., 81:279, 1981.

43. Rothkopf, M., Davidson, T., Lipscomb, K., et al.: Hemodynamic evaluation of the Carpentier-Edwards bioprosthesis in the aortic position. Am. J. Cardiol., 44:209,1979.

44. Sandza, J.G., Jr., Clark, R.E., Ferguson, T.B., et al.: Replacement of prosthetic heart valves: A fifteen-year experience. J. Thorac. Cardiovasc. Surg., 74:864, 1977.

45. Semb, B.K.H., Nitter-Hauge, S., and Hall, K.V.: The Hall-Kaster disc valve prosthesis: Clinical and hemodynamic observations in patients undergoing aortic valve replacement. J. Cardiovasc. Surg., 21:387, 1980.

46. Steind, D.W., Rahimtoola, S.H., Kloster, F.E., et al.: Thrombotic phenomena with nonanticoagulated, composite-strut aortic prostheses. J. Thorac. Cardiovasc. Surg., 71:680, 1976.

47. Syracuse, D.C., Bowman, F.O., Jr., and Malm, J.R.: Prosthetic valve reoperations: Factors influencing early and late survival. J. Thorac. Cardiovasc. Surg., 77:346, 1979.

48. Tandon, A.P., Whitaker, W., and Ionescu, M.I.: Multiple valve replacement with pericardial xenograft: Clinical and hemodydnamic study. Br. Heart J., 44:534, 1980.
49. Thompson, R., Ahmed, M., Seabra-Gomes, R., et al.: Influence of preoperative left ventricular function on results of homograft replacement of the aortic valve for aortic regurgitation. J. Thorac. Cardiovasc. Surg., 77:411, 1979.
50. Triestman, B., and El-Said, G.: Valvular aortic stenosis and coronary artery disease. Cardiovasc. Dis., 2:193, 1975.
51. Wallace, R. B., Londe, S.P., and Titus, J.L.: Aortic valve replacement with preserved aortic valve homografts. J. Thorac. Cardiovasc. Surg., 67:44, 1974.
52. Williams, J.B., Karp, R.B., Kirklin, J.W., et al.: Considerations in selection and management of patients undergoing valve replacement with glutaraldehyde-fixed porcine bioprostheses. Ann. Thorac. Surg., 30:247, 1980.
53. Wortham, D.C., Tri, T.B., and Bowen, T.E.: Hemodynamic evaluation of the St. Jude Medical valve prosthesis in the small aortic annulus. J. Thorac. Cardiovasc. Surg., 81:615, 1981.

75. PNEUMOTHORAX
L. DOUGLAS COWGILL, M.D.

1. **What are the major etiologic categories of pneumothorax?**
(1) Spontaneous. (2) Traumatic: often associated with bleeding (hemopneumothorax). (3) Iatrogenic: attempted central line placement; post pleurocentesis/post pleural or needle lung biopsy; ventilator barotrauma, especially using PEEP; postoperative thoracic procedures.

2. **Who are likely candidates for spontaneous pneumothorax?**
Three major types:
(1) Young (20 to 40 years of age); usually male (male-to-female ratio, 5 to 8:1); often tall, "asthenic" individuals with no history of pulmonary disease. Mortality low unless tension pneumothorax.
(2) Older (> 40 years) patients with chronic obstructive pulmonary disease, with significant mortality (up to 15 to 20%).
(3) Newborn infants: often immediately after delivery, especially in vaginal deliveries, when compressed chest suddenly expands. Also related to hyaline membrane disease in premature infants, and with barotrauma from ventilators.
Several "minor" or infrequent categories:
(1) Certain pulmonary or connective tissue diseases: tuberculosis, pneumonia, lung abscess, histiocytosis X, scleroderma, Marfan's syndrome, Ehlers-Danlos syndrome, hydatid cyst, metastatic neoplasm.
(2) Perimenstrual pneumothorax (catamenial): always on right, from 72 hours before to 72 hours after onset of menses. Etiology unclear, but possibly related to thoracic endometriosis implants and/or diaphragmatic pores or defects.
(3) Postemetic esophageal perforation (Boerhaave's syndrome): usually left-sided; may confuse underlying diagnosis; true surgical emergency.

3. **What are the most common symptoms?**
Pain and dyspnea; less commonly, cough and hemoptysis. The pain simulates that of other thoracic conditions: myocardial infarction, aortic dissection, pulmonary embolism, esophageal perforation, and empyema.

4. **What are the most common signs?**

1.   Examination usually normal in small pneumothorax. ("Chest meant to be seen and not heard".)
2.   For larger pneumothorax: ipsilateral decreased breath sounds, decreased tactile fremitus, increased tympany and resonance.
3.   For tension pneumothorax: same as for larger pneumothorax, plus signs of shock, cyanosis, and contralateral tracheal deviation.
4.   Posttraumatic: often includes subcutaneous emphysema.

5.   How is diagnosis made?

Chest x-ray. Standard posteroanterior film is usually diagnostic: hyperlucent area with completely absent lung markings in the periphery of hemithorax.
1.   Expiration film helpful for small pneumothorax; with expiration, decreased lung volume and increased lung density results in relative increase in size and lucency of pneumothorax.
2.   Decubitus film (affected side up) also helpful for small pneumothorax; free air accumulates along uppermost part of chest. This may be particularly helpful in differentiating from giant bulla.
3.   Air-fluid level occasionally present, especially posttraumatically (blood).
4.   Rib fractures and subcutaneous emphysema often present posttraumatically.
5.   Mediastinal shift with tension.

6.   Can one be "fooled" by chest x-rays?

Yes.
1.   If negative but history is suggestive, delayed film (4 to 12 hours) may be diagnostic.
2.   If "positive," may be confused with skin folds, scapular or rib margins, or especially a giant bulla.

7.   Why is recognition of giant bullae important, and what is the coin test?

If pneumothorax is mistakenly diagnosed, placement of a chest tube will often rupture existing thin-walled bullae, resulting in bronchopleural fistula that will require operative closure in the high-risk patient with advanced COPD.

The coin test attempts to differentiate bullae from pneumothorax: coin pressed against the anterior chest, when tapped with another coin, results in auscultating "metallic" ring posteriorly with pneumothorax, a sign that is absent in patients with large bullae . Nevertheless, chest x-ray is still the most helpful determinant between the two disorders. With experience, bullae characteristics such as bilaterality and multiple unilateral hyperlucencies usually can be recognized.

8.   What is tension pneumothorax and why is it particularly important to recognize?

If air accumulating in the pleural cavity reaches a pressure high enough to shift mobile structures (mediastinum, opposite lung) away from that side, a tension pneumothorax results. This occurs in 2 to 3% of all pneumothoraces. Most often the patient is on a ventilator, where the constant positive pressure may allow continued accumulation of air. If the pleural opening has a "check valve," closing it on expiration and preventing egress of air will result in tension pneumothorax.

Signs: patient in extremis, shock with distended neck veins (similar to tamponade or cardiogenic shock), heart sounds, and tracheal deviation to the opposite side. It may occur bilaterally, in which case tracheal shift is not present.

Treatment must begin immediately, as pathophysiology includes both respiratory (from compression of normal lung) and, more importantly, circulatory (due to mediastinal shift, increased intrathoracic pressure, and severely reduced venous return to the heart) compromise.

9. **How does one estimate percent size of pneumothorax?**
Assuming the size of the ipsilateral pleural cavity to be 100%, subtract estimated size of ipsilateral lung volume (e.g., if ipsilateral lung volume is 75% of pleural cavity volume, patient has a 25% pneumothorax). Generally the size of the pneumothorax is underestimated, as lung volume decreases with the cube of the radius (i.e., loss of 50% diameter of lung from edge to hilum is much more than 50% loss of volume).

10. **May pneumothorax occur bilaterally?**
Yes: synchronously in 5% and asynchronously in about 10%.

11. **May pneumothorax recur?**
With one spontaneous pneumothorax, approximately 20 to 30% chance of recurrence. With a second recurrence, greater than 50% chance of a third.

12. **Which patients are at greatest risk once pneumothorax occurs?**
    1. Those at extremes of age: older patients with advanced COPD (15 to 20% mortality); neonates, especially premies.
    2. Those with severe underlying disease, particularly adolescents with cystic fibrosis, COPD with giant bullae.
    3. Any patient with tension pneumothorax.
    4. Intraoperative pneumothorax.
    5. When associated with chest vascular injury that results in air embolism.
    6. When associated with sucking chest wound.

13. **Why is intraoperative pneumothorax especially dangerous?**
Not only is the deleterious effect of pneumothorax added to the standard morbidity associated with surgery, but:
    1. Pneumothorax is often tension-type as a result of positive-pressure ventilation.
    2. If occurs during "one-lung anesthesia" to ventilated lung during thoracic procedure, ventilation may be interrupted totally.
    3. May be missed, as patient's sudden deterioration during surgery often ascribed to hypovolemia, myocardial ischemia, etc.
Several situations predispose patients to intraoperative pneumothorax:
    1. Combined chest-abdominal trauma: If admission chest x-ray film is normal and patient requires abdominal exploration, surgeon should be wary of instituting anesthesia (positive-pressure ventilation) without chest tube to side of chest trauma.
    2. Following placement of central lines (subclavian, internal jugular) prior to induction: In all patients requiring central line and thoracotomy, line should be placed on side of thoracotomy for this reason.

14. **Blebs, which are the most common cause of spontaneous pneumothorax in the 20 to 40-year-old age group, almost always occur apically and usually in tall "asthenic" men. Why? Are they congenital or acquired?**
Originally thought to be caused by tuberculosis (also prone to occur apically), blebs are now thought to be due to the increased negativity of the intrapleural presure at the apex of the pleural cavity. Canine studies have shown, in the up-

right position, that apical pleural pressure is considerably more negative than that at the base. In addition, the weight of the lung results in a natural downward shift of lung mass, and consequently a smaller volume of lung must fill a space with excessive negative pressure. The greater the superoinferior dimension (i.e., in tall individuals), the greater the "pull." In this situation, alveolar disruption probably occurs during growth spurts in adolescence, resulting in nonepithelial-lined apical blebs that subsequently rupture from excessive pressure.

15. **What is the treatment of pneumothorax?**
Generally, placement of chest tube is indicated for initial episodes of documented pneumothorax, regardless of etiology (spontaneous, traumatic, or iatrogenic).

16. **Is tension pneumothorax treated differently?**
Preferably yes. As the major difference is its requirement for emergent decompression, two points should be stressed:
   1. Immediate decompression can safely be performed with insertion of large-bore (14 to 18 gauge) needle into chest. Delay in acquiring chest tube with necessary instruments may be fatal.
   2. For the same reason, chest x-ray in an appropriate clinical setting is not indicated prior to needle placement, as this causes needless, risky delay. Diagnosis of tension pneumothorax should be clinical, not radiologic.
   3. Chest tube can then be inserted when the patient has been stabilized.

17. **Can any pneumothorax be observed?**
Most would agree that a small pneumothorax (less than 15%, apical) may safely be watched if the patient is not in a high-risk group (emphysema, cystic fibrosis, neonate, on ventilator). Pneumothorax requires hospitalization and close follow-up.

18. **If observation is chosen, will any maneuver hasten resolution?**
Only approximately 1.25% of air in stable pneumothorax will reabsorb each day with the patient breathing room air. Placing the patient on oxygen by nasal prongs will possibly hasten resolution, as oxygen is more soluble than the nitrogen it replaces. Also, the nitrogen that remains has a greater pleural-capillary gradient, favoring its absorption.

19. **Is needle aspiration, plombage, or toxin instillation ever indicated instead of chest tube placement?**
See Controversies.

20. **Where should the chest tube be placed? What size? How many?**
For pneumothorax alone, a small (18 to 20 gauge) anterior chest tube with the tip in the apex of the pleural cavity is optimal. The major argument against high (second intercostal space) anterior chest tube placement is cosmetic, and for this reason the trend is toward more lateral, inferior tube placement. Proportionally smaller chest tubes may be used in children.
   For hemothorax, tube should be larger (36 to 40 gauge) and directed posteriorly to allow drainage in the supine position. One tube is sufficient unless the volume of air leak is so great that the lung won't expand with a single tube, or if the anticipated volume of bleeding postoperatively requires more than one tube to keep the chest evacuated and the lung expanded.

21. **Is suction needed on chest tube, as opposed to water seal?**
Only for bleeding or an ongoing air leak. In absence of this, air will evacuate through water trap, and unless the patient has bronchopleural fistula (ongoing air leak), the lung will expand without suction.

22. **Does a "bubbling" chest tube prove the presence of broncho-pleural fistula?**
No. Common causes of bubbling, preventing reexpansion of the sealed lung, are the following: improper position of the chest tube (last hole outside the chest wall); leak in the system (e.g., at connection of the chest tube apparatus); nonocclusive suture or dressing where chest tube enters the chest (comparable to a sucking chest wound); elevation of the chest tube apparatus above the patient; "trapped lung" (i.e., collapsed lung with empyema, patient may not have bronchopleural fistula but will require decortication for expansion).

23. **What are the potential problems with chest tube placement?**
1. Discomfort, especially on insertion but also afterward.
2. Bleeding, most often from the chest wall, especially intercostal if the tube is inserted in inferior rather than superior margin of rib; infrequently the chest tube is placed below the diaphragmatic margin, into the spleen or liver, in which case bleeding is serious.
3. Lung injury and additional site for air leak.
4. Infection (empyema).
5. Creation of pneumothorax if removed improperly.

24. **What are indications for surgery for spontaneous pneumothorax?**
1. Recurrence is the most common indication. Virtually all recommend surgery after the second recurrence and many following the first.
2. Persistent bronchopleural fistulas require surgery: (a) If the air leak continues, particularly when associatied with severe lung pathology (blebs, bullae, or cystic fibrosis. (b) Occasionally, the leak may continue even though the lung has adhered to the chest wall. In this situation, if the patient tolerates tube clamping without dropping lung, he can presumably tolerate removal of the chest tube even though the fistula has not closed, as the fistula is too small to overcome fusion of the lung to the chest wall. (c) Postoperative pulmonary procedures often have prolonged air leaks. Patience is usually rewarding here, as most will eventually close, while reexploration often aggravates the amount of air leak.
3. Bilateral pneumothorax.
4. Associated ongoing bleeding.
5. Massive air leak after chest trauma: generally indicates ruptured bronchus.
6. Secondary to esophageal perforation, secondary to primary malignancy.
7. Certain occupations: airline pilot, deep sea diver, etc.

25. **What operation is performed?**
Three maneuvers are important: (1) correction of underlying lung pathology (stapling apical blebs, etc.), particularly at the site of leak; (2) "pleurodesis" (see Controversies) creates severe inflammatory reaction of parietal and, to a lesser extent, visceral pleura, usually by vigorous abrasion but occasionally chemically induced, resulting in their fusion; (3) placement of appropriately positioned (apical) chest tubes to pull lung up to chest wall.

CONTROVERSIES

26. **Are measures other than chest tube placement effective?**
Usually not. Although needle aspiration may rarely expand the lung if the leak has sealed, generally it will not and adds needless delay as well as a slight risk of bleeding and lung puncture in attempting to insert the needle. Plombage (extrapleural administration of material such as paraffin to collapse the parietal

pleura onto lung) is unecessary and prevents return to previous pulmonary function. Instillation of toxins (talc, quinacrine, tetracycline, etc.) through chest tube into pleural cavity has been effective, but unless the patient is strictly nonsurgical, it should be avoided, as it is usually ineffective as well as very painful.

27. Timing of operative intervention?

How many recurrences? Most now operate after the second pneumothorax (i.e., first recurrence), as greater than a 50% chance of there being another, and mortality with surgery is less than 1% in young spontaneous group.

How long should one treat bronchopleural fistula before operating? See the guidelines outlined above. The major dilemma is in those with such advanced COPD that surgery constitutes significant risk of morbidity and mortality. Unfortunately, this is also the group that may least tolerate prolonged bronchopleural fistula (e.g., those with cystic fibrosis). No evidence of improvement after 1 week should suggest failure of the chest tube.

28. Can any surgical maneuver decrease the recurrence rate of 2 to 3%?

Yes, pleurectomy. This is a true controversy. Advocates claim nearly 0% recurrence if parietal pleura, particularly apical, is removed, whereas critics cite increased incidence of postoperative bleeding relative to pleurodesis (> 5% : 2-3%) and difficulty reentering chest if subsequent thoracotomy becomes necessary.

29. Does a postresectional "space" pneumothorax require obliterative treatment (usually thoracoplasty)?

Not usually. Currently most surgeons will observe a patient with a "space problem" after resection (remaining lung does not fill the pleural cavity), provided there is no evidence of infection, as it has increasingly been recognized that they are usually well tolerated and often resolve with time. Historically, however, a persistent post-resectional space, especially following tuberculosis surgery, was obliterated by thoracoplasty to avoid the highly morbid tuberculous empyema that occasionally resulted from empty apical "spaces." As noted, the trend is nonoperative now when infection is absent.

A related issue involves phrenic nerve "crush" or "pinch" at the time of lobectomy, trading decreased pulmonary function for obliteration of the apical space by elevation of the diaphragm and immobility. Currently, most surgeons preserve all ventilatory function possible and thus spare the phrenic nerve.

BIBLIOGRAPHY

1. Adkins, P.C., and Smyth, P.C.: Bilateral simultaneous spontaneous pneumothorax. Dis. Chest, 37:702, 1960. A good description of cause and management of uncommon presentation of pneumothorax.
2. Baker, W. L., Faber, L.P., Ostermiller, W.E., and Langston, H.T.: Management of persistent bronchopleural fistulas. J. Thorac. Cardiovasc. Surg., 62:393, 1971. Impressive experience of large thoracic surgery practice, which describes method of closing postresectional fistulas with muscular flaps.
3. Bernstein, A., Wagaroddin, M., and Shah, M.: Management of spontaneous pneumothorax using a Heimlich flutter valve. Thorax, 28:386, 1973. Describes use of one-way flutter valve attached to chest tube, allowing patient ambulation and avoiding problems with collection apparatus.
4. Burks, J.W.: Open thoracotomy in the management of spontaneous pneumothorax. Ann. Surg., 177:798, 1973. Review of indications and timing of operative intervention for pneumothorax.

5. Cattoneo, S.M., Sirak, H.D., and Lassen, K.P.: Recurrent spontaneous pneumothorax in the high-risk patient. J. Thorac. Cardiovasc. Surg., 66:467, 1973. Series that emphasizes higher mortality in certain risk groups, and use of intrapleural administration of quinacrine to achieve pleurodesis.

6. DeVries, W.C., and Wolfe, W.A.: The management of spontaneous pneumothorax and emphysema. Surg. Clin. North Am., 60:851, 1980. Good review article, with comparative discussion of emphysema and giant bullae.

7. DesLauriers, J., Beaulicu, M., Despres, J.P., et al.: Transaxillary pleurectomy for treatment of spontaneous pneumothorax. Ann. Thorac. Surg., 30:569, 1980. Description of technique and results of pleurectomy, with subsequent discussion debating pros and cons.

8. Lavrier, A.M., Tyers, F.O., Williams, G.H., et al.: Intrapleural instillation of quinacrine for treatment of recurrent spontaneous pneumothorax. Ann. Thorac. Surg., 28:146, 1979.   Describes technique and results of nonoperative method of obtaining pleurodesis.

9. Luck, S.R., Raffensperger, J.G., Sullivan, H.J., and Givson, L.E.: Management of pneumothorax in children with chronic pulmonary disease. J. Thorac Cardiovasc. Surg., 74:834, 1977. Describes severity of pneumothorax in cystic fibrosis, and frequent requirement of operative intervention.

10. Munin, P., and Vert, P.: Pneumothorax. Clin. Perinatol., 5:335, 1978. Good review article of special considerations: neonatal pneumothorax.

11. West, J.B.: Distribution of mechanical stress in the lung: A possible factor in localization of pulmonary disease. Lancet, 1:839, 1971. Uses study of intrapleural pressure in dogs to explain occurrence of blebs at apices.

---

76. EMPYEMA
MICHAEL JOHNSTON, M.D.

---

1. **What is an empyema?**
An infection in the pleural space.

2. **What is the most common cause of empyema?**
Pneumonia in approximately 75% of patients.

3. **What criteria have been used to differentiate an empyema from a pleural effusion?**
Bacteria seen on Gram stain, positive culture, turbid fluid, and a pH less than 7.2.

4. **The *sine qua non* in treating an empyema is to ensure proper drainage of the infected pleural space.   What constitutes effective drainage?**
This mainly depends on the characteristics of the empyema fluid, although the age of the patient, the causative organism, and the toxicity of the patient must all be considered.   In general, thoracentesis may be adequate if the fluid is serous. Insertion of a chest tube is required when fluid is thick and purulent. If the fluid is loculated or if a chronic empyema with lung entrapment is present, a decortication is often necessary.

5. **The main surgical principles espoused in treating closed space infections are proper drainage and obliteration of the cavity.   How is the infected empyema space managed in the rigid confines of the thoracic cavity?**

The preferred means of obliterating a well-drained empyema cavity is by reexpansion of the collapsed lung. If this is impossible either because the lung has been destroyed or surigically removed, collapse of the chest (thoracoplasty) may be indicated.

6. **Postpneumonectomy empyema represents a most difficult management problem, because of the large cavity involved. What are the steps in the present day management of this infection?**
    (1) If the patient is toxic on presentation, immediate chest tube insertion. (2) After the patient is stabilized or in a patient who is stable on presentation, rib resection and open, dependent drainage of the cavity (Eloesser flap procedure). (3) Daily irrigation of the cavity with a mild antiseptic solution for 3 to 6 months. (4) Surgical closure of the chest wall opening after filling the cavity with an appropriate antibiotic solution. This management of postpneumonectomy empyema is referred to as the Clagget technique and is successful in 40 to 60% of the patients.

7. **Under what two conditions should an empyema not be surgically drained?**
    Pure tuberculous empyema and poststaphylococcal pneumonia empyema in children.

BIBLIOGRAPHY

1. Clagett, O.T., and Gelaci, J.E.: A procedure for the management of postpneumonectomy empyema. J. Thorac. Cardiovasc. Surg., 45:141, 1963.
2. DeMeester, T.R.: The pleura. In Sabiston, D.C., and Spencer, R.C. (eds.): Gibbon's Surgery of the Chest, 4th ed. Philadelphia, W.B. Saunders Co., 1983.
3. Samson, P.C.: Empyema thoracis. Ann. Thorac. Surg., 112:210, 1971.

77. LUNG CANCER
MICHAEL JOHNSTON, M.D.

1. **How do patients with lung cancer present?**
    Eighty percent have primary lung symptoms (cough, 25%; hemoptysis, 30%, and dyspnea, 11%). Fifteen percent are asymptomatic and have a mass discovered in the lung on routine chest x-ray. The rest have symptoms related to regional or systemic disease.

2. **Describe the "typical" lung cancer patient on presentation.**
    The patient is a male in his late 50's or early 60's with a long history of cigarette smoking. He is thin, barrel-chested, and has a chronic "smoker's" cough which recently has become more productive and possibly with a small amount of blood. He may have lost weight recently and his appetite has decreased. He also may have noticed a recent decrease in exercise tolerance.

3. **How extensive is the disease at diagnosis?**
    Fifty percent have metastatic spread (bloodstream) of lung cancer. The rest are about equally divided between patients with regional spread of cancer and those with cancer localized to the primary site.

4. **What are the major WHO histologic cell types and their approximate incidence in the United States?**
    Epidermoid or squamous carcinoma, 35%; adenocarcinoma, 35%; small cell carcinoma, 20%; and large cell carcinoma, 10%.

5. **In a patient in whom lung cancer is strongly suspected based on history, physical examination, and chest x-ray, what are the next steps in management?**
    Noninvasive and invasive staging procedures to determine the extent of metastatic, regional nodal, and primary tumor involvement.

6. **What constitutes an "adequate" metastatic work-up of a patient with a diagnosis of non-small cell lung cancer?**
    History, physical examination, liver function tests, and alkaline phosphatase and serum calcium levels. Further specific studies such as CT scan, nuclear medicine scans, etc., are necessary only if specific organic abnormalities are found on the initial screening. Routinely performing further x-ray and nuclear medicine studies indiscriminately on all patients with lung cancer cannot be justified.

7. **Why is a distinction made between small cell lung cancer and non-small cell lung cancer?**
    The biology and natural history of the non-small cell lung cancers (squamous, adeno, and large cell carcinomas) are similar. Between 30 and 60% of patients will have local or regional disease on presentation. These tumors usually metastasize to regional lymph nodes within the mediastinum before spreading systemically, and all of these cell types are uniformly resistant to chemotherapy. In contrast, nearly 100% of patients with small cell lung cancer have distant metastases on diagnosis. Recently, however, small cell cancer has been found to be sensitive to a number of chemotherapeutic agents. Long-term results now show a significant favorable impact on survival when chemotherapy is used in the treatment of this disease.

8. **Cure rate after lung resection for non-small cell lung cancer is directly related to the size of the surgical resection (i.e., cure after pneumonectomy is greater than after lobectomy). True or false?**
    False. Incidence or cure and local recurrence are based on whether all surgical resection margins are clear of tumor and the status of the nodal metastases. The magnitude of the surgical resection should be based only on the size and location of the primary cancer.

9. **In determining if the patient is a candidate for surgical resection, the status of the mediastinal lymph nodes is of prime importance. What methods are available to evaluate this critical area?**
    Noninvasive studies include chest x-ray, chest CT scan, and gallium scanning. The CT scan is the most sensitive and specific of these and accurately reflects the status of the mediastinal nodes in up to 80% of patients. Since size alone is the determinant of metastatic involvement, microscopic metastases will be reflected as a false-negative result whereas large inflammatory nodes will result in a false-positive. Surgical staging by either mediastinoscopy or mediastinotomy will give histologic confirmation of nodal status by direct biopsy. There is an 80 to 95% accuracy, less than 3% morbidity, and approximately 30% of the patients will be spared a thoracotomy. Patients with small peripheral lung cancers probably do not require surgical staging if the mediastinum is normal on chest x-ray since the yield is very low.

10. How is mediastinoscopy performed and which nodal groups are accessible for biopsy?

Through a small suprasternal incision, the pretracheal space is developed and followed into the middle mediastinum. Hilar, paratracheal, and subcarinal lymph nodes can routinely be visualized and biopsied.

11. Other than its use as a surgical adjuvant, what roles does radiation therapy play in the management of patients with lung cancer?

Radiation therapy is often used to control the primary tumor in patients with small cell lung cancer along with combination chemotherapy. It also is very beneficial for palliation in patients with locally advanced lung cancer who develop bronchial obstruction, hemoptysis, pain from chest wall invasion, or the superior vena caval syndrome.

12. With lung cancer now being the most common malignant disease, are screening tests available that might be useful in detecting early tumors?

No. In three large mass screening studies in which high-risk groups, mostly middle-aged male smokers, underwent periodic chest x-rays, sputum cytologies, or both, the number of new lung cancers found was too small to make the screening economically feasible. However, a high percentage of the cancers discovered were of an earlier, more curable stage than what is normally seen.

CONTROVERSIES

13. When are patients with non-small cell lung cancer and nodal metastases considered as candidates for surgical resection if there are no signs of distant metastases?

The standard of practice in most communities is that patients with positive hilar nodes (N-1) are still surgically resectable whereas those with mediastinal node metastases (N-2) are unresectable for cure. Several uncontrolled studies (Kirsh, Naruke, Pearson, and Martini) report up to 35% 5-year survival rates in highly selected patients with N-2 disease. These patients usually have nodal metastases only in the low, ipsilateral, paratracheal nodes or in the subaortic nodes when the primary lesion is in the left upper lobe.

14. What adjuvant therapy has proved efficacious after surgical resection of non-small cell lung cancer and for which types of tumor should it be given?

Most studies show no proven efficacy for any type of adjuvant therapy in stage I or stage II disease. Postoperative radiation therapy has been advocated by some in patients with resected N-2 disease, especially those with squamous cell carcinomas. Many clinicians would disagree with these studies and as yet there are no published, well-controlled clinicial trials to substantiate this claim. In patients with lung cancers invading chest wall, especially in the superior sulcus (Pancoast tumor), preoperative radiation therapy may offer some advantage. Neither chemotherapy or immunotherapy has been shown to be effective adjuvants.

BIBLIOGRAPHY

1.   Firmin, R.K., Azariades, M., Lennox, S.C., et al.: Sleeve lobectomy (lobectomy and bronchoplasty) for bronchial carcinoma. Ann. Thorac. Surg., 35:442, 1983.
2.   Friedman, P.J., Feigin, D.S., Liston, S.E., et al.: Sensitivity of chest radiography, computed tomography, and gallium scanning to metastasis of lung carcinoma. Cancer, 54:1302, 1984.

3.   Minna, J.D., Higgins, G.A., and Glatstein, E.J.: Cancer of the lung. In DeVita, V.T., Hellman, S., and Rosenberg, S.A. (eds): Cancer: Principles and Practice of Oncology. Philadelphia, J.B. Lippincott, 1978.

4.   Naruke, T., Suemasu, K., and Ishikawa, S.: Lymph node mapping and curability at various levels of metastasis in resected lung cancer. J. Thorac. Cardiovasc. Surg., 70:832, 1978.

5.   Paulson, D.L.: Carcinomas in the superior pulmonary sulcus. J. Thorac. Cardiovasc. Surg., 70:1095, 1975.

6.   Pearson, F.G., DeLarue, N.C., Ilves, R., et al.: Significance of positive superior mediastinal nodes identified at mediastinoscopy in patients with resectable cancer of the lung. J. Thorac. Cardiovasc. Surg., 83:1, 1982.

7.   Pearson, F.G., Nelems, J.M., Henderson, R.D., and DeLarue, N.C.: The role of mediastinoscopy in the selection of treatment for bronchial carcinoma with involvement of superior mediastinal lymph nodes. J. Thorac. Cardiovasc. Surg., 64:382, 1972.

8.   Pilch, Y.H., Rigler, L.G., and Selecky, P.: Current and future concepts of lung cancer. Ann. Intern. Med., 834:93, 1975.

78. SOLITARY PULMONARY NODULE
MICHAEL JOHNSTON, M.D.

1.   What is meant by a "solitary pulmonary nodule"?
An asymptomatic, usually spherical lung mass located in the periphery of the lung. It is invariably discovered on a chest x-ray obtained for other reasons and shows no radiographic evidence of extension outside the lung, nor are there concomitant hilar or mediastinal abnormalities noted on the chest x-ray.

2.   What is the chance of a solitary pulmonary nodule being malignant?
In a patient under 40 with no known previous malignancies, it is very rare. In patients over 50 with no previously known lung nodules, the change of the solitary pulmonary nodule representing a primary cancer is approximately equal to the patient's age.

3.   How is an undiagnosed solitary pulmonary nodule approached surgically?
The lesion is first wedge-resected, usually using one of the automatic stapling devices through a limited posterolateral thoracotomy. The nodule is then sent for immediate frozen section diagnosis. If benign, no further resection is indicated; however, if the mass is malignant and thought to be of primary lung origin, a lobectomy with hilar and mediastinal node sampling or dissection is usually performed.

4.   What is the expected survival rate following resection of a malignant solitary pulmonary nodule?
If the tumor is a primary, non-small cell lung cancer and is smaller than 3 cm in diameter with no evidence of nodal metastases, survival is between 60 and 80% at 5 years. In patients with either hilar (N-1) nodal metastases or primary lesions greater than 3 cm in diameter (T-2), 5-year survival decreases to between 40 and 60%.

5. It is often difficult to distinguish histologically between a primary and a metastatic lesion of the lung when a resected solitary pulmonary nodule is found to be an adenocarcinoma. How extensive should the postoperative work-up be in an effort to discover an occult primary adenocarcinoma somewhere else in the body?
Stool guaiac and a urinalysis.

CONTROVERSY

6. Should an attempt be made to obtain a tissue diagnosis prior to surgical resection of a solitary pulmonary lung nodule?
Most clinicians would agree that fiberoptic bronchoscopy with transbronchial biopsy under fluoroscopic control should be attempted on all lesions that can be visualized under fluoroscopy. If this does not provide a histologic diagnosis, many clinicians would attempt a percutaneous aspiration needle biopsy of the lesion. If the nodule is malignant, the chance of a positive cytologic diagnosis with the aspiration needle biopsy is very good, approximately 80%. However, in 20 to 30% of patients who undergo needle aspiration biopsies, adequate tissue for diagnosis will not be obtained. In those two groups, those with a positive diagnosis of malignant disease and those with inadequate tissue obtained, the vast majority will be subjected to exploratory thoracotomy. In the best series in the literature the diagnosis by aspiration needle biopsy of a benign lesion will be wrong in approximately 15 to 20% of patients.

BIBLIOGRAPHY

1. Higgins, G.A., Shields, T.W., and Keehn, R.J.: The solitary pulmonary nodule. Arch. Surg., 110:570, 1975.
2. Martini, N., and Beattie, E.J.: Results of surgical treatment in stage I lung cancer. J. Thorac. Cardiovasc. Surg., 74:499, 1977.
3. Ray, J.F., Lawton, B.R., Magnin, G.E., et al.: The coin lesion story: Update 1976. Chest, 70:332, 1976.

---

79. DISSECTING AORTIC ANEURYSM
DAVID CAMPBELL, M.D.

---

1. Why is the term "dissecting aortic aneurysm" really incorrect in the acute dissection?
The correct term should be dissecting aortic hematoma since the lesion is not an aneurysm at all but rather a dissection of blood between the middle and outer layers of the media of the aorta.

2. How is the diagnosis made?
An index of suspicion is the most important factor since there is no one common feature among patients presently with aortic dissections. In any patient who presents with severe "knife-like ripping" chest and back pain, the diagnosis of aortic aneurysm should be considered.

3. Once the diagnosis is entertained, how should the patient be managed?

Besides aortic dissection, the other diagnosis to be strongly considered is acute myocardial infarction in a patient who presents with severe chest and back pain. Therefore, the patient should be placed in an intensive care unit, monitored closely, and stabilized. Two thirds of patients may be hypertensive and blood pressure must be controlled. An electrocardiogram will often rule out an infarction but not always since some aortic dissections can tear off a coronary artery and thus have acute infarction as part of the process.

4.   What is the most significant diagnostic clue?
The presence of a new aortic diastolic murmur, indicating aortic regurgitation. Neurologic findings including paraplegia and hemiplegia may be present as well. Hypertension is also common as well as differential blood pressures in the four extremities owing to the measurement of blood flow from the dissecting hematoma encircling the blood vessel and constricting it or from actually cleaning off the takeoff of the subclavian or femoral vessels.

5.   What chest x-ray findings are helpful in diagnosis?
Widened mediastinum and loss of aortic knob silhouette.

6.   How is the diagnosis confirmed?
As soon as posible after stabilization, an aortogram should be obtained to confirm the diagnosis, the type of dissection (the location of the intimal tear), and the extent of immobility of the major branches of the aorta.

7.   What are the types of dissection?
Type A: involves ascending aorta and/or the descending aorta. Type B: involves only the descending aorta.

8.   Why is the type of dissection important?
Type A, or ascending, dissections (i.e., those involving the ascending aorta, though the tear may be anywhere in the aorta) should usually undergo *early* surgical correction. Type B, or descending, dissections (no involvement of the ascending aorta) may be managed medically or surgically (see Controversies).

9.   What is the key to   medical management?
The blood pressure should be lowered to the 100 to 110 mm Hg range (diastolic) using a combination of sodium nitroprusside and propranolol. Propranolol is particularly important since it decreases the contractility of the myocardium (DP/DT), thereby decreasing the shearing force and preventing propagation of the dissection down the aorta.

10.   Can Arfonad be used instead of propranolol/nitroprusside?
No!

11.   What are the principles of surgical management?
        TYPE A:
        1.   To close off the hematoma by obliterating the false lumen both proximally and distally.
        2.   To restore competency to the aortic valve.
        3.   To exclude the aortic tear.
        4.   To restore flow to any branches of the aorta which have been sheared off and receive blood flow from a false lumen.
        5.   To protect the heart during these maneuvers and possibly restore coronary blood flow if a coronary has been sheared off.

Technique: This is done with cardiopulmonary bypass, moderate hypothermia, and potassium cardioplegia to protect the heart, and usually a Dacron interposition graft in the ascending aorta. Whether to replace the aortic valve or repair it is controversial.

TYPE B:

1. To close off the hematoma by obliterating the false lumen both proximally and distally.

2. To restore blood flow to branches of the aorta fed by the false channel.

Technique: Can be done using partial cardiopulmonary bypass, Gott shunt, or the Crawford technique, in which the aorta is cross clamped and the graft is sewn in as far as possible (see Controversies).

12. What are the operative complications?

1. Hemorrhage (10 to 20%). Very common because of the use of heparin and the poor quality of the aortas, which do not hold suture well.

2. Renal failure (21%).

3. Pulmonary insufficiency (30% higher in type B repair).

4. Paraplegia. Often present prior to operation. As a surgical complication, it usually occurs only with type B.

5. Acute myocardial infarction or low cardiac output (5 to 40%), chronic dissection repairs (6 to 20%).

6. Bowel infarction (5%).

7. Death (8 to 25%). Higher for acute than for chronic dissections. Higher for type A than type B.

13. Describe the Gott shunt.

A Gott shunt is a hollow plastic tube tapered at both ends; it has an internal coating of TDMA-C bound with heparin, which allows blood to flow through the shunt without clotting. One end is placed in the aorta proximal to the aneurysm and the other is placed distal to the aneurysm. This allows removal or repair of the aneurysm without interrupting the flow of blood beyond the aneurysm.

14. What are the long-term results?

Of those who survive operation, two thirds will be dead in 7 years due to cardiac and cerebral causes.

CONTROVERSIES

15. Surgical or medical management of type B dissections?

Type B–Initial Surgical Management: For:

1. Approximately 25% of these patients initially treated medically need an operation eventually.

2. Operative mortality is much less today (20%) than in the past.

3. Medical managment has the same in-hospital mortality (20%).

Type B–Initial Medical Management: For:

1. Avoids unnecessary operation and its attendant cost and complication rate.

16. Management of aortic insufficiency in type A dissections.

Replace Aortic Valve:

1. Easy (valved conduits now available).

2. Eliminates aortic insufficiency completely.

3. Should always be done in patients with Marfan's syndrome.

Repair Aortic Valve:
    1. With construction, when done correctly, need to replace the valve at a later time is 5 to 10% in some series.
    2. Avoids need for anticoagulation, which is necessary when a mechanical valve is used to replace the aortic valve.

17. Repair of type B dissections.

Partial femoro-femoral or aortofemoral bypass: For:
    1. Allows unloading of the heart.
    2. Allows distal perfusion to avoid ischemia.
    3. Allows as much time as is needed to complete anastomosis.
Against: requires heparinization.

Gott shunt: For:
    1. Allows unloading of the heart.
    2. Allows distal perfusion to avoid ischemia.
    3. Does not require heparinization.
    4. Allows as much time as is needed to accomplish the anastomosis.
Against: can injure the aorta in placement.

Simple aortic cross clamping: For:
    Fast.
Against: Placement of the graft has to be done in less than 30 minutes or the complication rate, particularly paraplegia, increases significantly.

BIBLIOGRAPHY

1.   Appelbaum, A., Karp, R. B., and Kirklin, J.W.: Ascending vs. descending aortic dissections. Ann. Surg., 183:296, 1976.

2.   Attar, S., Fardin, R., Ayella, R., and McLaughlin, J.S.: Medical versus surgical treatment of acute dissecting aneurysm. Arch. Surg., 103:568, 1971.

3.   Collins, J.J., and Cohn, L.H.: Reconstruction of the aortic valve. Correcting valve incompetence due to acute dissecting aneurysm. Arch. Surg., 106:35, 1973.

4.   Crawford, E.S., Palamara, A.E., Saleh, S.A., and Roehm, J.O. F., Jr.: Aortic aneurysm: Current status of surgical treatment. Surg. Clin. North Am., 59:597, 1979.

5.   Daily, P.O., Trueblood, H.W., Stinson, E.B., et al.: Management of acute aortic dissections. Ann. Thorac. Surg., 10:237, 1970.

6.   Doroghazi, R.M., Slater, E.E., and DeSanctis, R.W.: Medical therapy for aortic dissections. J. Cardiovasc. Med., 6:187, 198l.

7.   Griepp, R.B., Stinson, E.B., Hollingsworth, J.F., and Buehler, D.: Prosthetic replacement of the aortic arch. J. Thorac. Cardiovasc. Surg., 70:1051, 1975.

8.   Hirst, A.E., Jr., Johns, V.J., Jr., and Kime, S.W., Jr.: Dissecting aneurysm of the aorta: A review of 505 cases. Medicine, 37:217, 1958.

9.   Hunter, J.A., Dye, W.S., Javid, H., et al.: Abdominal aortic resection in thoracic dissection. Arch. Surg., 111:1258, 1976.

10.   Kolff, J., Bates, R.J., Balderman, S.C., et al.: Acute aortic arch dissection: Reevaluation of the indications for medical and surgical therapy. Am. J. Cardiol., 39:727, 1977.

11.   Kouchoukos, N T., Karp, R.B., Blackstone, E.H., et al.: Replacement of the ascending aorta and aortic valve with a composite graft: Results in 86 patients. Ann. Surg., 192:403, 1980.

12.   Meng, R.L., Najafi, H., Javid, H. et al.: Acute ascending aortic dissection–surgical management. Circulation, 64(Suppl. 2):23l, 1981.

13.   Miller, D.C., Stinson, E.B., Oyer, P.E., et al.: Operative treatment of aortic dissections. Experience with 125 patients over a sixteen-year period. J. Thorac. Cardiovasc. Surg., 78:365, 1979.

14.   Najafi, H.: Aneurysm of the cystic medionectrotic aortic root–a modified surgical approach. J. Thorac. Cardiovasc. Surg., 66:71, 1973.

15. Najafi, H., Dye, W.S., Javid, H., et al.: Acute aortic regurgitation secondary to aortic dissection: Surgical management without valve replacement. Ann. Thorac. Surg., 14:474, 1972.

16. Najafi, H., Dye, W.S., Javid, H., et al.: Aortic insufficiency secondary to aortic root aneurysm and/or dissection. Arch. Surg., 110:1401, 1975.

17. Prokop, E.K., Wheat, M.W., Jr., and Palmer, R.F.: Hydrodynamic forces in dissecting aneurysms. Circ. Res., 27:131, 1970.

18. Reul, G. J., Jr., Cooley, D.A., Hallman, G. H., et al.: Dissecting aneurysm of the descending aorta. Improved surgical results in 91 patients. Arch. Surg., 110:632, 1975.

19. Rosenberg, H.L., and Mulder, D.G.: Dissecting thoracic aneurysms. Arch. Surg., 105:19, 1972.

20. Weldon, C.S., Connors, J.P., and Martz, M.N.: Use of saphenous vein to extend and relocate coronary arteries: Clinical experience during extensive reconstructive operations of the aortic root. Arch. Surg., 114:1330, 1979.

21. Wheat, M.W., Jr.: Treatment of dissecting aneurysms of the aorta. Current status. Prog. Cardiovasc. Dis., 16:87, 1973.

22. Wheat, M.W., Jr., and Shumacker, H.B., Jr.: Dissecting aneurysm. Problems of management. Chest, 70:650, 1976.

23. Wheat, M.W., Jr., Palmer, R.F., Bartley, T.B., and Seelman, R. C.: Treatment of dissecting aneurysms of the aorta without surgery. J. Thorac. Cardiovasc. Surg., 50:364, 1965.

24. Wolfe, W.G., and Moran, J.F.: The evolution of medical and surgical management of acute aortic dissection. (Editorial.) Circulation, 56:503, 1977.

25. Wolfe, W.G.: Acute ascending aortic dissection. Ann. Surg., 192:658, 1980.

80. HYPERTROPHIC PYLORIC STENOSIS
FRITZ M. KARRER, M.D.

1. What is the incidence of hypertrophic pyloric stenosis?
It occurs from 1 to 300 to 1 in 900 births. Males outnumber females 4 to 1. It has been said to occur more often in firstborns but this has been questioned. A definite familial tendency is seen.

2. What is the typical presentation?
Most are healthy infants who initially feed normally. Vomiting begins, at first occasionally, but then progresses to projectile vomiting following each feeding. The emesis is always nonbilious but may contain some blood or "coffee-grounds" owing to esophagitis. After vomiting, the baby is again hungry and will refeed immediately. Over time, dehydration and malnutrition worsen. Not infrequently, the infant's formula has been changed from one to another during this period.

3. What are the physical findings?
These infants are dehydrated to varying degrees. The abdomen is not distended but occasionally gastric peristalsis can be seen through the abdominal wall. The pyloric tumor or "olive" is palpable in 75 to 90% of cases depending on the persistence of the examiner. Ten percent have inguinal hernias and 2 to 8% have mild icterus.

4. How is the diagnosis made?

In the majority, the "olive" is palpable on physical examination. This, in combination with a suggestive history, is sufficient to make the diagnosis. If doubt exists, ultrasonography in experienced hands is highly accurate in confirming the presence of a pyloric tumor. A barium examination is also diagnostic when typical findings of a "string" sign, the "shoulder" sign, or "pyloric tit" are seen.

5. **What electrolyte abnormalities are likely to be encountered?**
Findings of hyopkalemic hypochloremic metabolic alkalosis are classic for pyloric obstruction. Adequate fluid resuscitation with one half normal saline and added potassium is essential *preoperatively*.

6. **What procedure is recommended for hypertrophic pyloric stenosis?**
The Fredet-Ramstedt pyloromyotomy is accepted as the procedure of choice. Medical management, although effective in some patients, has a higher failure rate and requires longer hospitalization than surgical therapy. For the pyloromyotomy, we prefer a transverse incision over the right rectus. The pylorus is delivered and a superficial incision made longitudinally over the pylorus in an avascular area. The muscle fibers are carefully split down to the mucosa. The mucosa can then be seen to bulge up through the myotomy from the duodenum to the stomach. The duodenum should be milked toward the pylorus and inspected for any leak.

7. **What should be done if a leak is identified?**
If the duodenum has been violated, usually the mucosa can be closed with a few fine sutures. If the myotomy has been compromised by this closure, it should be sutured closed and a second myotomy made parallel to, but 90 degrees away from, the original.

8. **When and how can feedings be started postoperatively?**
Gastric ileus persists for 12 to 18 hours after the procedure, but usually feedings of 5% dextrose and water or electrolyte solutions are tolerated within 6 to 8 hours postoperatively. These should be given as frequent, small amounts (15 to 30 ml every 2 hours). The amount and strength of formula can be gradually advanced over the next 24 hours. Small amounts of vomiting are not unusual and should not cause alarm unless persistent. In any case, reoperation should not be considered for at least 2 weeks.

BIBLIOGRAPHY

1. Benson, C.D., and Hight, D.W.: Stomach and duodenum. In Welch, K.G. (ed.): Complications in Pediatric Surgery: Prevention and Management. Philadelphia, W. B. Saunders, 1982. The section on hypertrophic pyloric stenosis describes all of the potential pitfalls and complications, their prevention and management.
2. Blumhagen, J.D., and Noble, H.G.S.: Muscle thickness in hypertrophic pyloric stenosis: Sonographic determination. A.J.R., 140:2211, 1983. Eighty-six of 93 patients with pyloric stenosis were diagnosed by abdominal sonograms. The diagnosis was based on a muscle wall thickness of 4 mm or greater. This resulted in a 8% false-negative rate and no false positives.
3. Day, L.R.: Medical management of pyloric stenosis. J.A.M.A., 207:948, 1969. Eleven of sixteen patients responded to a medical regimen of fasting and gastric lavage, followed by administration of scopolamine and slow advancement of oral feedings requiring an average of 9 days of hospitalization. The results of surgical therapy are far superior, making this article of historical interest only.

4.   Pollock, W.F., and Norris, W.J.: Dr. Conrad Ramstedt and pyloromyotomy. Surgery, 42:966, 1957. Ramstedt's reflections on his original case of pyloric stenosis and the development of the technique which bears his name is included in this extremely interesting historical article.

5.   Redo, S.F.: Pyloric obstruction. In Principles of Surgery in the First Six Months of Life. Hagerstown, Maryland, Harper and Row, 1976. Excellent review of the presentation, diagnosis, management, and complications of pyloric stenosis.

6.   Spicer, R.D.: Infantile hypertrophic pyloric stenosis: A review. Br. J. Surg., 69:128, 1982. Very complete summary of the history, epidemiology, presentation and management of hypertrophic pyloric stenosis. The re-examination of the various etiologic theories is particularly thorough.

7.   Spitz, L., and Batcup, G.: Hematemesis in infantile hypertrophic pyloric stenosis: The source of the bleeding. Br. J. Surg., 66:827, 1979. Gastritis, long held as the source of bleeding in hypertrophic pyloric stenosis, was not found in any of 13 patients endoscoped in this series. Significant esophagitis was seen in all 13.

8.   Wooley, M.M., Felsher, B.F., Asch, M.J., et al.: Jaundice, hypertrophic pyloric stenosis, and glucuronyl transferase. J. Pediatr. Surg., 9:359, 1974. The authors found 32 of 396 patients (8.1%) with pyloric stenosis to have clinical jaundice (serum bilirubin > 2 mg/dl). Investigation of 5 such infants revealed reduced glucuronyl transferase activity. Hyperbilirubinemia cleared in all following pyloromyotomy.

81. NEONATAL INTESTINAL OBSTRUCTION
LUIS A. MARTINEZ-FRONTANILLA, M.D., and
ALEJANDRO M. HERNANDEZ-CANO, M.D.

1.   Which are the common types of neonatal bowel obstruction?
     1.   Atresia at any level from duodenum to rectum. Rare at the large bowel level.
     2.   Obstructions of the duodenum related to intestinal malrotation and/or abnormal fixation (midgut volvulus or Ladd's bands).
     3.   Ileal obstruction due to meconium ileus.
     4.   Obstruction at the level of the colon due to Hirschsprung's disease, small left colon syndrome, or meconium plug syndrome.
     5.   Obstruction at the anorectal level due to congenital atresia (imperforate anus).
     6.   Congenital intraabdominal bands, neonatal intussusception, and obstructions related to Meckel's diverticulum are much less common.

2.   Do all atresias of the alimentary canal share a common etiology?
No. Probably there are different entities. Anorectal and esophageal atresia may have a similar background. They may be part of a broad constellation of abnormalities (VACTER syndrome). Duodenal atresias may be related to Down's syndrome. Some jejunoileal atresias result from an acquired form of in utero mesenteric artery occlusion or other vascular accidents. These are rarely associated with other syndromes or anomalies; exceptions to these are the association with cystic fibrosis in 10% of cases of jejunoileal atresia, and the family occurrence of "apple peel" jejunal atresia.

3.   What is the clinical presentation of neonatal intestinal obstruction?
Vomiting, usually bilious, commonly in the first week of life. Depending on the level of obstruction: abdominal distention, obstipation, or failure to pass meconium.

4. **How is an infant with neonatal intestinal obstruction properly studied and diagnosed?**
    Careful physical examination including aspiration of the stomach with a nasogastric tube. Rectal examination. A two-way plain x-ray film of the abdomen. If the obstruction appears located at the duodenal or high jejunal level, a limited contrast study of the upper gastrointestinal tract should follow. If the obstruction appears to lie beyond the upper jejunum, a barium enema is probably indicated next. Gastrografin may be the appropriate contrast medium if meconium ileus is suspected (see Controversies).

5. **How are jejunoileal atresias classified?**
    1. Membrane or diaphragm type: There is interruption of the intestinal lumen which can also be partial. There is external continuity of the intestine.
    2. Cord type: A string of solid tissue is interposed between the atretic ends of the intestine.
    3. Gap type: Loss of tissue between the atretic ends. Multiplicity and combinations of these three types can occur in the same patient.
    4. "Apple peel" type: Described next.

6. **What is "apple peel" jejunal atresia?**
    A severe form of atresia with loss of significant length of intestine. Only a short segment of jejunum remains proximal to the atresia. The distal intestine, totally separated, is represented by the entire colon and a coiled segment of terminal ileum, the vascular supply of which is a marginal artery derived from the middle colic artery. These infants have a worse prognosis than infants with the other varieties of jejunal atresia. Familial incidence and association with other malformations have been reported.

7. **How is intestinal malrotation diagnosed?**
    By the demonstration on a contrast x-ray film of the gastrointestinal tract of an abnormal position and configuration of the duodenum or the cecum (barium enema or upper gastrointestinal rays; see Controversies).

8. **What is meconium ileus and how is it diagnosed?**
    It is a neonatal gastrointestinal manifestation of cystic fibrosis. The meconium is extremely thick and plugs the ileum, producing an intraluminal obstruction. The diagnosis is made with a contrast study of the lower gastrointestinal tract or intraoperatively.

9. **Is the sweat test useful in the diagnosis of meconium ileus?**
    Only retrospectively, since the test is inaccurate in the neonatal period when this disease manifests.

10. **What is the treatment for neonatal intestinal obstructions?**
    For the majority, the treatment is surgical (either bypass or removal of the obstruction). Some cases of meconium ileus resolve with the administration of Gastrografin enema, and most cases of small left colon syndrome and meconium plug syndrome resolve spontaneously.

11. **What are the surgical options?**
    1. Duodenojejunal anastomosis bypassing or resecting a duodenal atresia.
    2. For jejunoileal atresia: "End-to-back" anastomosis. Frequently requires resection of a proximal segment (see Controversies).

3. For meconium ileus: Evacuation of the inspissated meconium through an opening in the ileum. Further treatment of the intestine is described under Controversies.

4. For malrotation-related obstructions: Detorsion of the midgut volvulus, if present, followed by division of all adhesions and bands between the cecum and over the duodenum (Ladd's bands).

5. For Hirschsprung's disease and imperforate anus: See corresponding chapters.

12. **What are possible complications of operations to correct intestinal obstruction in the neonate?**
The stretched out and dilated intestine proximal to an atresia may fail to provide peristaltic function after the anastomosis, frequently requiring reoperation with either resection or enteroplasty to reduce the diameter of the intestine. Short-gut syndrome and anastomotic leak are also possible complications.

CONTROVERSIES

13. **Are contrast studies of the gastrointestinal tract necessary, or are plain films sufficient to make the diagnosis?**
On many occasions plain x-ray films of the abdomen may give a high suspicion of a diagnosis, particularly in duodenal atresia. This, added to the small risk that a contrast study may represent for the infant, weighs in favor of avoiding contrast studies. However, a barium enema or upper gastrointestinal radiographic study done by a radiologist familiar with neonates may provide useful information such as malrotation, Hirschsprung's disease (and level of transition); meconium ileus, or transient colonic obstructions. Some of these may respond to medical treatment or dictate different surgical approaches or priorities.

14. **Upper versus lower gastrointestinal x-ray films for the diagnosis of malrotation.**
Traditionally a barium enema had been the x-ray of choice to show the malposition of the cecum. However, this can be challenged, since occasional malrotation of the midgut with volvulus can occur with a normally rotated cecum. An upper gastrointestinal study may have also the advantage of showing other possible causes of upper intestinal obstruction.

15. **Primary versus deferred anastomosis for jejunoileal atresia.**
Frequently the dilated proximal loop of jejunum leading to the atresia has a very impaired peristaltic action. This has been the reason why diverting the intestinal flow as cutaneous enterostomies has been used as a temporizing method of treatment. However, employing the techniques of resection of the dilated intestine or plication to reduce its diameter with primary anastomosis has been shown to overcome this problem.

16. **Primary anastomosis versus some form of cutaneous enterostomy for meconium ileus.**
Although primary anastomosis after evacuation of the thick obstructing meconium has been used by some authors, most pediatric surgeons favor some type of enterostomy. These vary from a Bishop-Coop (end-to-side) chimney, to the Santulli (side-to-end) chimney, or a Mickulicz enterostomy. There are minor variations in the end result, and the controversy is merely a matter of personal preference.

BIBLIOGRAPHY

1. Benson, C.D., Loyd, J.R., and Smith, J.D.: Resection and primary anastomosis in the mangagement of stenosis and atresia of the jejunum and ileum. Pediatrics, 26:265, 1960.
2. deLorimer, A.A., Fonkalsrud, E.W., and Hays, D. M.: Congenital atresia and stenosis of the jejunum and ileum. Surgery, 65:819, 1969.
3. Grosfeld, J.L.: The small intestine. In Ravitch, M.M., Welch, K.J., Benson, C.B., et al.: (eds.): Pediatric Surgery, Vol. 2. Chicago, Year Book, 1979, p. 933.
4. Louw, J.H., and Barnard, C.N.: Congenital intestinal atresia: Observations on its orgin. Lancet, 2:1065, 1955.
5. Nixon, H.H.: Intestinal obstruction in the newborn. Arch. Dis. Child., 30:13, 1955.
6. Santulli, T.V., and Blanc, W.A.: Congenital atresia of the intestine: Pathogenesis and treatment. Ann. Surg, 154:939, 1961.
7. Simpson, A.J., Leonidas, J.C., Krasna, I.H., et al.: Roentgen diagnosis of midgut malrotation: Value of upper gastrointestinal radiographic study. J. Pediatr. Surg., 7:243, 1972.

82. TRACHEOESOPHAGEAL MALFORMATIONS
LUIS A. MARTINEZ-FRONTANILLA, M.D.

1. **Which are the common types of congenital tracheoesophageal malformations?**
Single or combined forms of esophageal atresia and tracheoesophageal fistula. The fistula may connect the trachea with one or either atretic ends of the esophagus.

2. **What are the possible combinations?**
Esophageal atresia without fistula.
Esophageal atresia with tracheoesophageal fistula to the proximal pouch of the esophagus.
Esophageal atresia with fistula to the distal pouch.
Esophageal atresia with two fistulas, one to each esophageal pouch.
Tracheoesophageal fistula without atresia, the so-called H type.

3. **What is the relative incidence of each variety?**
Very unequal. The most frequent one is the combination of esophageal atresia with tracheoesophageal fistula to the distal atretic pouch of the esophagus (85%).

4. **Are there other anomalies associated with tracheoesophageal fistulas?**
In over 30% of the cases there are associated anomalies of other organs and systems. The most frequent ones are cardiovascular malformations, followed by gastrointestinal ones consisting of imperforate anus and duodenal atresia.

5. **What is the VACTER syndrome?**
A "package" of multisystem malformations of which the esophageal ones are most important. VACTER is an acronym descriptive of the malformations: *Vertebral, Anorectal, Cardiac, TracheoEsophageal, Renal,* and limb (usually on the radial side of the upper extremity). Two or more of these varieties should be

present to constitute the syndrome. The importance of this syndrome is that the presence of one malformation can lead to the suspicion and investigation of others, which are possibly fatal if unrecognized.

6.   What is the clinical presentation?
Usually related to inability to swallow (in cases of atresia). Excess salivation: "mucousy baby." Episodes of coughing and cyanosis in the first 2 to 3 days of life. In cases of pure fistula the symptoms present later and resemble those of aspiration pneumonia.

7.   How is the diagnosis made?
Clinically. Most times the diagnosis is confirmed by the inability to pass a nasogastric tube beyond a distance of about 12 cm from the nose. This should be accompanied by a plain x-ray film of the entire baby ("Babygram").

8.   What information is obtained from a Babygram?
    The position of the nasogastric tube is observed.
    Vertebral and other skeletal anomalies are noted.
    Status of the lungs: pneumonia, lobar collapse, etc.
    Intestinal gas pattern: increased in cases of fistula and absent in atresia without a fistula to the distal pouch; typical "double-bubble" if associated with duodenal atresia; abnormal in more distally located intestinal atresia which may be associated.

9.   Is the use of x-rays with contrast material in the upper esophageal pouch indicated?
The use of air as contrast is safe and can be helpful. The use of liquid contrast (barium or Gastrografin) carries a high risk of aspiration and pneumonia. It should be reserved for cases of unclear diagnosis and it should be done under fluoroscopy using a very small amount of contrast material (less than l ml) (see Controversies).

10.   What is the treatment for these malformations?
The ultimate goal is to interrupt the fistula and to restore esophageal continuity. It varies for the different combinations.

11.   How is the most common variety (esophageal atresia with distal tracheoesophageal fistula) treated?
The definitive treatment consists of surgical division of the tracheoesophageal fistula and anastomosis of the atretic esophagus. This can be achieved in a primary or a staged fashion. The creation of a tube gastrostomy can be part of the treatment (see Controversies). Indications for staging are severe prematurity and/or pneumonia, deterioration during the initial stages of surgical treatment, and technical difficulties to approximate the ends of the esophagus. The stages consist of gastrostomy, ligature of the fistula via throacotomy, and esophageal anastomosis or replacement.

12.   Discuss the treatment of other varieties of esophageal atresia with tracheoesophageal fistula.
Atresia without fistula to the distal pouch or without fistula at all usually presents the difficulty of a long gap between the atretic ends of the esophagus. For these varieties the approach of delayed esophageal repair is used. A gastrostomy is created early in all of these infants. This is used for feedings. A period of observation and/or instrumental stretching of the atretic pouches of about 8 weeks follows. The esophageal gap is reevaluated radiographically. A thoracot-

omy can be then peformed and anastomosis attempted. If still unsuccessful, further treatment is delayed until the infant is approximately 1 year old, at which time the esophageal gap is bridged with a piece of colon or stomach (see Controversies).

13. **Which are the complications of these operations?**
Immediate: Anastomotic leak, empyema, and pneumothorax. Delayed: Esophageal stricture requiring most often dilatations and occasionally reoperation; food impaction can occur repeatedly at the level of the anastomosis; fistula recurrence; gastroesophageal reflux, which may require surgical treatment; cases in which interposition of other organs to replace the esophagus are required are more complicated.

14. **What are the results of the treatment of congenital esophageal atresia with tracheoesophageal fistula?**
The mortality can be heavily increased by two factors: prematurity and presence of major associated anomalies. In the absence of these factors, survival currently approaches 100%. In the long term, most patients require esophageal dilatations and some reoperation. These problems tend to disappear after the first few years of life.

CONTROVERSIES

15. **Use of contrast x-rays in the diagnosis of esophageal atresia.**
This procedure provides the most reliable confirmation of diagnosis, may demonstrate a proximal fistula, and may differentiate a traumatic pseudodiverticulum of the esophagus. Most pediatric surgeons, however, avoid contrast procedures because of the danger of aspiration.

16. **Primary versus staged repair in premature babies with or without pneumonia or other malformations.**
Creation of a gastrostomy tube followed by a period of observation has the advantage of providing an opportunity to treat or evaluate associated conditions or of allowing time for some aggravating conditions to improve. However, it carries a risk of continuous soiling of the lungs with gastric acid through the fistula. Currently, there is a tendency toward earlier definitive treatment in smaller and smaller babies as pediatric anesthesia, neonatal intensive care, and nutritional support have improved in recent years.

17. **Gastrostomy.**
Some surgeons prefer to use gastrostomy selectively as part of the treatment of these fistulas, avoiding its use particularly in term babies with no associated conditions. Advantages of gastrostomy are access to gastric decompression, access to feeding, and access to retrograde dilatation in case of stricture.

18. **Colon versus gastric or jejunal interposition for long-gap atresia of the esophagus.**
The ideal organ to replace the esophagus is still to be found. The use of both colon and reverse or direct gastric tube are plagued with complications. Most pediatric surgeons seem to favor the former. For these reasons, all attempts should be made to reapproximate and repair the patient's esophagus, leaving interpositions as the very last resort.

19. **Transpleural versus extrapleural thoracotomy.**
Transpleural approach is easier technically. However, anastomotic leaks are better tolerated after extrapleural operations.

BIBLIOGRAPHY

1. Holder, T.M., Cloud, D.P., Lewis, G.E., Jr., et al.: Esophageal atresia and tracheo-
    esophageal fistula. A survey of its members by the Surgical Section of the American
    Academy of Pediatrics. Pediatrics, 34:542, 1964.
2. Myers, M.A., and Aberdeen, E.: The esophagus. In Ravitch, M.M., Welch, K.J., Benson,
    C.D., et al. (eds.): Pediatric Surgery, Vol. 1. Chicago, Year Book, 1979. p.446.

---

83. HIRSCHSPRUNG'S DISEASE
LUIS A. MARTINEZ-FRONTANILLA, M.D.

---

1. **What is Hirschsprung's disease?**
    A form of distal intestinal obstruction of functional type caused by lack of
    peristaltic activity of the area of affected intestine.

2. **Which histologic changes can be demonstrated in the affected
    intestine?**
    Absence of ganglion cells in the submucosal and myenteric plexus. Also
    increased nerve fibers in the same area.

3. **What is the location and extent of the disease?**
    It always affects, at least, the lower rectum. From there it extends to a variable
    distance in a continuous involvement (see Controversies). In more than 75% of
    cases, the extent is confined to the left colon. In less than 10% of patients, it
    involves the entire colon.

4. **How is the diagnosis made?**
    Clinical suspicion. Usually a lifelong history of constipation that goes back to the
    nursery (90% of newborn infants have their first bowel movement within 48 hours
    of birth). Poor growth and development. Distended, prominent abdomen.
    Rectal ampulla usually empty, as opposed to patients with psychogenic
    constipation.

5. **How is the diagnosis confirmed?**
    The most reliable modality is a rectal biopsy usually done transanally. Anorectal
    manometry has been used by some authors as an acceptable alternative (see
    Controversies).

6. **What is the role of a barium enema in the diagnosis?**
    To reinforce the clinical suspicion and to help determine the area of transition
    between normal and aganglionic intestine. It should not be used as a definitive
    diagnostic modality.

7. **Which are the complications of untreated Hirschsprung's disease?**
    Chronic constipation, failure to thrive, acute enterocolitis, intestinal perforation,
    and death.

8. **Describe the treatment of Hirschsprung's disease.**
    Surgical. Usually staged starting with a diverting colostomy at a site uninvolved
    with the disease (verified by biopsy). This is followed several months later by a
    definitive operation that either removes or bypasses the affected area of the
    intestine. Occasionally in very short segment Hirschsprung's disease, an
    anorectal myectomy (removal of a posterior strip of muscularis) can be curative.

9. **Which are the accepted surgical techniques for definitve treatment?**

Swenson: removal of the entire affected area and anastomosis of the normal intestine near the anal level.

Soave: Endorectal pull-through preserving the external layer of the affected rectum into which the normal intestine is telescoped.

Duhamel: "back-to-back" anastomosis of uninvolved end of the intestine to the rectum down to the anal level.

10. **What are possible complications of these operations?**

Rectal stenosis with constipation, recurrent obstruction and enterocolitis, soiling or diarrhea, and genitourinary neurologic dysfunction.

11. **What are the results of these operations?**

Excellent results with normal intestinal function in 75 to 90%.

CONTROVERSIES

12. **"Skip area" of aganglionosis.**

There have been occasional reports of patients with more than one area without ganglion cells separated by a normal segment of intestine, or an area of aganglionosis proximal to the rectum with normal ganglion cells distally. The difficulties in diagnosis and treatment in these instances are obvious. The existence of this variant is, however, strongly disputed by most pediatric surgeons.

13. **Rectal biopsy versus manometry to confirm the diagnosis.**

Both modalities seem to give equally good results, and preference and accuracy seem to vary according to the experience of the authors. Rectal biopsy is more widely accepted.

14. **Primary versus staged surgical treatment.**

Diverting colostomy as a first stage is the treatment of choice for newborn infants and patients with severe enterocolitis as the presenting event. Currently most patients fall into this category. A small number of older patients with only mild or chronic symptoms who can be adquately decompressed can be treated primarily with one of the accepted definitive procedures.

BIBLIOGRAPHY

1. Aaronson, I., and Nixon, H.H.: A clinical evaluation of ano-rectal pressure studies in the diagnosis of Hirschsprung's disease. Gut, 13:138, 1972.
2. Kleinhaus, S., Boley, S.J., Sheian, M., et al.: Hirschsprung's disease: A survey of the members of the Surgical Section of the American Academy of Pediatrics. J. Pediatr. Surg, 14:588, 1979.
3. MacIver, A. G., and Whiteside, R.: Zonal colonic aganglionosis, a variant of Hirschsprung's disease. Arch. Dis. Child., 47:233, 1972.
4. Sieber, W.K.: Hirschsprung's disease. In Ravitch, M.M., Welch, J.J., Benson, C.B., et al.: (eds.): Pediatric Surgery, Vol. 2. Chicago, Year Book, 1979, p. 1035.
5. Swenson, O., Sherman, J.O., and Fisher, J.H.: Diagnosis of congenital megacolon: An analysis of 501 patients. J. Pediatr. Surg., 8:587, 1973.
6. Tiffin, M.E., Chandler, F.R., and Faber, H.K.: Localized absence of the ganglion cells in the myenteric plexus in congenital megacolon. Am. J. Dis. Child., 59:1071, 1940.
7. Tobon, F., and Schuster, M.: Megacolon: Special diagnostic and therapeutic features. Johns Hopkins Med. J., 135:91, 1974.

84. INTUSSUSCEPTION
FRITZ M. KARRER, M.D.

1. **Intussusception is most common at what age?**
Approximately 80% occur between 2 months and 2 years of age.

2. **What is the etiology of intussusception?**
Ninety percent of cases are idiopathic. In most, lymphoid hyperplasia of the terminal ileum is found. Upper respiratory infection is a common antecedent problem in many infants and may play a significant role in the development of intussusception. The incidence of other lesions acting as the lead point for an intussusception increases with age. The common lead points include Meckel's diverticulum, intestinal polyps, duplications, and lymphosarcoma.

3. **What is the most common type of intussusception?**
Ileocolic is by far more common than colo-colonic or ileo-ileal. The latter two are more frequently associated with lead points.

4. **Which is the intussusceptum and which is the intussuscipiens?**
The advancing telescoping inner part is known as the intussusceptum and that segment into which it is telescoped, the outer part, is the intussuscipiens.

5. **How do these children present?**
Intussusception occurs most often in previously healthy, well-nourished infants. Classically, the intussusception is heralded by sudden onset of abdominal pain. This sharp, crampy pain causes the child to cry out, double up, and draw up the legs, and is frequently accompanied by sweats. The pain subsides within a short time and the infant appears well again, only to recur. Vomiting and fever follow. Bloody, "currant jelly" stools are classically described but are not universally seen. In fact, the triad of abdominal pain, vomiting, and rectal bleeding is present in only 15% of cases. Physical findings vary considerably depending on the duration and severity of the illness. A variable degree of dehydration and abdominal distention is seen. An abdominal mass, sausage-shaped, in the right upper quadrant or mid-upper abdomen is palpable in about one half of patients. Dance's sign, an absence of viscera in the right lower abdomen, is noted in some patients. On rectal examination, grossly bloody or guaiac-positive stools are seen, or occasionally, the intussusception is palpable.

6. **How is the diagnosis confirmed?**
Plain radiographs of the abdomen showing partial or complete small bowel obstruction are suggestive but barium enema is most useful for diagnosis. The "coiled spring" and "fist" signs are classic for intussusception.

7. **What are the therapeutic options?**
Once the diagnosis is established, there is a choice of treatment between operation and hydrostatic reduction using barium enema. In experienced hands, barium enema reduction is successful in 50 to 80% of patients and should be attempted. Contraindications to hydrostatic reduction include findings of peritonitis, free intraperitoneal air, complete bowel obstruction, or clinical shock. Duration of symptoms for more than 24 hours or patient age over 6 years are relative contraindications.

8. **What are the limitations to be followed for reduction by barium enema?**

The hydrostatic reduction of intussusception should be attempted only after the following conditions: (1) The patient should be prepared for operation, i.e., an intravenous line should be started and rehydration begun; blood should be obtained for complete blood cell count, electrolyte studies, type, and crossmatch; a nasogastic tube should be in place if significant obstruction is present. (2) The barium reservoir should not be elevated more than 1 meter above the table height. (3) Reflux of barium freely into the terminal ileum is required to be certain of the reduction.

9. **What should be the operative approach?**
    If barium enema fails or is not attempted for reasons discussed above, the patient should be operated upon expeditiously to prevent ischemic necrosis. A right-sided transverse incision is preferred. The intussusception can often be reduced by gentle milking from the distal end against the leading edge. No traction should be applied proximally. If any portion of the intussusception is nonviable or irreducible, it should be resected with primary anastomosis except in the face of perforation and advanced peritonitis.

BIBLIOGRAPHY

1. Eklof, O. A., Johanson, L. and Lohr, G.: Childhood intussusception: Hydrostatic reducibility and incidence of leading points in different age groups. Pediatr. Radiol., 10:83, 1980. The authors report an 85% success rate of hydrostatic reduction in 658 patients. Those patients < 1 or > 5 years of age had the lowest rate of success. Older patients had the highest incidence of lead points.

2. Hutchison, I. F., Olayiwola, B., and Young, D.G.: Intussusception in infancy and childhood. Br. J. Surg., 67:209, 1980. Two hundred nine cases of intussusception over a 10-year period are reviewed. Hydrostatic reduction was attempted in only 27%, and successful in over half. Of the remainder undergoing laparotomy, 21% required resection with end-to-end anastomosis. The incidence of resection increased with the longer duration of symptoms.

3. Ravitch, M.M.: Intussusception. In Ravitch, M.M., Welch, K.J., Benson, C.D., et al. (eds.): Pediatric Surgery, 3rd ed. Chicago, Year Book, 1979. This well-illustrated chapter contains an extensive review of the history, epidemiology, and diagnosis of intussusception. The discussion of the therapeutic options including hydrostatic reduction is excellent.

4. Ravitch, M.M.: Intussusception in Infants and Children. Springfield, Illinois, Charles C Thomas, 1959. This is a classic monograph on the entire spectrum of intussusception, including the history of the early use of hydrostatic pressure for reduction.

5. Rosenkrantz, J.G., Cox, J.A., Silverman, F.N., et al.: Intussusception in the 1970's: Indications for operation. J. Pediatr. Surg., 12:367, 1977.

6. Wayne, E.R., Campbell, J.B., and Burrington, J.D.: Management of 344 children with intussusception. Radiology, 107:597, 1973. In this large series, 266 of 344 patients had barium enemas and 66% were successfully reduced. Five patients with lymphosarcoma acting as the lead point were seen, all over age 6. Exploratory laparotomy is recommended for children over age 6, even if hydrostatic reduction is successful.

85. CONGENITAL DIAPHRAGMATIC HERNIA
FRITZ M. KARRER, M.D.

1. **What is the most common type of congenital diaphragmatic hernia?**
    Posterolateral, foramen of Bochdalek hernias are far more common than foramen

of Morgagni hernias. Eighty to ninety percent are left-sided. The anterior (foramen of Morgagni) hernias are rarely symptomatic in the neonatal period.

2. **What signs and symptoms suggest this diagnosis?**

These infants often present with progressive respiratory distress with severe dyspnea, retractions, and cyanosis. The abdomen is scaphoid since much of the abdominal contents are located in the chest. The mediastinum is shifted, usually to the right, and the heart sounds are heard over the right chest. The ipsilateral chest is usually dull to percussion, breath sounds are diminished, and bowel tones may be heard. As the bowel becomes distended with air, further mediastinal shift may result in impaired venous return and hypotension. Some patients have insufficient pulmonary function to survive and expire very soon antenatally. Others have minimal pulmonary dysfunction and may escape diagnosis until days or months after birth.

3. **How is the diagnosis confirmed?**

The chest radiograph demonstrates multiple loops of air-filled intestine within the hemithorax. If, however, films are obtained very early, prior to any air entering the bowel, a confusing pattern of mediastinal shift, cardiac displacement, and a completely opaque hemithorax may be seen. Insertion of a nasogastric tube, injection of air, and repeat chest radiographs should confirm the diagnosis.

4. **What therapeutic measures should be performed prior to operation or transport?**

Insertion of an orogastric or nasogastric tube placed to continuous suction will prevent further distention of the bowel with air or fluid. Endotracheal intubation will also reduce bowel insufflation caused by mask ventilation or crying. Since the lungs are hypoplastic, the ventilatory pressures should be kept low (< 30 mm Hg) to prevent pneumothorax. Venous access should be obtained and fluids administered to maintain perfusion and metabolic acidosis corrected.

5. **What is the preferred operative approach?**

While some controversy exists over whether the transabdominal or transthoracic approach is preferable, the transabdominal is superior for the following reasons. The reduction of the viscera into the abdomen is simplified and, hence, the diaphragm can be repaired with unobstructed vision and without undue tension. The abdomen can be stretched to facilitate closure. Malrotation with or without obstruction can be recognized. Placement of a gastrostomy is possible. The transthoracic approach is preferable for older children (> 1 year of age) or for repair of recurrent diaphragmatic hernias. In these situations, adhesions are more easily taken down and a better diaphragmatic closure achieved with excellent exposure.

6. **What problems may be expected postoperatively and how can they be treated or prevented?**

Even after successful diaphragmatic repair, the infant is in danger of sudden deterioration and rapid death. The lung is still hypoplastic and may be incapable of providing sufficient oxygenation. The risk of alveolar rupture and life-threatening pneumothorax is high. It is most efficient to paralyze these babies in the early postoperative period and to ventilate them at high rates with the lowest airway pressures possible that provide adequate oxygenation and ventilation. These infants have a tendency to develop increasing pulmonary vascular resistance and persistent fetal circulation (PFC). This can be documented by simultaneous sampling of preductal (radial) and postductal (umbilical artery) arterial blood gases. If PFC develops, pulmonary vasodilators such as tolazoline (Priscoline) sometimes produce dramatic improvement. Hypoxia, acidosis, and hypercarbia are potent vasoconstrictors; therefore, the oxygen delivery should be liberal, ventilator rates high, and metabolic acidosis prevented by maintaining perfusion with adequate intravenous fluids or blood, and appropriate administration of bicarbonate.

7.   What is the expected outcome?
If the infant developed respiratory distress in the first 24 hours after birth, the mortality remains near 50%. Other factors influencing survival include the gestational age of the baby, the severity of pulmonary hypoplasia, and the development of PFC.

8.   What new techniques are on the horizon for treatment of congenital diaphragmatic hernia?
Extracorporeal membrane oxygenation (ECMO) can be used to provide adequate oxygen delivery and the time necessary to advance pulmonary function to a level compatible with survival. The technique requires intensive monitoring and special training but its use is becoming more widespread. The possibility of prenatal repair is being explored but awaits refinements so that premature labor can be avoided and techniques to diagnose the lesion early enough to allow lung growth and affect the outcome can be perfected..

BIBLIOGRAPHY

1.   Bloss, R.S., Aranda, J.V., and Beardmore, H.E.: Congenital diaphragmatic hernia: Pathophysiology and pharmacologic support. Surgery, 89:418, 1981. This article provides an excellent review and update of the recent advances in the area of pulmonary vascular physiology and pharmacologic manipulation.

2.   Cohen, D.E., and Reid, J.S.: Recurrent diaphragmatic hernia. J. Pediatr. Surg., 16:42, 1981. Thirteen cases of recurrence following repair of congenital diaphragmatic hernia are reviewed. A transthoracic approach utilizing an intercostal flap for repair is recommended.

3.   Collins, D.L.: Complications of surgery for diaphragmatic defects. In DeVries, P.A., and Shapiro, S.R. (eds.): Complications of Pediatric Surgery. New York, Wiley Medical, 1982. This text focuses primarily on the complications encountered in pediatric surgery. The chapter on diaphragmatic defects is of great assistance in identifying potential complications and how they might be avoided, but also provides insight into future developments.

4.   Gross, R.E.: Congenital hernia of the diaphragm. In Surgery of Infancy and Childhood. Philadelphia, W. B. Saunders, 1953. This classic textbook is highly readable and informative. The section on diaphragmatic hernia is not only of historical interest but contains many "surgical secrets" of its own.

5.   Hardesty, R. L., Griffith, B. P., Debski, R. F., et al.: Extracorporeal membrane oxygenation: Successful treatment of persistent fetal circulation following repair of congenital diaphragmatic hernia. J. Thorac. Cardiovasc. Surg., 81:556, 1981. Two of three infants with diaphragmatic hernias developed persistent fetal circulation and were successfully managed with ECMO after other modalities failed.

6.   Harrison, M. R., and deLorimier, A.A.: Congenital diaphragmatic hernia. Surg. Clin. North Am., 61:1023, 1981. This review provides an excellent section on the pathophysiology of congenital diaphragmatic hernia and the preliminary work on prenatal correction.

7.   Holder, T.M., and Ashcraft, K.W.: Congenital diaphragmatic hernia. In Ravitch, M.M., Welch, K.J., Benson, C.D., et al. (eds.): Pediatric Surgery. Chicago, Year Book, 1979. This is the standard textbook in pediatric surgery. This section is very thorough and includes a historic review.

8.   Redo, S.F.: Principles of Surgery in the First Six Months of Life. Hagerstown, Maryland, Harper and Row, 1976. This volume covers the congenital anomalies and problems encountered in infancy which require surgical intervention in a well-organized systematic manner.

9. Weiner, E.S.: Congenital posterolateral diaphragmatic hernia: New dimensions in management. Surgery, 92:670, 1982. The author compares pharmacologic manipulation with ECMO. No significant improvement in survival was found with the addition of pharmacologic treatment. ECMO is advanced as an alternative until more effective pharmacologic agents are developed.

10. Wesenberg, R.L.: Congenital diaphragmatic hernia. In The Newborn Chest. Hagerstown, Maryland, Harper and Row, 1973. This book deals solely with the roentgenographic study of the neonatal chest. Approach to interpretation, diagnosis and technique is invaluable.

86. IMPERFORATE ANUS
STEPHEN K. GREENHOLZ, M.D., and JOHN R. LILLY, M.D.

1. **What are the two basic types of imperforate anus and how do you tell the difference between them?**
    The two types of imperforate anus are "high" and "low." Presence of a perineal or forcette (in girls) fistula indicates a low type. Meconium present on urinalysis, demonstration of a rectourinary fistula on cystogram, or inability to visualize a vaginal fistula in girls all point to a high-type imperforate anus. The use of upside-down films (invertograms) to demonstrate rectal gas above or below arbitrary lines through pelvic bones is controversial.

2. **How does surgical treatment differ in the high and low types of imperforate anus?**
    Patients with a low imperforate anus are treated by anoplasty , whereas those with a high imperforate anus require colostomy and later a pullthrough operation.

3. **Are there other important clinical distinctions between patients with a high and low type of imperforate anus?**
    Patients with a high imperforate anus have a major incidence of associated malformations. Genitourinary and cardiac anomalies in particular should be sought out. In patients with a low imperforate anus, the incidence of associated malformations is quite low.

4. **What are the chances for normal continence in the two types of imperforate anus?**
    In patients with a low imperforate anus, continence should be normal after a properly performed anoplasty. Only about half of the patients with a high imperforate anus have normal continence after a pullthrough operation. The other half have only fair to poor continence.

CONTROVERSY

5. **Upside-down films.**
    The upside-down film has been used for years to distinguish between a high and low type of imperforate anus. Arbitrary lines are drawn between the pubis, sacrum, and bony trochanters. If rectal gas has gone beyond these lines, the patient is thought to have a low imperforate anus; if not, a high imperforate anus is diagnosed. There are many pitfalls with this examination. For example, rectal propulsion may push the rectum distal to the line in cases of high imperforate anus. Again, x-ray examination too soon after birth may not have permitted the

intestinal gas to descend to its nadir, giving a false impression of a high imperforate anus in patients with low imperforate anus. In general, external examination, urinalysis, and cystogram are safer methods to distinguish between these two basic types of imperforate anus.

BIBLIOGRAPHY

1.   Kiesewetter, W.B., and Chang, J.H.T.: Imperforate anus: A five to thirty year follow-up perspective. In Rickham, P.P., Hecker, W.C., and Prevot, J. (eds.): Progress in Pediatric Surgery. Munich, Urban & Schwarzenberg, 1977.
2.   Stephens, F.D.: Congenital rectal fistulae and their sphincters. Aust Paediatr. J., 1:107-110, 1965.

87. ABDOMINAL TUMORS
ALEJANDRO M. HERNANDEZ-CANO, M.D., and JOHN R. LILLY, M.D.

1.   **What are the two major malignant abdominal tumors in young children?**
Wilms' tumor and neuroblastoma.

2.   **What is the primary site of origin for Wilms' tumor and for neuroblastoma?**
Wilms' tumor originates in the kidney. Neuroblastoma originates in tissue derived from the neural crest, i.e., adrenal gland, sympathetic ganglion.

3.   **How may you clinically distinguish between these two retroperitoneal tumors?**
Both tumors most often present with an asymptomatic abdominal mass but Wilms' tumor rarely grows large enough to cross the abdominal midline to the opposite side. Neuroblastoma not infrequently will do so. Because of catecholamine excretion, many patients with neuroblastoma will have systemic symptoms such as transient skin flush and diarrhea. Finally, the average age at presentation is somewhat younger for patients with neuroblastoma (1 to 2 years) than it is for those with Wilms' tumor.

4.   **What are the major sites for metastases for Wilms' tumor? For neuroblastoma?**
Pulmonary and hepatic metastases are the usual sites checked before operation in a child with Wilms' tumor. Neuroblastoma often metastasizes to the bone marrow. Bone marrow analysis is usually done before operation in a child with neuroblastoma.

5.   **What is the primary treatment for these two tumors?**
Surgical extirpation.

6.   **Does adjunctive therapy (chemotherapy or radiotherapy) have a significant role in management?**
Since the advent of chemotherapy and radiotherapy, the cure rates for Wilms' tumor have increased dramatically. On the other hand, the cure rate for neuroblastoma has changed little despite adjunctive therapy.

7. **Does the prognosis of these tumors depend on patient's age at operation?**
    Yes, especially for neuroblastoma. For example, neuroblastoma in infants under 6 months of age has a 90% cure rate even with widespread metastases; neuroblastoma in older children (over 5 years of age) have cure rates less than 50%.

CONTROVERSY

8. **Adjunctive therapy.**
    Adjunctive therapy is often given to patients with unresectable neuroblastoma. Prolongation of life is reported. However, the overall cure rate is not changed.

BIBLIOGRAPHY

1. Grosfeld, J.L., and Baehner, R.L.: Neuroblastoma: An analysis of 160 cases. World J. Surg., 4:29-38, 1980.
2. Johnson, D.G.: Treatment of Wilms' tumor in children. World J. Surg., 4:5-13, 1980.

88. CONGENITAL CYSTS AND SINUSES
ROBERTA J. HALL, M.D., and JOHN R. LILLY, M.D.

1. **What is a thyroglossal duct cyst?**
    A thyroglossal duct cyst is a malformation caused by failure of normal obliteration of the migration tract (from the foramen cerum to the normal location in the neck) of the thyroid gland.

2. **Why should a thyroglossal duct cyst be excised?**
    It may be become infected. Once infected, the cyst must be incised and drained and excision postponed until infection is resolved.

3. **Is there thyroid tissue in the cyst?**
    Not infrequently, small nests of thyroid tissue are present in the cyst. Unusually, the cystic mass may represent the entire thyroid gland. If the thyroid gland cannot be palpated in its normal location, a thyroid scan should be obtained. If the thyroid gland is located in the cyst, the thyroid should be surgically relocated, autotransplanted, or have no operative treatment.

4. **What is the major complication of excision of a thyroglossal cyst?**
    Recurrence. The incidence of recurrence can be kept quite low if excision of the center of the hyoid bone (through which the thyroglossal duct cyst passes) is routinely done.

5. **What is a branchial cleft cyst?**
    Branchial cleft cysts are malformations formed because of incomplete obliteration of the first and second (and rarely, the third) branchial clefts.

6. **How do branchial cleft cysts present clinically?**

The malformations occur in front of the ear or under the mandible (first branchial cleft) or along the anterior border of the sternocleidomastoid muscle (second branchial cleft). They present as a cysts, sinuses, or fistulas. If there is an opening (sinus of fistula), a clear or mucoid secretion may exit from it. Occasionally, the cyst becomes infected, requiring incision and drainage.

7. **Where do the first and second branchial cleft cysts originate?**
   The first branchial cleft originates at the external auditory canal; the second, at the tonsillar fossa. The surgeon must be prepared to trace these malformations to their origin to avoid recurrence.

8. **What are the major operative hazards of branchial cleft cyst excision?**
   The facial nerve is in the proximity of the first branchial cleft; the second branchial cleft often runs in the bifurcation of the carotid artery.

9. **Why should branchial cleft cysts be excised?**
   Most eventually become infected. Like thyroglossal duct cyst, excision must then be postponed until infection has resolved.

CONTROVERSY

10. **Treatment of lingual thyroid?**
    Patients with lingual thyroids, in which the thyroid is completely in the mouth (nondescent), may be treated by complete thyroid excision, with or without autotransplantation, or by conservative means. In the latter case, thyroid extract is given indefinitely to cause the lingual thyroid to shrink and to maintain a relatively small size.

BIBLIOGRAPHY

1. Buckingham, J.M., and Lynn, H.B.: Branchial cleft cysts and sinuses in children. Mayo Clin. Proc., 49:172-175, 1974.
2. Knight, P.J., Hamoudi, A.B., and Vassy, L.E.: The diagnosis and treatment of midline neck masses in children. Surgery, 93:603-611, 1983.
3. Telander, R.L., et al.: Thyroglossal and branchial cleft cysts and sinuses. Surg. Clin. North Am., 57:779, 1977.

NOTES

NOTES

NOTES